The Evidence-Based Primary Care Handbook

Dedicated to Gundi, Laura and Julia

The Evidence-Based Primary Care Handbook

Edited by

Mark Gabbay FRCGP Dip Psychotherapy DFFP

Senior Lecturer in General Practice
University of Liverpool
Liverpool, UK

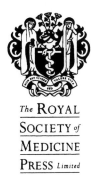

The ROYAL
SOCIETY *of*
MEDICINE
PRESS *Limited*

© 1999 Royal Society of Medicine Press Ltd

Published by the Royal Society of Medicine Press Ltd
1 Wimpole Street, London W1G 0AE, UK
Tel: +44 (0)20 7290 2921
Fax: +44 (0)20 7290 2929
E-mail: publishing@rsm.ac.uk
Website: www.rsmpress.co.uk

Reprinted 2005

British Library Cataloguing in Publication Data
A catalogue record for this book is available from the British Library

ISBN: 1-85315-415-6

Distribution in Europe and Rest of World:
Marston Book Services Ltd
PO Box 269
Abingdon
Oxon OX14 4YN, UK
Tel: +44 (0)1235 465500
Fax: +44 (0)1235 465555
Email: direct.order@marston.co.uk

Distribution in the USA and Canada:
Royal Society of Medicine Press Ltd
c/o Jamco Distribution Inc
1401 Lakeway Drive
Lewisville, TX 75057, USA
Tel: +1 800 538 1287
Fax: +1 972 353 1303
Email: jamco@majors.com

Distribution in Australia and New Zealand:
Elsevier Australia
30–52 Smidmore Street
Marrikville NSW 2204, Australia
Tel: +61 2 9349 5811
Fax: +61 2 9349 5911
Email: service@elsevier.com.au

Typeset by Phoenix Photosetting, Chatham, Kent

Printed and bound in Great Britain by Marston Book Services Limited, Oxford

▶ Contents

Section 3: Evidence-Based Primary Care in Practice

▶ List of Contributors

Jackie Bailey Senior Research Associate, Department of Epidemiology and Public Health, University of Newcastle upon Tyne, Newcastle upon Tyne

Peter Bundred Reader in Primary Care, Department of Primary Care, University of Liverpool, Liverpool

Judith Cantrill Clinical Senior Lecturer, School of Pharmacy and Pharmaceutical Sciences and National Primary Care Research and Development Centre, University of Manchester, Manchester

David Chappel Lecturer, Department of Epidemiology and Public Health, University of Newcastle upon Tyne, Honorary Senior Registrar in Public Health Medicine, Gateshead and South Tyneside Health Authority, Newcastle-upon-Tyne

Mike Crilly Senior Lecturer, Department of Public Health, University of Liverpool, Liverpool

Rumona Dickson Co-ordinator, Research Synthesis, Research Support and Development Unit, University of Liverpool, Liverpool

Chris Dowrick Professor of Primary Medical Care, Department of Primary Care, University of Liverpool, Liverpool

Yenal Dundar Visiting Lecturer in Primary Care, Department of Primary Care, University of Liverpool, Liverpool and Assistant Professor, Department of Family Medicine, University of Kocaeli, Izmit, Turkey

Martin Eccles Professor of Clinical Effectiveness, Centre for Health Services Research, University of Newcastle upon Tyne, Newcastle-upon-Tyne

Aneez Esmail Senior Lecturer in General Practice and Head of School of Primary Care, University of Manchester, Manchester

Peter Fink General Practitioner, Secretary of Local Medical Committee and Primary Care Group Board Member, Manchester

Lucy Frith Lecturer in Medical Ethics, Department of Primary Care, University of Liverpool, Liverpool

Mark Gabbay Senior Lecturer in General Practice, Department of Primary Care, University of Liverpool, Liverpool

Alan Gibbs Lecturer in Medical Statistics, University of Manchester, Manchester

Trevor Gibbs Director of Community Studies, Department of Primary Care, University of Liverpool, Liverpool

Stephen Gillam Director, Primary Care Programme, King's Fund Development Centre, London

Tony Gosden Research Associate, National Primary Care Research and Development Centre, University of Manchester, Manchester

Peter Griffiths General Practitioner and Primary Care Group Board Member, Liverpool

Alastair McColl Lecturer in Public Health Medicine, Health Care Research Unit, Wessex Institute for Health Research and Development, University of Southampton, Southampton

Frances Mair Senior Lecturer in General Practice, Department of Primary Care, University of Liverpool, Liverpool

Carrie Morrison Primary Health Care, Médecins Sans Frontières, London

Steve Rose Information Services Manager, National Primary Care Research and Development Centre, University of Manchester, Manchester

Matthew Sutton Research Fellow, National Primary Care Research and Development Centre at Centre for Health Economics, University of York, York

Ajay Thapar Lecturer in General Practice, School of Primary Care, University of Manchester, Manchester

Mary Patricia Tully Research Fellow, School of Pharmacy and Pharmaceutical Sciences, University of Manchester, Manchester

Anna van Wersch Senior Lecturer Health Psychology, Newcastle Centre for Health Services Research University of Newcastle, Newcastle upon Tyne, and School of Social Sciences, University of Teesside, Teesside

▶ Preface

As professionals, we seek to ensure our patients get the best deal. There are many means to achieve this. By availing ourselves of the most reliable and up-to-date knowledge, we can free up our intellectual capacity to utilise our communication, examination and other diagnostic skills. We can also discuss clinical management problems with greater confidence, and make the most effective referral and commissioning choices.

It is our belief that evidence is not just for doctors: it is relevant to all members of the primary care team and its philosophical approach is likely to benefit decision making and standards of care throughout services. We have tried to ensure that the book is relevant to a wide range of health-care professionals. Furthermore, the contents reflect a diversity of opinions and give space to evidence-based health's critics, to enable readers to gain a wider perspective. The authors are familiar with primary care, as clinicians and/or researchers, and we hope this is apparent to readers.

This book cannot hope to provide a complete guide and is not intended to. The aim is to introduce concepts, some familiar, some less so. At times the arguments may be controversial. The subject is by its essence challenging, however. It is also important to know where we are working in the absence of 'best evidence', which may indicate a gap aching to be filled by research, or the inapplicability of available evidence to the case in hand.

The first section of the book provides a basic introduction to the evidence-based approach. It aims to introduce practitioners to the principles of evidence-based practice. Its chapters include an overview and critique, guides to reading, literature searching, continuing education and ethical concerns. We also include chapters on guidelines, dissemination, evidence for nurses, patient perspectives, and statistics. Section 2 focuses on issues of particular relevance to planners and primary care groups, and includes chapters on commissioning, prescribing issues and health economics. The section concludes with a chapter describing one practice's experience using evidence-based approaches to answering questions triggered by daily work.

This leads into the final section in which the book attempts to practise what it preaches, by providing worked examples of evidence applicable to common primary care issues. This, strictly speaking, goes against the grain, as by their very nature textbooks risk becoming yesterday's news. Clearly, the 'answers' we provide are only true at the time they were written. The reader can follow the workings outlined, and see if the same conclusions can still be drawn. They can also be used as exemplars, demonstrating the routine approach as well as some strategies for coping with the exceptions and problems in the process of searching for and analysing evidence. They are not intended to be comprehensive systematic reviews, but we hope we have summarised the best current evidence relevant for primary care at the time of writing.

I am often taken aback when firmly held beliefs from my training and 'experience' are laid to rest when I search for the evidence. There are a number of examples in this book of information that is new to me, and will change my practice. I suspect that if you read this book, you are likely to find it challenging, informative, and relevant. I hope we have succeeded in making it interesting and readable as well. Only you can judge that.

Mark Gabbay

July 1999

▶ Acknowledgements

Professor J Gabbay and Dr Mike Crilly for comments on earlier drafts of Chapter 1; members of the District Stroke Group who helped put together the technical document discussed in Chapter 12; Matt Sutton, Dr Peter Bower, Professor Martin Roland and Nicola Mead for their comments on earlier drafts of Chapter 14; Dr Yenal Dundar and Dr James McGuire for their help with the searches described in Chapter 21; Stuart Barton and Alan Haycox for their advice and help with the literature searches described in Chapter 26; Gene Feder for his help and advice in the preparation of Chapter 30.

SECTION 1

GENERAL ISSUES IN EVIDENCE-BASED PRIMARY CARE

▶ 1

Why Evidence-Based Health?

Mark Gabbay

The basic premise

The work of the primary care team largely centres on the problems of patients and their families, carers and dependants. This often throws up questions about diagnosis, prognosis and treatment. Whilst there may be an easy answer that is almost second nature, sometimes no obvious solution is to hand and the answer needs to be searched for. The process of discovering these answers, and checking their validity and appropriateness for a particular situation, is what this book is all about. The ability to access and consider the best available evidence is a powerful ally for primary health-care teams and primary care commissioning groups in a climate of stressed and limited resources. Our main motivation in writing this book is to catalyse primary care staff into considering, and hopefully adopting, this approach. We are not suggesting that lack of evidence of effectiveness is the same as evidence of ineffectiveness. However, when there is evidence of ineffectiveness, or evidence of something better, safer or more cost effective, should we not try and find out about it so that it enters our databank when we consider our options?

Issues about quality

As governments seek to ensure value for taxpayers' money, the professions, in turn, must try and ensure that the outcome and quality measures on which their work is judged, are based on the best available, regularly updated, evidence. Such an approach is advocated in McColl *et al*'s recent paper (1998) which outlines the evidence underpinning the suggested NHS quality measures for primary care. On the basis of reliable evidence, they propose a different list of measures. Martin Roland's (1999) McKenzie lecture at the RCGP identified the development of valid, reliable and relevant measures of quality as a priority for the professions in primary care. We need to consider how we may best use evidence to help primary care set priorities, judge performance and ensure access. A recent round-table discussion organised by the Royal Society of Medicine looked at the relationship between primary care and evidence-based health (EBH), and its relevance for emerging primary care groups (PCGs) (Harrison 1998). The belief was that the PCG framework provided a real opportunity to enhance the adoption of care based on best evidence in light of the needs of individual patients and populations.

Clinical governance

The UK government white paper (Secretary of State for Health 1998) *A First Class Service, Quality in the New NHS* establishes clinical governance as an integral component of health services (Roland *et al* 1999). This is a framework encompassing an overarching theme designed to safeguard high standards of care and enhanced quality. The four main components are:

▶ structures to ensure clear lines of responsibility and accountability;

▶ quality improvement programmes;

▶ risk management;

▶ support frameworks to identify and improve poor performance.

Evidence-based practice is identified as one of the main facets of the quality improvement programme. It should be enhanced and supported by the National Institute for Clinical Excellence (NICE). Set up in early 1999, the NICE is expected to carry out 30–50 evidence appraisals per year of the most significant new and existing health interventions. Structures will also be in place to ensure that such evidence is incorporated into everyday practice at local and national levels. It seems that in the UK NHS at least, evidence-based practice is at the forefront of developments (such as the introduction of NHS-wide clinical governance frameworks) and quality monitoring.

As professionals we should ensure we understand what evidence is, what it is not, or perhaps cannot or should not be, and how we can make best use of it. We need to understand its limitations, and how we can best integrate it into our work and thinking. This book is designed to help primary care team members through this process. It sets out to explain the fundamentals and present practical examples. It also outlines the limitations of the evidence-based approach and some of the arguments against it.

Competing demands

Primary care teams, and GPs in particular, work in an environment of competing priorities and demands. They must seek ways to resist being overwhelmed by 'evidence' sent from a range of sources. The vast array of recommended guidelines and protocols, often sent unsolicited, purporting to be based on evidence, research or expert opinion (in any combination) overflow from many in-trays (Hibble *et al* 1998).

The prescribing dilemmas are manifold (see Chapter 15). Newdick (1998) outlined the conflicts surrounding the legal position of GPs in the NHS. It remains unclear whether their first priority is to work within the restrictions of resource allocations or if such an approach risks potential contravention of their terms of service. Published evidence at least gives us something to fall back on, particularly if it comes out against a particular therapeutic approach.

There are dangers however. 'Best evidence' is almost exclusively population based, whereas most clinical decisions are about individuals. Furthermore, there is a wealth of topics and problems where evidence is inconclusive, missing or based on 'less robust' data and methodologies. There are many who would challenge the view that the 'randomised controlled trial (RCT) is the only true gold standard of evidence'. What is important is that the most appropriate methodology is used, perhaps in combination with others, to answer the research question. Green and Britten (1998) have presented a sound argument for the importance of qualitative research evidence, particularly within primary care, patient experiences, service development and other management and quality topics.

The patient focus

Evidence-based medicine (EBM) has been often said to start and end with the patient. More recently the concept has been extended to decisions about managing health resources, but the focus of the concept of EBM remains patient based. You should be cautious about the rationing of resources being solely based on 'the strength of evidence'. Health care is a complex matrix of needs, demands and intervention options. The most appropriate choices may not be restricted to those with the strongest evidence. When considering alternatives it is also important to distinguish between the extent to which decisions may be influenced by:

▶ lack of evidence of effectiveness;

▶ evidence about the relative effectiveness of alternatives;

▶ evidence of ineffectiveness.

Clinicians deal with people, and this focus needs to be maintained. One should, however, retain that thirst for knowledge that epitomises early professional training. Practitioners are well placed to evaluate newly acquired knowledge in the setting of their clinical experience; the danger is that the experience seeks to reaffirm old assumptions and knowledge, and is not challenged and informed by regular updating from the wealth of good research. Proponents of the practice of EBM espouse the ideal of clinicians who keep abreast of what is best in relevant research and who are able to modify their practice in the light of the evidence they seek to help them answer their questions.

Lag and resistance

It is sad that despite considerable attempts to disseminate good clinical research evidence into common conditions, which if implemented could make considerable differences to morbidity and mortality, the professions are slow to adopt the new information. We accept that we deal with the idiosyncrasies of the individuals in their community but we also have a responsibility to the wider population. We agree that primary care often involves a complex matrix of clinical, social and psychological problems, under increasing resource stresses, and does not readily fall into the classical medical model approach that would facilitate an evidence-based approach. But, when there is an opportunity to question what we do, or to negotiate with patients or other professionals, we should endeavour to have some confidence that what we are saying is valid and remains so in the light of recent discoveries and information.

What is evidence-based health?

Brief history

The classic paper introducing EBM (Evidence-Based Medicine Working Group 1992) described it as:

> *'The new paradigm ... de-emphasising intuition, unsystematic clinical experience, and pathophysiological rationale as sufficient grounds for clinical decision making and stresses the examination of evidence from clinical research.'*

It is perhaps overstating the case to describe it as a new paradigm (Couto 1998). Indeed, it appears to be a logical development of scientific medicine facing up to the social and political demands of its environment. Chapter 8 explores these philosophical issues in greater depth.

More recently EBM has been defined as:

> *'... the conscientious, explicit, and judicious use of current best evidence in making decisions about the care of individual patients. The practice of EBH means integrating individual clinical expertise with the best available external clinical evidence from systematic research.'* (Sackett et al 1996)

The term was first used at McMaster University Medical School in Canada in the 1980s to describe a clinical learning strategy developed around a problem-based learning approach (Rosenberg and Donald 1995). However the philosophical origins extend back to mid-19th century Paris and before (Sackett *et al* 1996).

The approach involves searching and appraising information derived from research, which clinicians can use to help them make decisions about the care of individual patients. The original focus was clinical medicine, but it now embraces all of health care, including public health and health economics. This wider definition is called EBH. The process seeks to close the gap between good research and good practice, both by incorporating research evidence into practice and identifying questions for researchers. These benefits are not confined to particular types of clinician; they are relevant to those practising and training at all levels of seniority. The rise in importance of EBH has critics, however (see below).

Application

The art and science of health care starts with a patient's (or population group's) problems and how they may best be prevented, diagnosed or managed. We are, therefore, as clinicians, constantly making decisions, using the information we gain from history taking, clinical examination and tests. We apply this to other information either retained in our memory, sought from the literature or from discussions with others. We then formulate solutions, based on a range of options, in negotiation with the patient. EBH is a way of enabling us to improve our decision making by providing the information from research that may aid us in our complex tasks. It does not seek to devalue clinical skills, personal experience, the relationship we have with our patients, or the knowledge we have about individual patients' circumstances or nuances. It does provide the means whereby the clinician can apply data gleaned from the scientific study of individual or groups of patients, and apply this to their patients. It has been asserted that:

'good doctors use both individual clinical expertise and the best available external evidence, neither alone is enough.' (Sackett *et al* 1996).

Writing about general practice, Sweeney (1996) concluded:

'GPs should develop EBM into another strength of General Practice'.

Thus, EBH can inform the clinical skills of obtaining a history, examination, investigations, problem formulation and patient management planning. As we seek to develop these skills, we should particularly emphasise those shown to be effective and perhaps discard those shown not to be. It can help us make appropriate referrals and improve our communication. However, there may be no good research evidence to help us decide about much of our work. It can help us make decisions about service management, planning and commissioning, across the skill mix. Surely prioritisation and rationing is better when informed by available evidence, rather than anecdote or prejudice.

Evidence-based health permeates through a variety of aspects of primary care (Reciuk and Walshe 1998):

- clinical practice;
- management, e.g. commissioning, service delivery planning, resources and skill mix;
- critical appraisal of relevant literature, solicited and otherwise;
- development of priorities and other aspects of policy;
- research activity, dissemination and education;
- service evaluation, e.g. audit criteria.

A clinical context

A bricklayer of 36 attends with low back pain, radiating down to the left knee, which has been present for 5 days. He has not knowingly injured his back, has rested in bed for the 5 days and taken an NSAID when the pain was at its worst, as was advised to him 4 years ago when he was off work for 6 weeks with a similar problem.

This case raises a number of questions.

- Concerning *diagnosis*:
  — what are the key points from the history, including worrying symptoms and signs?
  — how should I classify low back pain, particularly leg pain?

    — what are the key points of physical examination?
    — should I do any tests, and if so, what, when and in whom?

▶ What are my first *management plan* options and what if they do not work?

▶ What is the likely *prognosis*?

    An EBH approach seeks to provide reliable answers to such questions. Part of the skill is framing questions that can be answered from the literature (see Chapters 2 and 3). The evidence-based approach encompasses the process from devising questions, through searching the literature, understanding and appraising its contents, and then considering its applicability to practice.

Problems with other approaches

Traditional medical learning is based on didactic teaching and experiential work, including the art of diagnosis. In such a system, clinical problems are solved by reflecting on your own experience, applying the underlying basic medical sciences, consulting textbooks or asking local experts. Much of the information on which this traditional learning is based is derived from facts and opinions in textbooks. These may not be systematic in their review of the published literature, instead reflecting the bias of the authors.

Inadequacies of the expert 'review' article

Many doctors try to keep up to date by reading clinical review articles. Like textbooks, however, such articles are often subjective and reflect the opinion of their authors, who may select background reading to support their own perspective, fail to include important advances, and recommend approaches for which the evidence is equivocal (Taylor 1996). Furthermore, such reviews are unlikely to be fully referenced, and frequently fail to address the quality of the research used or how the papers were evaluated and their findings compared, e.g. whether the findings were weighted according to the strength of the research design. In contrast, a good meta-analysis or systematic review (see below for further explanation of these terms) should state clearly the breadth of the literature search, the criteria by which the papers reviewed were judged, and the statistical weighting of the findings in relationship to the 'strength of the evidence'. It is noticeable, however, that recently there has been a trend towards more comprehensive referencing in clinical review articles (Grubb and Fox 1998 is an example of this), although this is still uncommon in a number of 'professional' non-peer-reviewed publications.

Learning at the boss' side

The narrow perspective of teachers, limited often to their own experience, and that of a few colleagues, may lead to erroneous and potentially biased conclusions. Such views may be tainted by prejudice and subjective analysis, unchallenged by a comprehensive familiarity of the range of relevant and recent literature. A system of learning mainly from the 'experience' of senior colleagues, without cross-reference to good research literature, may be at risk of imparting defective knowledge. This is exacerbated in a system where there are difficulties in obtaining training posts in unfamiliar hospitals, as the insider is favoured for promotion, or in obtaining a variety of clinical training and experience across clinical specialities. In such circumstances the trainee is restricted to the opinions of a few and access even to biased views is constricted.

Some of the knowledge gained in training may thus be based on unsound evidence and false assumptions. The old adage of 'see one, do one, teach one', has often been applied to the gaining of practical surgical experience. This can be perhaps adapted to 'see one or two, remember it, call it clinical experience and teach it to others'. Indeed, perpetuating unsound or biased practice seems to be a risk we take as clinicians at the hands of some teachers, unless we are able critically to judge what we learn. This does not mean of course that clinical experience is not a vital component of the art of medicine, but that it is important that such experience is tested against scientific knowledge based on sound research, both clinical and biological, and in order to continue to keep such a perspective, clinicians need a system of keeping abreast of developments.

We should not restrict learning to knowledge gained from large-scale research trials either. We need to adopt a critical analytic approach, and seek the best available evidence and the most appropriate experience and learning sources. For example, case reports are a valuable way of illustrating the application of evidence, or of reporting the unusual or exceptional, but their limitation is that conclusions should be *generalised* with caution.

Criticisms of evidence-based approaches

It is important not to denigrate the value of the relationship between clinicians and their patients, and the *art of healing*. There has been a heated debate, particularly in the letter pages of *The Lancet* in November 1995 and the *British Medical Journal* in July 1996, between proponents and opponents of EBM. The main criticism against EBH is that it adds the rigidity of 'cookbook medicine' based on the biased opinions of western scientific medicine and statistics, at the expense of ignoring the art of medicine and individual patient and physician variation in experience and judgement. Others contest this interpretation:

> '... it requires a bottom up approach that integrates the best external evidence with individual clinical expertise and patients' choice, it cannot therefore result in slavish, cookbook approaches to individual patient care.'
> (Sackett et al 1996)

Proponents of EBH have no pretence that it can provide all the answers, but argue that it may help provide independently judged information that can aid clinical decision making.

Clearly EBM is only a means to inform and perhaps improve clinical decisions, not rigidly override all the other factors. Chapter 8 explores the ethics of evidence-based approaches in some depth. It is important that we maintain a critically aware perspective, rather than rushing headlong into this current fashionable approach, even if it does have strong governmental and establishment support.

Grahame-Smith (1998) argues that whilst EBH has its merits, there is a danger of over-simplification. Uncertainty is a reality in health care, which EBH cannot eradicate. Best evidence needs to be used in the context of the individual and his overall circumstances, or it can potentially promote poor care. He cites examples of patients receiving a series of evidence-based interventions, which are all individually justified and rational but are potentially dangerous in combination. He calls for a holistic approach, which can take into account the cumulative and interactive effects. Most would agree that EBH can only be an aid to, not a replacement for, critical evaluation and judgement pertaining to clinical challenges.

Carr-Hill (1998), meanwhile, cautions against the dangers of EBH in the context of a management-led NHS with performance targets to attain. He also mounts an attack on the process of conducting systematic reviews and the bias it introduces, which is only partly answered by the attempts to combat publication bias in the Cochrane approach (see Chapter 2). A spirited criticism of EBH has recently been published in a thematic issue of the *Journal of Evaluation in Clinical Practice* (e.g. Shahar 1998, Couto 1998, Miles *et al* 1998).

Randomised controlled trials cannot be developed for all dilemmas in medicine, and indeed would often be a poor approach to answering the research question. There is a danger, particularly in primary care settings, of a slavish categorising of the strengths of evidence, which seems innately biased towards a western scientific paradigm of truth, and militates against more social science-based or alternative approaches. A recent example of this was a request for information by an Internet discussion group for evidence about the outcomes of community drop-in centres, as such centres were the clear result of a needs assessment amongst the target community. One needs to consider whose outcomes are being assessed and according to whose criteria of success they are judged. Furthermore, what might be the effect on the community consulted for the needs assessment when their drop-in centre is not provided because of a lack of published RCT evidence of their effectiveness. The result of the discussion, however, was a useful summary of largely qualitative and participant-based research to inform the development of such a service, rather than calls for more RCTs and 'robust' outcome-based studies.

There is also a risk of being tempted towards a medical model approach to categorising health issues, rather than a psychosocial model or a more holistic paradigm. It is important, therefore, to be conscious of the risk that 'quantifiable' measures may be taken as judgements of 'quality'. Just because something can be measured, or readily researched for evidence, does not give it an innate priority over things less amenable to such approaches. A balance needs to be struck. It is also important to remember that demands are not necessarily the same as needs (Harris 1998, Stevens and Gabbay 1989).

Large parts of clinical work cannot be readily informed by current research and this highlights the need for further studies. It has long been asserted that only 15–20% of treatments are based on RCT evidence showing that benefit outweighs harm; however, Ellis *et al* (1995) found that up to 80% of hospital treatments on a medical ward were based on RCT evidence. Gill *et al* (1996) asserted similar figures for a general-practice based survey. Further comparable studies in psychiatry, paediatrics and surgery demonstrate that this level of evidence basis to interventions is common across many areas of practice (a summary of research on this is available on the SCHARR Internet site at http://www.shef.ac.uk/~scharr/. There is also research to support the notion that evidence-based practice enhances patient outcomes, but so far this has largely been restricted to specialist ischaemic heart disease interventions.

The way forward

A shift towards an increasing use of EBH principles in clinical practice may be seen as threatening and requiring the gaining of new skills and time. I hope that it is now clearer that the evidence-based approach is relevant to primary care. It has much to offer and is particularly timely as the locus of influence shifts to PCGs. By utilising its strengths, we can become more confident in individual and group decisions. However, we need to be aware of its limitations, particularly in community settings, where the issues are more likely to be vaguer and multidimensional. It is important to understand the concepts and process in order that they are not misused or misunderstood. Readers will differ in the extent to which they will embrace the approach, but they should not fear it. By explaining the framework and providing a variety of examples, this book seeks to provide knowledge and enable the development of skills. Thus, the book may provide the means to acquire appropriate skills and knowledge, which leaves the question of how you find the time to do this. The evidence practitioners obtain will help them work in more effective and more efficient ways. Thus, they may be able to save some time to seek the evidence to enable them to do this, or at least justify prioritising it in their schedule.

References

Carr-Hill R (1998). Evidence-based healthcare: flaws in the paradigm. *Journal of the Royal Society of Medicine* **91 (Suppl 35)**: 12–14.

Couto JS (1998). Evidence-based medicine: a kuhnian perspective of a transvestite non-theory. *Journal of Evaluation in Clinical Practice* **4**: 267–275.

Ellis J, Mulligan J, Rowe J, Sackett DL (1995). Inpatient general medicine is evidence based. *Lancet* **346**: 407–410.

Evidence-Based Medicine Working Group (1992). Evidence based medicine, a new approach to teaching the practice of medicine. *Journal of the American Medical Association* **268**: 2420–2425.

Gill P, Dowell AC, Neal RD, Smith N, *et al* (1996). Evidence based general practice: a retrospective study of interventions in one training practice. *British Medical Journal* **312**: 819–821.

Grahame-Smith D (1998). Evidence based medicine: challenging the orthodoxy. *Journal of the Royal Society of Medicine* **91 (Suppl 35)**: 7–11.

Green J and Britten N (1998). Qualitative research and evidence based medicine. *British Medical Journal* **316**: 1230–1232.

Grubb N and Fox K (1998). Aspirin in the prevention of myocardial infarction. *Prescriber* **5th October** : 115–121.

Harris A (Ed) (1998). *Needs to Know: A Guide to Needs Assessment for Primary Care*. London: RSM Publications.

Harrison S (Ed) (1998). Evidence-based medicine: its relevance and application to primary care commissioning. *Round Table Series* **59**. London: RSM.

Hibble A, Kanka D, Pencheon D, *et al* (1998). Guidelines in general practice: the new tower of Babel? *British Medical Journal* **317**: 862–863.

McColl A, Roderick P, Gabbay J, *et al* (1998). Performance indicators for primary care groups: an evidence based approach. *British Medical Journal* **317**: 1354–1360.

Miles A, Bentley P, Polychronis A, *et al* (1998). Recent progress in health services research: on the need for evidence-based debate. *Journal of Evaluation in Clinical Practice* **4**: 257–265.

Newdick C (1998). Primary care groups and the right to prescribe. *British Medical Journal* **317**: 1361–1365.

Reciuk E and Walshe K (1998). Evidence-based healthcare: a critical appraisal. *Journal of the Royal Society of Medicine* **91 (Suppl 35)**.

Roland M, Holden J, Campbell S (1999). *Quality Assessment for General Practice: Supporting Clinical Governance in Primary Care Groups*. Manchester: National Primary Care Research and Development Centre, University of Manchester.

Roland M (1999). Quality and efficiency, enemies or partners. *British Journal of General Practice* **49**: 140–143.

Rosenberg W, Donald A (1995). Evidence based medicine: an approach to clinical problem solving. *British Medical Journal* **310**: 1122–1126.

Sackett DL, Rosenberg WM, Gray JAM, *et al* (1996). Evidence based medicine: what it is and what it isn't. *British Medical Journal* **312**: 71–72.

Shahar E (1998). Evidence-based medicine: a new paradigm or the emperor's new clothers. *Journal of Evaluation in Clinical Practice* **4**: 277–282.

Secretary of State for Health (1998). *A First Class Service: Quality in the New NHS*. London: HMSO.

Stevens A and Gabbay J (1989). Needs Assessment: Needs Assessment. *Health Trends* **23**: 20–23.

Sweeney K (1996). How can evidence-based medicine help patients in general practice? *Family Practice* **13**: 489–490.

Taylor RJ (1996). Experts and evidence. *British Journal of General Practice* **46**: 268–270.

▶ 2

A Guide to Reading

Mark Gabbay

How to keep abreast of developments and new evidence

Research has shown a negative correlation between doctors' knowledge of up-to-date care and the number of years since qualification (Sackett and Haynes 1995). There has been a huge rise in the volume of literature in health care, and even if reading is restricted to a speciality several hours every day would be required to cover a reasonable breadth of published research which could potentially affect clinical decisions. Clearly, as generalists, specialists in family medicine cannot cover the literature relevant to their clinical workload unless they adopt a system for doing so.

We are overwhelmed with calls on our time from patients, management, administrators and colleagues, as well as being bombarded with vast amounts of research information, much of which is invalid, biased or irrelevant to our practice. We need to develop strategies to enable us to have sufficient, recent, valid information to aid our clinical decision making. This book aims to provide readers with a useful guide through this potential maze. Armed with relevant new information, you can be more confident in clinical decision making, and enabled to practise and learn with an enhanced enthusiasm for family medicine.

Muir Gray (1998) has suggested that knowledge needs to be systematically managed. This involves gathering evidence in a systematised and readily searched and retrieved manner, and disseminating it to relevant colleagues. He suggests this role be filled by a 'chief knowledge officer' in each health organisation, be it primary care, community or hospital trust. It certainly is a role primary care groups could consider developing.

Where to start and how to judge what is important

Clinicians cannot keep abreast of all the potentially relevant literature in their field. A filtering system needs to be used. A good start for the practising clinician (as opposed to the academic) is to restrict reading to that which is likely to alter practice.

One of the main problems for the busy clinician is finding the time to read and knowing where to start. Searching the vast array of literature sources can be very time consuming, and when relevant papers are found, judging their quality can be difficult. Fortunately, this task has been simplified by the publication of journals which specialise in scientifically rigorous review articles and judge the evidence available by strict criteria. The *British Medical Journal* launched *Evidence-Based Medicine* in autumn 1995. This scans a wide number of journals and summarises those papers which are methodologically rigorous and relevant to clinical practice. The journal draws on the work of the American College of Physicians journal club which performs a similar task for internal medicine. To these are added the most important clinical studies in general practice, obstetrics and gynaecology, paediatrics, psychiatry and surgery. BMJ Publishing is launching a book in 1999, which will come out twice a year, giving comprehensive reviews focusing on primary care hot topics, amongst others.

What determines the strength of evidence?

An obvious initial difficulty is how the average reader can judge the quality of articles and their scientific reliability. However, a basic strategy can be adopted. The strength of evidence refers to the extent to which you can rely on the conclusions of the research, and their potential for informing decision making. Chapter 3 highlights key references on how critically to assess published papers for their quality, validity and relevance, and an introduction to this process is described below.

The format of research articles will vary depending on the question being researched. Simply put, for articles on *diagnosis*, the most basic questions are:

▶ Was there a blind, independent comparison with a 'gold standard' diagnostic test?

▶ Did the sample studied include an appropriate spectrum of patients on whom such a test may be used in clinical practice?

For an article about *prognosis*:

▶ Were the patients studied well defined and at a comparable point in the disease's course?

▶ Were they followed through completely?

For *treatment* research we must know:

▶ Were subjects randomised and all properly accounted for at the end of the study?

▶ Were subjects, intervention providers and researchers 'blinded'?

These basic questions, and more detailed ones, can thus be used critically to assess the strength of evidence put forward in an article. This has led to the concept of 'levels of evidence', an example of which is that developed by the US Agency for Health Policy and Research and adapted by various other groups developing guidelines (see Chapter 4).

As an example, the strength of evidence on whether a particular treatment does more harm than good can be ranked in descending order for different types of clinical study as follows:

1. randomised controlled trial (RCT);
2. cohort study;
3. case-control study;
4. case series.

The strengths and weaknesses within such designs can also be assessed (Boxes 2.1–2.4).

Box 2.1. Criteria for judging the strength of an RCT

1. Were subjects randomly assigned to treatments using a rigorous method and was the process blinded?

2. How complete was follow-up?

3. Were subject outcomes assessed on an intention-to-treat basis?

4. Were the outcome evaluaters blinded to treatment allocation?

5. How comparable were the control and treatment groups?

6. Apart from intervention differences being studied, were there any other differences between the groups' treatment?

7. Was a sample size calculation made?

8. Are the statistical analyses used reasonable?

Box 2.2. Criteria for judging the strength of a cohort study

1. Are the exposed subjects reasonably representative?

2. Are the controls from an equivalent population?

3. Is the exposure defined and verified?

4. Were confounding factors accounted for?

5. Was a (dose response) relationship between exposure and outcome demonstrated?

6. Were the outcome assessors blinded to exposure?

7. Were sufficient numbers of affected and control groups followed up for long enough for outcome to be apparent?

8. Were drop out rates for case and control groups comparable?

A double blind RCT is considered the gold standard for the following reasons. In order to be confident that it is the treatment being studied and not other factors that is responsible for the 'treatment effects' observed, you need to be able to control for the 'confounding factors'. The process of randomisation means that as subjects are randomly allocated to different treatments or controls, there is an equal chance that confounding factors will be allocated to the treatment and control groups and should therefore cancel each other out. Blinding the research team, and if possible the clinicians and patients, too, as to which treatment the patient is receiving removes

---

Box 2.3.   Criteria for judging the strength of a case-control study

1. Has disease status been reliably assessed and confirmed?

2. Is there any selection bias?

3. Are the control and case groups comparable? Is it clear that controls are unaffected by the disease being studied?

4. Have potential confounders been accounted for?

5. Were both groups assessed in the same way?

6. Are the response rates and the characteristics of the non-responders comparable in the two groups?

7. Is case and control matching appropriate?

8. Are the statistical analyses appropriate?

Box 2.4.   Criteria for judging a longitudinal case series

1. Is it a random sample?

2. Are the subjects representative?

3. Are inclusion criteria defined and reasonable?

4. Are all the subjects assessed from similar stages in the disease?

5. Was there sufficient length of follow-up?

6. How were outcomes assessed—objectively?

---

other sources of bias. Otherwise, patients expected to do best may be allocated to the favoured treatment, and investigators may be able to bias their data.

Systematic reviews and meta-analyses

There is an increasing prevalence of published reviews compiling and comparing the results of different studies of the same subject. These seek to sift through the international literature, both published and not, looking for the best evidence about different treatments, tests, diagnostic and prognostic signs, etc. They should enable the clinician to read a comprehensive, evidence-based summary of the available research evidence. Such review articles should explain the basis of the search for evidence (search strategies used), the criteria upon which results were included or excluded from the paper, and the basis upon which the results from different studies were weighted (some evidence being considered more valid than others due to the trial design adopted). The criteria you should bear in mind when assessing reviews can be summarised as:

- the clarity of its objectives and question(s);

- details and thoroughness of the search: how systematic is it?;

- the criteria for including or excluding the evidence the literature search reveals;

- whether and how the methodology of the supporting research is assessed; whether the evidence is weighted, and if so, is it clear how and is it reasonable?;

- whether the authors' findings and conclusions seem reasonable in the light of their methodology and results;

- how the findings relate to your original question and clinical setting.

Statistical methods sometimes allow the results of different studies to be combined quantitatively, with larger studies receiving more weight (a *meta-analysis*). The reader can then see the combined treatment effect of a number of studies. If the design of the studies is too different for a statistical averaging out, the different studies will receive more or less qualitative weighting according to stated criteria which judge the strengths and weaknesses of the trial designs adopted and thus enable the reader to compare their conclusions (a *systematic review*).

The sifting of evidence to produce a worthwhile systematic review is an enormous task as it needs to include a widespread search in many languages, of published papers plus reports that may not have been widely disseminated (grey literature) and unpublished results. The latter are particularly important as journals tend not to publish negative results, which leads to what is called publication bias. This information is often obtained by computer and hand searches of the literature, and interviews with a number of researchers in the field in an attempt to unearth unpublished studies.

The Cochrane Centre, named after a British epidemiologist who had criticised the medical profession for not having 'organised a critical summary, by speciality or sub-speciality, updated periodically, of all relevant randomised clinical trials' (Cochrane 1979) was established in 1993 in Oxford, UK (Silagy and Lancaster 1993). This has now expanded into the Cochrane Collaboration which involves members from many countries in compiling such reviews. The Cochrane Collaboration in Primary Health Care was launched in 1993 and is co-ordinated from Australia. The important distinction between reviews published by the Cochrane Centre and other comparable organisations is that they are very widely based and quality controlled. Thus, the results can be said to have scientific validity.

Another approach is to conduct a systematic but less exhaustive review. This will become increasingly commonplace and is the approach frequently adopted by the NHS R&D centres (Stevens *et al* 1995). Chapter 3 includes a list of 'secondary sources' collating such systematic reviews.

The value of systematic reviews has been recently challenged by Edwards *et al* (1998). They argue that systematic reviews may underestimate the strength of evidence of relevant literature and they propose an alternative classification based on the message, not just the design. They use the analogy of a signal-to-noise ratio. It is argued to be a more flexible, balanced approach, and particularly relevant to primary care.

A framework for reading

The best way to read the literature is to base it around questions derived from clinical practice. You can keep a notebook for questions that occur in everyday practice and then search for evidence on which to inform future decisions around similar problems. The e mail discussion group 'evidence-based-health' has recently debated the most appropriate methodology for collecting such questions from everyday practice, to help identify the issues and prioritise reviews and research likely to be of greatest relevance to general practice.

Concerning the upper respiratory tract, you may wonder what criteria, if any, can be used to judge if antibiotics are likely to be of more benefit than harm. The questions would be:

▶ What signs and tests provide a validated guide as to whether the infection is likely to be bacterial or viral?

▶ What is the relative predictive strength of these tests?

▶ What are the benefits and risks of treating bacterial upper respiratory tract infections?

In this way the reading evolving from a literature search around these questions will have direct relevance to practice. Chapters 18–32 give examples of such questions from practice and the process of searching and evaluating the evidence.

However, you may also seek to keep abreast of developments in general which may alter practice. A basic guideline to the critical judgement of published literature was described above, and Chapter 3 cites references which approach this subject in greater detail.

READER system

A reasonably sophisticated basic guide is that described by MacAuley (1994, 1995) who outlined an acronym-based system that can be used by family physicians to keep abreast of the literature. The acronym is READER:

▶ R for *relevance*;

▶ E for *education* (behaviour modification);

▶ A for *applicability*;

▶ D for *discrimination* (quality).

This judgement process leads to:

▶ E for *evaluation* (a scoring system is included in the original article);

▶ R for *reaction* (the response to the evaluation).

This approach has been shown in a RCT to improve GPs' critical reading skills (MacAuley *et al* 1998).

Relevance

MacAuley suggests that time should be concentrated on reading articles likely to alter clinical practice ('**R**elevance'). Thus, for general practice, articles should be restricted to those with a primary care focus. The title and author details are a very useful initial screen. Thus, an article on diabetic complications of pregnancy, the title of which appears potentially relevant, may appear less so upon noting the author is a specialist in a regional hospital centre with no co-authorship from a GP.

Education

A quick scan of the title and summary will provide sufficient information to judge whether the article is likely to change behaviour (**E**ducation). If it does not challenge current practice or beliefs, reading it all may be ego boosting, but a poor use of valuable reading time; the summary is likely to be sufficient.

Applicability

The reported study needs to be relevant to the situation in which you practise, as it is only 'Applicable' if the findings can be applied to your own work; thus, it needs to describe a situation which is relevant. A rural GP may not feel an article dealing with homelessness in the inner city of sufficient relevance to their practice. Neither would an article describing the indications for different regimens of major tranquillisers for schizophrenics be useful if all such prescribing is initiated and reviewed by local hospital psychiatric departments. However, an article comparing the effectiveness of different regimens may enable the GP to develop a dialogue with such a department if it seems a regimen is preferred which the research asserts to be less effective than alternatives.

Discrimination

The reader needs to be able to **D**iscriminate between articles of differing validity. Although you should be able to rely on the process of peer review, papers of dubious validity do slip through the process. This is asserted to be increasingly likely as you descend through the hierarchy of clinical journals (Silagy and Lancaster 1993). Papers from academic departments are more likely to have been subjected to internal review before submission for publication. If a statistician is one of the authors, this should indicate that the reader can rely on the statistical validity of the presented results. Many journals use medical statisticians as referees and they should be able to identify inappropriate or incorrect statistical analyses.

Evaluation

MacAuley describes a scoring system that can be used to **E**valuate a paper by the above criteria and suggests responses that may be appropriate according to the score.

Reaction

The **R**eaction varies in descending order of importance from circulating the paper to all members of the practice team so that its findings can be immediately instigated, filing for easy access, noting the reference and brief summary in an index on cards or computer, or putting it in the bin.

There will of course be articles of interest to the reader which fall outside this system, but the purpose of reading them is different. In order to keep up with developments, clinicians do have to apply these critical appraisal skills to their reading.

What about specific reading?

In practice you often come up with questions when dealing with patients. Sometimes evidence is available in the literature which can help you answer such questions. However, the formulation of questions relevant to specific patients may be difficult, as patients often present a complex weave of inter-related problems, which may not be amenable to a ready dissection into specifics. This problem aside, there are a multitude of common clinical challenges which can be investigated, e.g. the use of antibiotics in upper respiratory tract infection (as described above), the examination, investigation and treatment of low back pain, or the treatment of congestive cardiac failure (all examples tackled later in this book). Ridsdale (1995) gives examples from her own practice of the sort of questions an average GP's work may pose, and discusses the evidence upon which answers may be drawn. Her book serves as both a source of information and inspiration as to how you can begin to adapt the principles of evidence-based health (EBH) in everyday practice. Greenhalgh's (1997) series of papers, which was expanded into a book, provides a user-friendly guide to making sense of research papers (see also Silagy and Haynes 1998, Ridsdale 1998).

The appliance of evidence-based science

You can begin to focus your reading to help in practical ways with your work and, using the principles described above, be more confident that the information you gain has some validity and is thus a sounder basis to aid decision making than much of traditional reading and teaching. Furthermore, you can begin to formulate questions to ask of the literature and thereby improve your practice and patient care. Patients often ask questions, e.g. on prognosis or treatment alternatives, and again EBH can provide the information to inform your response. There is increasing literature on the reliability and validity of particular clues in a patient's history, physical signs and the results of diagnostic tests.

Searching and retrieving literature is more difficult in primary care when there is no on-site access to a library or postgraduate centre and librarian. However, remote access via the Internet, and an increasing move towards electronic journals (sometimes restricted to abstracts) is a partial solution.

Keeping up to date by searching for the best current evidence should be an ultimately rewarding process, particularly if kept in perspective by linking it to real problems in practice. It should help reduce the stress of clinical decision making and discussing prognosis and treatment options with patients, and also raise the clinician's confidence and job satisfaction. Hopefully, readers of this book will feel more confident and willing to begin to explore how they may start, or indeed continue, on this journey.

References

Cochrane AL (1979). 1931–1971: A critical review with particular reference to the medical profession. In: *Medicines for the Year 2000.* London: Office of Health Economics.

Edwards AGK, Russell IT, Stott NCH (1998). Signal versus noise in the evidence base for medicine: an alternative to hierarchies of evidence? *Family Practice* **15**: 319–322.

Greenhalgh T (1997). How to Read a Paper, the Basis of Evidence Based Medicine. London: BMJ Publishing.

MacAuley D (1994). READER: an acronym to aid critical reading by general practitioners. *British Journal of General Practice* **44**: 83–85.

MacAuley D (1995). Critical appraisal of medical literature: an aid to rational decision making. *Family Practice* **12**: 98–103.

MacAuley D, McCrum E, Brown C (1998). Randomised controlled trial of the READER method of critical appraisal in general practice. *British Medical Journal* **316**: 1134–1137.

Muir Gray JA (1998). Where's the chief knowledge officer? To manage the most precious resource of all. *British Medical Journal* **317**: 832.

Ridsdale L (1995). Evidence-based general practice: a critical reader. London: WB Saunders and Co.

Ridsdale L (Ed) (1998). Evidence-based practice in primary care. London: Churchill Livingstone.

Sackett DL, Haynes RB (1995). On the need for evidence-based medicine. *Evidence-Based Medicine* **1**: 5–6.

Silagy C, Haynes A (Eds) (1998). Evidence based practice in primary care. London: BMJ Publishing.

Silagy C, Lancaster T (1993). The Cochrane collaboration in primary health care. *Family Practice* **10**: 364–365.

Stevens A, Colin-Jones D, Gabbay J (1995). 'Quick and clean': authoritative health technology assessment for local healthcare contracting. *Health Trends* **27**: 37–42.

►3

A Guide to Literature Sources

Steve Rose and Mark Gabbay

Introduction

Chapters 1 and 2 introduced the concept of evidence-based health (EBH) and reference was made to the huge rise in the volume of health-care literature which can create difficulties for doctors in keeping abreast of developments and new evidence. This increase, both paper based and electronic, presents both opportunities and threats to the would be EBH practitioner – opportunities in that there is a wealth of evidence to tap into; threats in that the task of finding the evidence may appear too daunting given the amount of information around and the time available to exploit it.

This chapter will assist those interested in applying best evidence to their work to overcome these obstacles by highlighting the main sources of evidence and giving advice on how to search for sources, both manually and electronically. To start with you need to have devised a question to ask of the literature. The first section of this chapter looks at how you can devise questions from clinical problems (in the widest sense), which are most likely to yield useful results from a search for the evidence.

Formulating answerable questions

Evidence-based health is clinically focused. Most patient contacts throw up questions for the clinician to answer. The practice of EBH seeks to provide the best evidence to support decision making. The art of asking answerable questions is crucial to successful forays into the process. Clinical contacts usually pose a need for information about diagnosis, prognosis or management. Often the questions are obvious, e.g. what is the starting dose of this new ACE inhibitor, and the answer readily to hand. However, on many occasions the questions will need some thought and the source of the best evidence to answer them may not be so readily available. Sackett *et al* (1997) devote a chapter of their book to the formulation of answerable questions. In it they classify eight areas from which clinical questions arise. These are summarised below:

► *Clinical findings*: the gathering and interpretation of clinical history and examination clues and signs.

► *Aetiology*: what may have caused the disease?

▶ *Differential diagnosis*: including its ranking by likelihood, potential severity and treatability.

▶ *Diagnostic tests*: their selection, interpretation and usefulness.

▶ *Prognosis*: what is the natural history of the disease and its complications and how can you estimate this patient's prognosis?

▶ *Therapy*: for which do the benefits outweigh the risks and costs?

▶ *Prevention*: what are the modifiable risk factors and what screening is appropriate?

▶ *Self improvement*: keeping up to date, improving clinical skills and increased efficiency.

Having outlined the potential sources of questions pertaining to a particular patient, you need to consider how to formulate an answerable question. Again Sackett *et al* (1997) address this, and consider there to be four essential elements:

▶ You need first to have a patient or particular clinically related problem in mind.

▶ Next, consider the potential answer, e.g. clinical finding, test, prognosis, treatment or prevention.

▶ Thirdly, if possible, consider a comparitor for the second part.

▶ Fourthly, specify the outcome you wish to consider.

Let us consider the clinical problem (that of back pain) from Chapter 1 to look at question formulation in practical terms.

A bricklayer of 36 attends with low back pain, radiating down to the left knee, which has been present for 5 days. He has not knowingly injured his back, he has rested in bed for the 5 days and taken an NSAID when the pain was at its worst, as was advised to him 4 years ago when he was off work for 6 weeks with a similar problem.

Now consider a series of clinical questions this poses, in terms of the list of eight categories above, and containing the four features described above.

Clinical findings
How useful is the finding of decreased straight leg raising (SLR) as a diagnostic test for a herniated intervertebral disc? How important is a contralateral restricted SLR? This can be compared to other neurological signs or vertebral tenderness, for example. Simply asking what signs and symptoms are diagnostic of a prolapsed disc would be much more difficult to search on. It needs breaking up into more specific questions and perhaps comparisons.

Aetiology
Are certain occupations related to increased incidence or relapse rates? Is a family history of low back pain related to incidence, severity or recurrence rates (three different questions)?

Differential diagnosis

Does the presence of radiating pain beyond the knee differentiate between neurological and mechanical low back pain? This may be easier to answer than what signs and symptoms differentiate between mechanical, neurological and malignant causes of low back pain.

Diagnostic tests

How useful is a plain X-ray of the lumbo-sacral spine compared to no X-ray? What are the indications for a plain X-ray?

Prognosis

It may be interesting to consider whether the prognosis of low back pain is dependant on the frequency and/or duration of recurrence, or whether the duration of symptoms is related to the prognosis. What is the likelihood of this patient getting back to work within 6 weeks? is another form of question which may be amenable to an EBH approach.

Therapy

You may wish to compare the efficacy of bed rest with specific exercises or graduated normal activity as the appropriate advice on mobilisation, or the most effective type (e.g. regular NSAID compared to PRN simple analgesia), dose and duration of drug treatments. This is more likely to lead to an answer than the vaguer question, what are the most effective treatments? You could look at other specific treatments such as acupuncture, manipulation, etc.

Prevention

Do back exercises prevent recurrence? Can the avoidance of poor lifting practices reduce the primary incidence in those at risk?

Self improvement

Am I better off reading an orthopaedic textbook or evidence-based guidelines on the diagnosis and management of low back pain?

There are of course other potential questions raised by this scenario, but there is not the space to explore them all in detail and illustrate how they may be honed to increase the likelihood and comparative ease of finding evidence.

From this example it is clear that a number of 'answerable' questions arise, so you need to consider how to prioritise them. This can be done in a number of ways, but consider particularly your interest in the answer, its relevance to the patient's care, your clinical practice as a whole, and the time it is likely to take to find the answer. Consider to what extent the outcome you are considering is relevant to patients; are the results applicable to real people?

Clinical presentations in family medicine are frequently more vague and multifactorial than those in specialised health care. This makes the formulation of questions less easy, and it is important not to confine yourself to considering only those problems which most readily fit the medical model which dominates much of the literature. However, it is important, perhaps, that those starting out in EBH begin with readily answerable questions to boost their confidence.

Perhaps you could practise developing questions from your clinical work for which EBH may provide the answer. The rest of this chapter will help you look for the evidence to answer the question. With practice you will improve your question development, but it is important to keep this all in context. The importance of a question is not necessarily related to the ease with which an answer can be found according to the principles of EBH.

Getting started

Familiarity with the concepts and ideas

Before looking at how you might identify sources of evidence, it may be useful to begin with sources that help anyone new to EBH become more familiar with the concepts discussed in Chapter 1. A useful starting point is the *Users' Guides to the Medical Literature*. Published in a number of volumes of the *Journal of the American Medical Association* by the Evidence-Based Medicine Working Group, this collection of articles covers issues such as: How to use articles, how to use an overview, how to use clinical practice guidelines, and how to use an article reporting variations in the outcomes of health services. A full bibliographic list to this series is included at the end of this chapter (Appendix 3.1). Another excellent introduction was published as a series of five articles in the *Canadian Medical Association Journal* between 15th April and 15th June 1994. These were written by the evidence-based care resource group (for details see Appendix 3.2).

Other useful paper-based resources looking at the theory and methodology around evidence-based practice are listed in Box 3.1.

Box 3.1. Useful articles on theory and methodology of EBM

➤ Chalmers I and Altman DG (1995). *Systematic Reviews*. London: BMJ Publishing.

➤ Crombie I K (1996). *The Pocket Guide to Critical Appraisal: A Handbook for Healthcare Professionals*. London: BMJ Publishing.

➤ Deeks J, Glanville J, Sheldon T (1996). *Undertaking Systematic Reviews of Research on Effectiveness: CRD Guidelines for Those Carrying Out or Commissioning Reviews*. York: University of York, NHS Centre for Reviews and Dissemination.

➤ Greenhalgh T (1997). *How to Read a Paper*. London: BMJ Publishing.

➤ Jadad AR (1998). *Randomised Controlled Trials: A User's Guide*. London: BMJ Publishing.

➤ Jones R, Kinmouth AL (1995). *Critical Reading for Primary Care*. Oxford: Oxford University Press.

Key journals

The number of titles in the biomedical sciences has burgeoned in recent years. For example SERLINE (Serials on Line), available on-line via Knight Ridder Datastar, records details of about 77 000 biomedical journal titles. For those without on-line connections, consult *Ulrich's International Periodicals Directory*, published by Bowker (last updated 1996). It can be searched by subject, enabling a comprehensive list of journals likely to contain relevant literature to be built up.

Even with the explosion of information technology, the Cochrane Collaboration Review Groups (contact details for key organisations mentioned in this chapter are given in Appendix 3.3) still hand search a large number of journal titles, specifically to identify randomised controlled trials (RCTs) which have not been recorded in commercial databases. For those without electronic access to bibliographic information, a selection of journals which are worth consulting on a regular basis is listed in Box 3.2. These have been selected because they:

▶ are peer reviewed;

▶ are likely to contain studies which include RCTs or at least controlled trials in their methodologies;

▶ include material relevant to primary health care.

It is by no means a comprehensive list of journals, but would be a useful starting point if developing collections.

Box 3.2.   Selected list of journals

▶ *British Medical Journal (BMJ)*. Published weekly by the British Medical Association, London.

▶ *British Journal of General Practice*. Published monthly by the Royal College of General Practitioners, London.

▶ *European Journal of General Practice*. Published quarterly by the European Society of General Practice/Family Medicine, Netherlands.

▶ *European Journal of Public Health*. Published quarterly by Oxford University Press, Oxford.

▶ *Family Practice: An International Journal*. Published bimonthly by Oxford University Press, Oxford.

▶ *Lancet*. Published weekly by The Lancet Ltd, London.

▶ *Journal of the American Medical Association (JAMA)*. Published weekly by JAMA & Archives Journals Reader Services Centre, London.

▶ *Journal of Epidemiology & Community Health*. Published bimonthly by BMJ Publishing, London.

▶ *Journal of Evaluation in Clinical Practice*. Published quarterly by Blackwell Science, Oxford.

▶ *Quality in Health Care*. Published quarterly by BMJ Publishing, London.

▶ *Medical Care*. Published monthly by Lippincott-Raven Publishers, USA.

Databases

Increasingly, published evidence in the form of journal articles and systematic reviews is available electronically. This information is accessed through either a major on-line host (e.g. Datastar or Dialog), or by compact disc (CD). Two major databases are MEDLINE and EMBASE and BMA members can access these free through the BMA library (see Rowlands (1998) for a guide).

MEDLINE

MEDLINE is produced by the National Library of Medicine (NLM) in the United States. Going back to 1966, information is indexed from approximately 3 700 biomedical journals worldwide. Although the database may be searched 'free text' by inputting directly a single word or phrase, NLM indexers have developed a sophisticated hierarchy of index terms known as Medical Subject Headings (MESH terms). These include main terms broken down into a number of subheadings. It is by developing a search strategy, using MESH terms, that the optimal results may be achieved. Since the early 1990s MESH terms have included not only subject terms but also index terms which denote the nature of the study being referenced, e.g. *randomised controlled trial* – the 'gold standard' in terms of evidence. RCTs, controlled clinical trials and clinical trials for example, can also be identified by combining subject MESH terms with a search of a designated 'Publication Type' field. Literature exists to assist database searchers unfamiliar with the structure and use of MESH and improve their searching skills (Lowe and Barnett 1994). The MESH terms are inputted by the indexers after reading the articles, and may thus be a more reliable indication of a paper's contents than the title (which may be enigmatic or humorous), or even key words or abstracts. Different interfaces are available for searching the MEDLINE database, such as OVID, Silver Platter, Grateful Med, etc. The databases are the same, but the process and sophistication of searching varies between the different interfaces.

A sophisticated search for identifying RCTs has been developed by Carol Lefebvre on behalf of the Cochrane Collaboration. However, if the search strategy in Box 3.3 were to be adopted (the examples are for the OVID interface), a high proportion of papers identified would be RCTs. There are inevitably compromises between high precision and missing relevant papers, and too many irrelevant papers (low precision) and comprehensive coverage.

The example in Box 3.3 is included to show the potential sophistication and sensitivity of a MEDLINE search. Few searchers will aspire to such levels of detail; those that do will probably seek the guidance of a librarian or other professional database searcher. Other strategies can be adopted to seek out systematic reviews and meta-analyses. Examples are given on the Centre for Evidence-Based Medicine web site in Oxford at: http://cebm.jr2.ox.ac.uk. The potential use of a MEDLINE search can be highlighted by the fact that since 1986 the number of RCTs indexed under the MESH term 'PRIMARY CARE' has increased 5-fold (Dickersin *et al* 1994).

Another recent development has been the availability of MEDLINE over the Internet. BMA members can access the BMA Library MEDLINE Plus Service

---

Box 3.3. Search strategy to identify RCTs

1. randomised controlled trial.pt.
2. randomised controlled trials.sh.
3. random allocation.sh.
4. double blind method.sh.
5. single blind method.
6. 1 or 2 or 3 or 4 or 5.
7. animal.sh.
8. human.sh.
9. 7 not (7 and 8).
10. 6 Not 9 (*this is the high precision lowest coverage strategy*).
11. clinical trial.pt.
12. exp clinical trials.sh.
13. (clin$ adj3 trial$). Ti,ab.
14. ((clin$ or double$ or treb$ or tripl$) adj3 (blind$ or mask$)). Ti,ab.
15. placebos.sh.
16. placebo$.ti,ab.
17. random.ti,ab.
18. research design.sh.
19. 11 or 12 or 13 or 14 or 15 or 16 or 17 or 18.
20. 19 not 9.
21. 20 not 10 (*this is a compromise position between precision and spread*).
22. comparative study.sh.
23. exp evaluation studies.sh.
24. follow-up studies.sh.
25. prospective studies.sh.
26. (control$ or prospectiv$ or volunteer$).ti,ab.
27. 21 or 22 or 23 or 24 or 25.
28. 27 not 9.
29. 28 not (10 or 21) (*this is the widest spread with least precision strategy*).
30. *Then add the terms relevant to your subject search.*
The following line would combine all 3 searches:
31. 30 and (10 or 21 or 29).

(In OVID, ti denotes title word, sh denotes MESH headings, $ is the truncation symbol, ab denotes abstract)

(includes both MEDLINE and EMBASE – see below) free of charge, whilst other Internet sites have compiled links to a variety of Internet addresses from where MEDLINE can be accessed free of charge (e.g. Dr Felix's free MEDLINE page: http//www.beaker.iupui.edu/drfelix). The NLM itself can be accessed via the web free of charge: http://igm.nlm.nih.gov/. you can then search either PubMed or the more sophisticated interface Grateful Med. Neither of these is as sophistcated as the commercial MEDLINE search engines such as Silver Platter or OVID.

EMBASE

Produced by Elsevier Science, EMBASE (Excerpta Medica) is another major bibliographic database covering the biomedical literature. Going back to 1974, information is indexed from approximately 3 500 journals. Although there are overlaps between MEDLINE and EMBASE, there are sufficient differences to make searching both sources worthwhile. For example, EMBASE has a particularly strong coverage of European literature and is also strong in the areas of drugs and toxicology. At the time of writing, the UK Cochrane Centre is working on developing a sensitive search strategy for the identification of RCTs in EMBASE.

Other databases

Perhaps not surprisingly, the Cochrane Collaboration features strongly in the production of other databases. Formally known as the Cochrane Database of Systematic Reviews, the *Cochrane Library* now includes four databases on one CD. You can look at the *Cochrane Library* via the web site: http://hiru.mcmaster.ca, which is the homepage of the health information research unit at McMaster University, Canada. The *Cochrane Library* includes the:

▶ *Cochrane Database of Systematic Reviews*. A regularly updated electronic journal of systematic reviews of research on the effects of health care. Includes both completed reviews and protocols from a number of Cochrane review groups worldwide.

▶ *Database of Abstracts of Review of Effectiveness (DARE)*. Produced by the NHS Centre for Reviews and Dissemination, University of York. A collection of structured abstracts and bibliographic references of reports of systematic reviews of the effects of health care. The reviews referenced on DARE have been quality assessed and the status of every review is made explicit in the database.

▶ *Cochrane Controlled Trials Register (CCTR)*. This register includes details of trials, not previously available on electronic databases, identified by hand searches of journals and conference proceedings, including non-English language publications, undertaken by members of the Cochrane review groups.

▶ *Cochrane Review Methodology Database (CRMD)*. A classified bibliography of books, special journal issues and articles on methodological aspects of systematic reviews.

The *Cochrane Library* is published by Update Software, Oxford. For an annual subscription of about £200, four updates are received on CD. The software is continually upgraded and improvements are being made with every issue. For example, the latest issues include an option for searching the databases using the MESH terms used on MEDLINE (see above). A useful training package for *The Cochrane Library* in the form of Powerpoint files and Word documents exists on the Internet at: http://www.cochrane.co.uk.

There are various organisations conducting health technology assessments. These usually involve a reasonably systematic review of the health intervention being assessed and are worth searching to see if an effectiveness review has been conducted of the subject you are interested in. Three useful web sites to visit are listed in Box 3.4.

Box 3.4.   Other useful web sites

- Wessex Institute for Health Research and Development:
  http://www.epi.bris.ac.uk/rd/publicat/dec/

- From the same Institute, the electronic publication, *Evidence Based Purchasing*, going back to 1994. This can be viewed and printed from:
  http://www.epi.bris.ac.uk/rd/publicat/ebpurch/index.htm

- Office of Health Technology Assessment, Centre for Health Services and Policy Research, University of British Columbia: http://www.chspr.ubc.ca/bcohta/

Secondary sources

Given the problems individuals are likely to face in tracking down the evidence, secondary sources are of particular importance because they summarise and review the primary evidence. They appear in paper format and/or electronically on the Internet. The appendix to this book presents a guide to the contents of these secondary sources that are most relevant for primary care teams. Some examples are given in Box 3.5.

Box 3.5.   Examples of secondary sources

- *Bandolier*: A newsletter of health care evidence produced monthly by the Oxford and Anglia NHS Executive, Research and Development Directorate, UK. Subscription to the printed version costs £30.00. It is available free of charge on the Internet at: http://www.jr2.ox.ac.uk:80/bandolier.

- *Evidence-Based Medicine*: Published by BMJ Publishing. This publication alerts clinicians to important advances in medicine, general and family practice by selecting from the biomedical literature those original and review articles whose results are most likely to be true and useful. These articles are summarised in value-added abstracts and commented on by clinical experts. Available on subscription.

- *Clinical Evidence*: To be launched by BMJ Publishing in 1999. It intends to be a journal in the form of a small book, updated 6 monthly. It aims to provide a readily accessible source of best evidence around a range of clinical topics, many of which will be particularly relevant to primary care. Work in progress can be viewed at: www.evidence.org.

- *Effective Health Care Bulletins*: Jointly produced by the Nuffield Institute for Health, University of Leeds, UK and the NHS Centre for Reviews and Dissemination, University of York, UK. Based upon systematic literature reviews, they cover a number of topics which have included: 'Implementing Clinical Practice Guidelines', 'Brief Interventions and Alcohol Use' and 'The Treatment of Depression in Primary Care'.

Journal clubs on the web

These aim to serve the same function as the paper-based secondary sources. Examples are given in Box 3.6.

Box 3.6.   Examples of web journal clubs

➤ *ACP Journal Club*: US based, its general purpose is to select from the biomedical literature key articles reporting studies and reviews, summarise them with 'value-added' abstracts and provide comments from clinical experts. Internet address: http://www.acponline.org/journals/acpjc/jcmenu.htm

➤ *Journal Club on the Web*. An experiment in implementing an on-line, interactive, general medical journal club which periodically summarises and critiques articles from the recent medical literature and collects and posts readers' comments. The articles are mainly from the *New England Journal of Medicine, Annals of Internal Medicine, JAMA* and the *Lancet*. Internet address: http://www.journalclub.org/

➤ *Journal of Family Practice Journal Club Web Page*. A feature of the *Journal of Family Practice* which each month reviews 7–10 important articles from the primary care literature. The goal is to identify articles which have the potential to change practice, critically appraise them and make recommendations for clinical practice. Editors review some 80 journals every month. Internet address: http://www.phymac.med.wayne.edu/jfp/jclub.htm

---

OMNI database

Another useful source of information is the OMNI (Organising Medical Networked Information) database. OMNI is the UK's gateway to high-quality biomedical Internet resources in medicine, biomedicine, allied health, health management and related topics. The OMNI Advisory Group on Evaluation Criteria has produced evaluation criteria for meriting inclusion on the database. For more information refer to web site: http://omni.ac.uk/

Does the Internet have the potential to change practice?

As noted above, key sources are appearing on the Internet. You can conduct MEDLINE and other searches, and journals such as the *BMJ* (www.bmj.com) and *JAMA* (http://www.ama-assn.org/sci-pubs/pubsrch.htm) are accessible, to varying extents, via the Internet.

Increasingly there is a wealth of information being produced specifically for this media. However, if there are difficulties in extracting relevant information from the wealth of hard copy and database sources of evidence, then these problems are greatly exacerbated on the Internet. There is little control as to what can be put onto the

Internet, which means that the quality of much of the information is open to question. This issue has been recently debated in the *BMJ* (Eysenbach and Diepgen (1998), Gray (1998), Bonati *et al* (1998), Arunachalam (1998)). Also, the Internet is not systematically indexed as is a major database such as MEDLINE. Therefore, it is impossible to construct a sensitive search strategy. Nevertheless, it is a resource worth pursuing.

Getting started

If you are part of a large academic network (e.g. the JANET network in the UK), then you will probably have access to the Internet through that network. For others, it is a case of obtaining a personal computer, a modem to connect to a telephone line and a contract with an Internet service provider (which are increasingly becoming free of charge). A number of publications give information for Internet novice users (Levine and Baroudi 1994).

Searching

In order to search (or surf as it is often referred to) the Internet you will also need access to a piece of software called a 'browser'. Examples include Netscape and Mosaic. Although it has been noted that the Internet is not indexed in the way that commercial databases have been, it is possible to formulate basic subject searches using search engines on the Internet. These are often referred to as Webcrawlers. They have been designed specifically to search the World Wide Web (WWW), a system for linking documents and services on the Internet via linked words, usually known as hypertext. These include Aliweb, Lycos and Harvest. Searching the WWW using these tools and inputting strings of words such as 'Evidence-Based Medicine', 'Evidence-Based health' or 'EBM', for example, will yield a number of web sites, but be prepared to retrieve far more information than you need or is relevant.

Just as it has been shown that access to paper-based secondary sources is useful in that they bring together, summarise and critique primary evidence, then identifying Internet pages that attempt to do the same is a useful way forward. Mention of Internet journal clubs has been made above. These were extracted from one Internet page – Netting the Evidence – which has been compiled by Andrew Booth at the School for Health and Related Research (ScHARR), at the University of Sheffield, UK. This one page brings together key resources, initiatives and organisations related to evidence-based practice on the Internet. It can be found at the Internet address: http://www.shef.ac.uk/uni/academic/R-Z/Scharr/ir/netting.html Examples of other useful web addresses to be found here are given in Box 3.7.

ScHARR has also produced a very helpful paper-based bibliography and resource guide, for £5, which brings together both Internet and paper resources (Booth 1997).

Box 3.7. Useful web addresses

▸ *Centre for Evidence Based Medicine*, Oxford, UK. Internet address:
http://cebm.jr2.ox.ac.uk

▸ *RAND Corporation*: A US-based non-profit institution that aims to improve health policy
through research and analysis. Internet address: http://www.rand.org/

▸ *EBM Searching Tutorial*. For those interested in searching skills in an EBH environment,
this is an interactive tutorial guiding the user through steps in query formulation and
searching. Internet address:
http://jeffline.tju.edu/CWIS/OAC/informatics/activities/ebm_info.html

▸ *Evidence-Based Topics*. Organised alphabetically by MESH heading with hypertext links
to the relevant WWW page. Internet address: http://www.ohsu.edu/bicc-
informatics/ebm/ebm_topics.htm

Accessing grey literature

Grey literature is usually characterised by its unavailability through normal book-
selling channels, its invisibility in bibliographies and the subsequent difficulties in
tracking it down (Padden 1995). Because of these characteristics, grey literature is
often regarded as ephemeral. However, it should not be dismissed, as some grey
literature may constitute important sources of evidence. Examples include research
in progress, conference proceedings, public health reports, annual reports, statistical series and publications by some professional organisations, e.g. the Royal Colleges.

Research in progress

Some literature is grey because it is as yet unpublished. However, when searching for
the evidence, it is as important to determine what is currently being done as well as
what has been done, especially if you are to avoid duplication of effort and make sure
that potential studies which may in future impact on the evidence base of knowledge
are identified. Two sources are worth mentioning in this context.

The National Research Register (NRR)
This is a register of research currently being funded by the Department of Health and
the NHS R & D Programme in the UK. It should eventually be available to all health
libraries in the UK. This register also contains details of ongoing research funded by
the Medical Research Council (MRC) and it also lists other potentially useful
registers, e.g. the *Directory of Registries of Clinical Trials*, which is also published
annually in the journal *Statistics in Medicine*.

The Database of Current Health Services Research (HSRproj)
This is a database of current health services research projects funded by government
agencies and private foundations in the USA. It is produced jointly by the NLM, the

Association for Health Services Research and the University of North Carolina at Chapel Hill. It is searchable using the NLM's Grateful Med software.

Other grey literature

Examples of some of the other sources of grey literature listed above may be found on SIGLE (The System for Information on Grey Literature in Europe). Dating back to 1981, this holds contributions from eight European countries and is produced by the European Association of Grey Literature Exploitation (EAGLE). It is available online or via CD-ROM.

Other strategies for searching grey literature can include:

▶ handsearching journals for details of newly published reports and current research in progress;

▶ developing effective networks with professional associations which are often the source of protocols and guidelines;

▶ the Internet.

One feature of the Internet not discussed above is electronic mail (e mail). Subscriptions (free) to specialist discussion lists can provide good opportunities for finding out about current research activities, either by keeping up with debates on the list or by posing specific questions. One such list, administered by Mailbase at the University of Newcastle, UK, is called Evidence-Based-Health. To join, send an e mail to: mailbase@mailbase.ac.uk, with a text message 'Join Evidence-based-health [first name] [Last Name]'. A list of all such open mailbase lists can be found on http://www.mailbase.ac.uk. They can be browsed by subject by going to http://www.mailbase.ac.uk/category.html and selecting the subjects you are interested in. You can also search for lists by keyword: go to http://www.mailbase.ac.uk/search.html, or click the search button at the bottom of any of the mailbase pages, and then type the keywords in the 'search for a list' box. A search can also be done via e mail by sending the command: lists to mailbase@mailbase.ac.uk. A list of approximately 2200 mailbase lists will result, so we would advise that you instead send the command: find lists searchterm, substituting the appropriate search term such as 'medical'. A list of discussion lists relevant to EBH can also be viewed at: http://www.shef.ac.uk/~scharr/ir/email.html. The same page can also be accessed through the ScHARR netting the evidence guide by looking at D for discussion lists, then selecting the hypertext link for the email.html page.

Conclusion

Hopefully, the reader will now feel able to have a go at formulating some questions and then searching for the answers. Try and keep it simple to start with and be patient. It can be very rewarding and of considerable practical benefit. Furthermore, it can be interesting and stimulating, and form the basis of debate and professional relationships and learning groups.

It is beyond the scope of one chapter to detail all sources which may be relevant to the implementation and practice of EBH in the primary care setting. Indeed, to try and do so would inflict on the reader the problem of information overload. Instead, this chapter has attempted to capture the main sources of information, both paper based and electronic, which have a bearing on the subject, and to suggest ways in which these sources may best be interrogated.

References

Arunachalam S (1998). Assuring quality and relevance of Internet information in the real world. *British Medical Journal* **317**: 1501–1502.

Bonati M, Impicciatore P, Pandolfini C (1998). Quality on the Internet. *British Medical Journal* **317**: 1501.

Booth A (1997). *The ScHARR Guide to Evidence Based Practice*. Sheffield: University of Sheffield.

Dickersin K, Scherer R, Lefebure C *et al* (1994). Identifying relevant studies for systematic reviews. *British Medical Journal* **309**: 1286–1291.

Eysenbach G, Diepgen TL (1998). Towards quality management of medical information on the Internet: evaluation, labelling, and filtering of information. *British Medical Journal* **317**: 1496–1500.

Gray JA (1998). Hallmarks for quality of information. *British Medical Journal* **317**: 1500.

Levine JR, Baroudi C (1994). *The Internet for Dummies*, 2nd edn. Foster City, CA: IDG Books.

Lowe HJ, Barnett GO (1994). Understanding and using the medical subject headings (MESH) vocabulary to perform literature searches. *Journal of the American Medical Association* **271**: 1103–1108.

Padden S (1995). Grey literature in health care. In: Carmel M (Ed) *Health Care Librarianship and Information Work*, 2nd edn. London: Library Association Publishing.

Rowlands JA (1998). Using the BMA library's MEDLINE Plus service. *Practitioner* **5th Nov:** 31–35.

Sackett DL, Richardson WS, Rosenberg W, *et al* (1997). Evidence-based medicine: how to practice and teach EBM. Edinburgh: Churchill Livingstone.

Appendix 3.1

Users' Guides to the Medical Literature Series

▶ Anon (1996). Erratum: Users' guides to the medical literature. IX. A method for grading healthcare recommendations: *Journal of the American Medical Association* **274**: 1800–1804; **275**: 1232.

▶ Guyatt GH, Rennie D (1993). Users' guides to the medical literature. *Journal of the American Medical Association* **270**: 2096–2097.

▶ Guyatt GH, Sackett DL, Cook DJ (1993). Users' guides to the medical literature. II. How to use an article about therapy or prevention: A. Are the results of the study valid? *Journal of the American Medical Association* **270**: 2598–2601.

▶ Guyatt GH, Sackett DL, Cook DJ (1994). Users' guides to the medical literature. II. How to use an article about therapy or prevention: B. What were the results and will they help me in caring for my patients? *Journal of the American Medical Association* **271**: 59–63.

▶ Guyatt GH, Sackett DL, Sinclair JC *et al* (1995). Users' guides to the medical literature. IX. A method for grading health care recommendations. *Journal of the American Medical Association* **274**: 1800–1804.

▶ Hayward RS, Wilson MC, Tunis SR *et al* (1995). Users' guides to the medical literature. VIII. How to use clinical practice guidelines. A. Are the recommendations valid? *Journal of the American Medical Association* **274**: 1630–1632.

▶ Jaeschke R, Guyatt G, Sackett D L (1994). Users' guides to the medical literature. III. How to use an article about a diagnostic test: A. Are the results of the study valid? *Journal of the American Medical Association* **271**: 389–391.

▶ Jaeschke R, Guyatt GH, Sackett DL (1994). Users' guides to the medical literature. III. How to use an article about a diagnostic test: B. What are the results and will they help me in caring for my patients? *Journal of the American Medical Association* **271**: 703–707.

▶ Laupacis A, Wells G, Richardson S *et al* (1994). Users' guides to the medical literature. V. How to use an article about prognosis. *Journal of the American Medical Association* **272**: 234–237.

▶ Levine M, Walter S, Lee H *et al* (1994). Users' guides to the medical literature. IV. How to use an article about harm. *Journal of the American Medical Association* **271**: 1615–1619.

▶ Naylor CD, Guyatt GH (1996). Users' guides to the medical literature. X. How to use an article reporting variations in the outcomes of health services. *Journal of the American Medical Association* **275**: 554–558.

▶ Naylor CD, Guyatt DH (1996). Users' guides to the medical literature. XI. How to use an article about a clinical utilization review. *Journal of the American Medical Association* **275**: 1435–1439.

▶ Oxman AD, Sackett DL, Guyatt GH (1993). Users' guides to the medical literature. I. How to get started. *Journal of the American Medical Association* **270**: 2093–2095.

▶ Oxman AD, Cook DJ, Guyatt GH (1994). Users' guides to the medical literature. VI. How to use an overview. *Journal of the American Medical Association* **272**: 1367–1371.

▶ Richardson WS, Detsky AS (1995). Users' guides to the medical literature. VII. How to use a clinical decision analysis. A. Are the results of the study valid? *Journal of the American Medical Association* **273**: 1292–1295.

▶ Richardson WS, Detsky AS (1995). Users' guides to the medical literature. VII. How to use a clinical decision analysis. B. What are the results and will they help me in caring for my patients? *Journal of the American Medical Association* **273**: 1610–1613.

▶ Wilson MC, Hayward RS, Tunis SR *et al* (1995). Users' guides to the medical literature. VIII. How to use clinical practice guidelines. B. What are the recommendations and will they help you in caring for your patients? *Journal of the American Medical Association* **274**: 1630–1632.

Appendix 3.2

Canadian Medical Association Journal evidence-based care series
- Evidence-Based Care Resource Group (1994). Evidence-based care: 1. Setting priorities: how important is this problem? *Canadian Medical Association Journal* **150**: 1249–1254.
- Evidence-Based Care Resource Group (1994). Evidence-based care: 2. Setting guidelines: how should we manage this problem? *Canadian Medical Association Journal* **150**: 1417–1423.
- Evidence-Based Care Resource Group (1994). Evidence-based care: 3. Measuring performance: how are we mananging this problem? *Canadian Medical Association Journal* **150**: 1575–1579.
- Evidence-Based Care Resource Group (1994). Evidence-based care: 4. Improving performance: how can we improve the way we manage this problem? *Canadian Medical Association Journal* **150**: 1793–1796.
- Evidence-Based Care Resource Group (1994). Evidence-based care: 5. Lifelong learning: how can we learn to be more effective? *Canadian Medical Association Journal* **150**: 1971–1973.

Appendix 3.3

Contact details for key organisations
- Bandolier: Editorial Office, Pain Relief Unit, The Churchill Hospital, Oxford, OX3 7LJ, UK.
- Cochrane Collaboration: A number of Cochrane Centres internationally make up the collaboration. The UK Cochrane Centre, Summertown Pavilion, Middle Way, Oxford, OX2 7LG, UK.
- European Association of Grey Literature Exploitation (EAGLE): Bureau Jupiter, Postbus 90407, DIL-2509 LK, The Hague, Netherlands.
- Knight Ridder Information Ltd: Haymarket House, 1 Oxendon Street, London, SW1Y 4EE, UK.
- National Library of Medicine (NML): Library Operations, 8600 Rockville Pike, Bethesda, Maryland 20894, USA.
- NHS Centre for Reviews and Dissemination: University of York, Heslington, York, YO1 5DD, UK.
- ScHARR: Information Resources, Regent Court, 30 Regent Street, Sheffield, S1 4DA, UK.
- Update Software Ltd: Summertown Pavilion, Middle Way, Oxford OX2 7LG, UK.

▶4

Clinical Practice Guidelines and Primary Care

Jackie Bailey and Mark Gabbay

Introduction

Chapters 1–3 provide an overview of evidence-based health (EBH) and its potential benefits for primary care, and a guide to searching for that evidence. This and the next linked chapter explore one way in which evidence can be practically implemented and disseminated into everyday clinical work by means of *clinical guidelines*. Clinical guidelines need not of course be evidence based, but as has been argued earlier in this book, unless they are their clinical value and justification may be considerably diminished.

This chapter aims to provide an introduction for those considering developing guidelines, based on best evidence, and those wishing to adapt existing ones for local use. It should also help readers critically judge guidelines in use, or proposed for use. Perhaps most importantly, Chapter 5 discusses the issue of ensuring that good quality guidelines are practical, known about and used.

What are guidelines?

Clinical guidelines, which may be defined as:

> *'systematically developed statements to assist practitioner decisions and patient decisions about appropriate health care for specific clinical circumstances'* (Field and Lohr 1990)

can be important aids to support busy GPs by making evidence-based health care practical and by reducing inappropriate variations in practice (Berg 1997). Well developed and appropriately implemented guidelines have been shown to improve clinical practice and patient outcome (Grimshaw and Russell 1993; Thomas et al 1998a,b). Siriwardena (1995) reported that many GPs have produced in-house guidelines and have positive attitudes about their effectiveness and benefits. Unfortunately, few guidelines are presented in a form that enables GPs quickly to access them for use with individual patients at the time of a consultation, and clearly based on best available relevant evidence. Currently, primary care teams receive an abundance of guidelines, many of which are of poor quality and from an unclear evidence base (Benech *et al* 1996, Hibble *et al* 1998). Primary care team members need to be able critically to appraise guidelines to ensure they are useful, valid, reliable and relevant to local needs.

Problems with guidelines

Some of the problems with guidelines are similar to those described for EBH (see Chapter 1). If guidelines are promoted as 'gold standards', then there are medico-legal implications surrounding their use (Benech *et al* 1996, Hurwitz 1994), as failure to follow them may leave a clinician open to accusations of poor practice. However, following guidelines of a poor standard may actually enhance medico-legal risks (Hurwitz 1998). Guidelines may represent factional interests, e.g. as a way of promoting particular drug treatments. It is important to acknowledge that there is rarely an absolute truth in medicine, particularly in primary care. Best available evidence is open to interpretation and clinicians may come to different conclusions using the same evidence.

Other concerns about guidelines are that they will lead to 'cookbook medicine', reduce clinical freedom (Rappolt 1997) and stifle innovation. Problems highlighted by Berg (1997) are that guidelines may represent the process of medical care as a formal, rational process where there are clear, single answers; in reality medical decision making is much more complicated than this and rife with uncertainty. Onion and Walley (1998) have recently written a discussion paper comparing what they term the 'scientific' and 'practical' schools of guideline development, and call for a middle way. The same journal carries six responses to their paper. Those intending to embark on the process of developing guidelines would find the debate informative.

Barriers to using guidelines (see Fig. 4.1)

Clinicians may perceive guidelines as threatening their sense of competence. The result of negotiation with patients about their health management may conflict with the guideline. There may also be financial disincentives and administrative constraints to guideline implementation. Other barriers to guideline development, dissemination and implementation include those related to information management. Searching for and identifying evidence takes time and skill (see Chapter 3) and research findings are often poorly presented leading to difficulties in interpreting published evidence; furthermore, there may be problems dispersing relevant literature (Watkins *et al* 1999).

Why bother with guidelines?

Grimshaw and Russell (1993) reviewed the literature on guidelines and reached the general conclusion that guidelines may be an effective way to promote evidence-based change. The majority of studies reviewed showed statistically significant effects of guidelines on both processes and outcomes of care, although the magnitude (clinical importance) of these effects has been questioned (Eve *et al* 1996). Benech *et al* (1996) stated that:

> 'guidelines are rarely used if they are provided unsupported and without direct relevance to the clinical situation.'

Success depends on the process by which guidelines are developed, disseminated, implemented and monitored (Anon 1994), and this process, which involves protracted

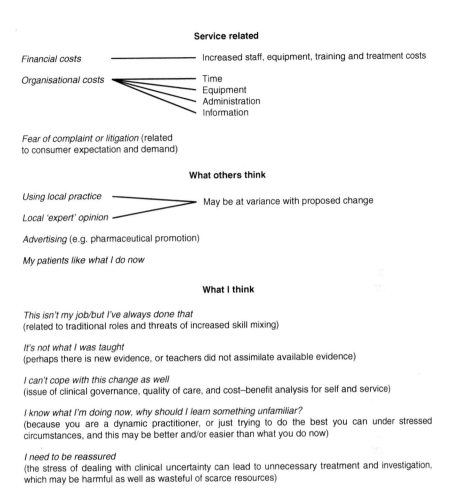

Service related

Financial costs ———————— Increased staff, equipment, training and treatment costs

Organisational costs ——— Time
Equipment
Administration
Information

Fear of complaint or litigation (related to consumer expectation and demand)

What others think

Using local practice ———
May be at variance with proposed change
Local 'expert' opinion ———

Advertising (e.g. pharmaceutical promotion)

My patients like what I do now

What I think

This isn't my job/but I've always done that
(related to traditional roles and threats of increased skill mixing)

It's not what I was taught
(perhaps there is new evidence, or teachers did not assimilate available evidence)

I can't cope with this change as well
(issue of clinical governance, quality of care, and cost–benefit analysis for self and service)

I know what I'm doing now, why should I learn something unfamiliar?
(because you are a dynamic practitioner, or just trying to do the best you can under stressed circumstances, and this may be better and/or easier than what you do now)

I need to be reassured
(the stress of dealing with clinical uncertainty can lead to unnecessary treatment and investigation, which may be harmful as well as wasteful of scarce resources)

Fig. 4.1. Barriers to using guidelines.

negotiation and agreement, may itself be the impetus for change at a local level (Eve et al 1996).

Individuals who participate in guideline development may find the exercise rewarding and educationally very valuable. If the development is carried out according to the recommendations outlined below, the result is likely to be of considerable benefit to clinicians and their patients. However, in many ways, this first process is easier than that of raising awareness about the guideline and ensuring it is of practical benefit and widely used. Chapter 5 contains a detailed overview of strategies to disseminate and implement guidelines.

Development of guidelines

Developing a clinical guideline is a major undertaking and requires enthusiastic effort from already busy clinicians and others (Onion *et al* 1996). Figure 4.2 illustrates the stages of the development process, including dissemination and implementation. Topics for guidelines must be carefully chosen. Enthusiasm is required to develop and later disseminate and implement them. This enthusiasm is enhanced and sustained when the clinical problem being investigated is considered important and relevant, perhaps when audit has identified a need for consensus and consistency to improve the quality of clinical care. Start with areas likely to yield high clinical gain as successful implementation will result in enthusiasm for more guidelines once clear benefits can be identified. It is likely to be more rewarding to start by focusing on areas of interest and less frustrating where the search for evidence is likely to be reasonably straightforward.

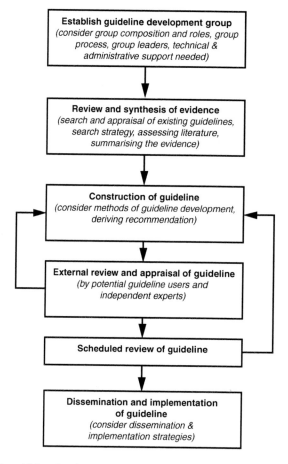

Fig. 4.2. Steps in guideline development, appraisal and implementation.

Grimshaw *et al* (1995) reported that the validity of guidelines relates to three key factors:

▶ the composition of the guideline development panel and its processes;

▶ the identification and synthesis of evidence;

▶ the method of guideline construction.

However, as there is little empirical evidence concerning guideline development, uncertainty exists about how best to optimise these factors.

Guideline development groups

Guidelines may be produced locally or nationally and usually involve a 'consensus' group (Grol 1993). The composition of the group varies, but may include patients or their representatives, health-care professionals who are going to use the guidelines, and other professionals and independent experts. The focus of the guidelines should influence the number of group members and the balance of disciplines needed.

> 'Primary health-care professionals should be in the majority when a guideline is being developed predominantly for management of patients within primary care.' (Grimshaw *et al* 1995)

When guidelines intended to be used in primary care are produced by hospital specialists, from their perspective, there is a distinct risk that they will fail to be relevant or useful (e.g. Little and Williamson (1996)). Administrative and technical support is needed to ensure success in the development of guidelines, including support to identify and synthesise evidence and present it effectively.

Review and synthesis of evidence

The best method of identifying and synthesising the evidence is by systematic review (see Chapter 2) using explicit search strategies and inclusion criteria. However, guidelines have a broader scope than systematic reviews (Grimshaw *et al* 1995), and rigorous evidence may not be available for all issues covered by them. The evidence may vary in scientific rigour, or not be available at all. Collective evaluation of the evidence will ensure that the guideline is applicable in practice whilst retaining scientific validity. Developers will need to assess the generalisability of the findings to the target patient population. Therefore, an important role for the guideline development group is to assess the relevance of research evidence to the clinical issues addressed. Most guideline developers choose to produce documents containing a mixture of evidence-linked and consensus recommendations (RCGP 1995). It is important that the guideline clearly states where clinical uncertainty exists and what grading the evidence has (see Chapter 2). Eccles *et al* (1996) present their approach to evidence grading as applied to the development of primary care guidelines. All seem to derive from work initially carried out by the Canadian Medical Association in the late 1970s.

Methods of guideline development

Guideline development and adaptation can take place at national, regional or local levels.

Informal consensus

This is the method of guideline development most frequently used in the UK. It involves a panel of experts formulating a series of recommendations, with or without a systematic review of the literature (RCGP 1995). Although inexpensive and relatively quick, the means whereby guideline panels reach their recommendation is not apparent (Eccles *et al* 1996).

Formal consensus

This involves consensus development conferences and/or Delphi[1] groups providing a more structured approach to the generation of recommendations, with reviews of the evidence where available. These methods are used primarily for areas without good research evidence.

Evidence linking

This requires an explicit link between the recommendations and the quality of the supporting evidence. Systematic reviews of the evidence are used as the basis of the recommendations and the quality and thus strength of that evidence is graded. This more transparent approach enables the guideline user to make an informed choice about whether to comply with recommendations (Eccles *et al* 1996). A detailed description of how a group produced evidence-based guidelines at a local district level has recently been published (Stokes *et al* 1998).

Where should you start?

As guideline development is a time- and resource-consuming task, the local adaptation of national and regional guidelines may be an appropriate strategy. This prevents inefficient repetition of these tasks in each locality. Local adaptation allows the guidelines to be amended considering local needs and resources (RCGP 1995) and may follow the same methods as described above. The educational benefit is maintained as the local adaptation groups will still have plenty of learning opportunities without feeling overwhelmed with re-inventing wheels. The crucial concern when starting out in guideline development and implementation is to avoid an initial failure, which would be demoralising. The first part of the process is to look at the process within the team and identify a guideline review and implementation group. This may be confined to the practice or involve others in primary care or local trusts, public health or the MAAG,[2] for example.

One way to initiate the process of 'testing the water' about evidence would be to critically review the current guidelines adopted within the practice. The extent to which they refer to evidence could be investigated, as well as the strengths and weaknesses of that evidence. This is covered in the next section.

[1] The Delphi technique is 'a method for the systematic collection and aggregation of informed judgements from a group of experts on specific questions or issues. Repeat rounds of this process can be carried out until full consensus is reached' (Reid (1988)). See also Jones and Hunter (1995).
[2] Medical audit advisory group or other body to support audit and clinical governance, clinical standards, etc.

A more ambitious project would involve the introduction of a new guideline, or the replacement of a current one with a clearer, relevant, evidence-based model. It is advisable to start with an area of clinical care that is accepted to be a problem area, perhaps identified by an audit. A list of these can be drawn up and then prioritised in terms of the mortality, morbidity and disability caused by the respective clinical problems the guidelines would seek to address. Next, consider whether a feasible, effective intervention is available to modify or prevent the clinical problem, within your setting.

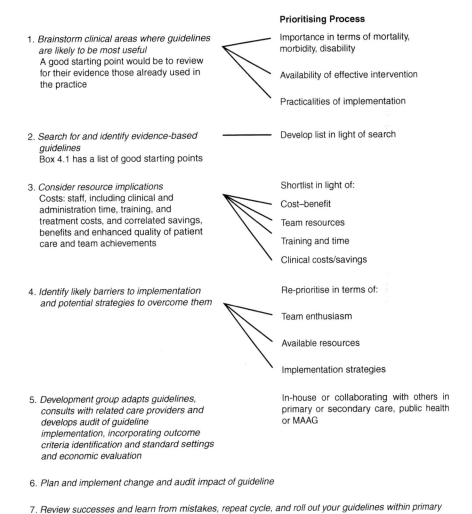

Prioritising Process

1. *Brainstorm clinical areas where guidelines are likely to be most useful*
   A good starting point would be to review for their evidence those already used in the practice

   Importance in terms of mortality, morbidity, disability

   Availability of effective intervention

   Practicalities of implementation

2. *Search for and identify evidence-based guidelines*
   Box 4.1 has a list of good starting points

   Develop list in light of search

3. *Consider resource implications*
   Costs: staff, including clinical and administration time, training, and treatment costs, and correlated savings, benefits and enhanced quality of patient care and team achievements

   Shortlist in light of:

   Cost–benefit

   Team resources

   Training and time

   Clinical costs/savings

4. *Identify likely barriers to implementation and potential strategies to overcome them*

   Re-prioritise in terms of:

   Team enthusiasm

   Available resources

   Implementation strategies

5. *Development group adapts guidelines, consults with related care providers and develops audit of guideline implementation, incorporating outcome criteria identification and standard settings and economic evaluation*

   In-house or collaborating with others in primary or secondary care, public health or MAAG

6. *Plan and implement change and audit impact of guideline*

7. *Review successes and learn from mistakes, repeat cycle, and roll out your guidelines within primary care group and beyond. The point is to try and avoid major failures and disappointments!*

Fig. 4.3. A staged approach to introducing an evidence-based guideline.

The next stage is to identify evidence-based guidelines suitable for local adaptation for as many of the listed topics as possible. The list can then be re-prioritised in the light of this search. After this the group can anticipate potential barriers to implementing the guidelines for each of the remaining clinical areas on the short list, and consider the strategies to, and feasibility of, overcoming them. Revise the short list again.

Next, the process is to consider the resource implications for each of the remaining guidelines, both savings and costs (financial, training and personnel), and the anticipated gains in the quality of patient care. Now, with the final re-prioritisation, the order for introduction of the guidelines can be agreed. Some topics may drop off the list altogether, others will be delayed until the team feels more experienced and confident.

The group is now ready to review the identified guidelines, adapt and implement them. At this stage plan the audit process to review the implementation and outcomes. The process is summarised in Figure 4.3.

Appraisal and review of guidelines

Guidelines need to be tested by targeted users and appraised as to their practical usability and content (Grimshaw et al 1995). Testing should occur towards the end of guideline development by sending a draft to a number of potential users and independent experts. Various appraisal tools exist, including that developed by the Agency for Health Care Policy and Research (AHCPR) (Institute of Medicine 1992)

Table 4.1. Desirable attributes of clinical guidelines.

Attribute	Explanation
Validity	Guidelines are valid if, when followed, they lead to the health gains and costs predicted for them
Reproducibility	Guidelines are reproducible if, given the same evidence and methods of guideline development, another guideline group produces essentially the same recommendations
Reliability	Guidelines are reliable if, given the same clinical circumstances, another health professional interprets and applies them in essentially the same way
Representative development	Guidelines should be developed by a process that entails participation by key affected groups
Clinical applicability	Guidelines should apply to patient populations defined in accordance with scientific evidence or best clinical judgement
Clinical flexibility	Guidelines should identify exceptions to their recommendations and indicate how patient preferences are to be incorporated in decision making
Clarity	Guidelines must use unambiguous language, precise definitions, and user friendly formats
Meticulous documentation	Guidelines must record participants involved, assumptions made, and evidence and methods used
Scheduled review	Guidelines must state when and how they are to be reviewed (under two separate circumstances – the identification or not of new scientific evidence or professional consensus)

(Taken from Grimshaw and Russell (1993) who adapted it from Institute of Medicine (1992)) and examining the guidelines according to attributes highlighted in Table 4.1 (a full critical appraisal instrument can be accessed at: http://www.sghms.ac.uk/phs/hceu/form.htm).

Appraising the evidence and making recommendations are difficult in practice. You rarely find several studies (with a rigorous design) testing the same hypothesis with the same outcomes measured. Drawing conclusions may require expert analysis, e.g. taking into account the effect of sample size on clinical significance, etc. Input from health economists or statisticians may also be very useful.

Examples of guidelines

There are numerous examples of actual guidelines developed in primary care (see Box 4.1). The reader may find these a useful place to start. Using the criteria described above, judge the relative merits and quality of these guidelines. It may be a useful exercise to get a group together to study them and consider how the more promising ones may be adapted and modified for local use. Box 4.2 lists some that may provide a worthwhile starting point.

Box 4.1.   Sources of guidelines

▷ *Search strategies in MEDLINE*
  Guideline, practice guideline, consensus development conference (all publication types)
  Practice guidelines (MESH heading)

▷ *Agency for Health Care Policy and Research Guidelines*
  http:// text.nlm.nih.gov/ftrs/dbaccess/ahpcr

▷ *Canadian Medical Association Clinical Practice Guidelines Infobase*
  http://www.cma.ca/cpgs/index.html

▷ *Scottish Intercollegiate Guideline Network*
  http://www.show.scot.nhs.uk/sign/clinical.htm

▷ *ScHARR Introduction to Evidence-Based Practice on the Internet. Netting the Evidence*
  http://www.shef.ac.uk/~scharr/ir/netting.html

▷ *Guidelines Database Project*
  www.ihs.ox.ac.uk/guidelines

▷ *Royal College of General Practitioners UK*
  http://www.rcgp.org.uk

▷ *Prodigy*
  http://www.schin.ncl.ac.uk/prodigy

▷ *Dutch College Guidelines*
  They can be contacted at nhgmail@nhg.knmg.nl and www.knmg.nl the web site of the Royal Dutch Medical Society, incorporating the Dutch College of General Practice. Their address is: NHG, Lomanlaan 103, 3526 XD Utrecht, The Netherlands

---

Box 4.1.   Sources of guidelines – *contd.*

▶ *North of England Evidence Based Guidelines Project*
Centre for Health Services Research, University of Newcastle, Newcastle upon Tyne NE2 4AA, UK

▶ *NHS Executive South and West R&D Directorate Development and Evaluation Committee*
http://www.epi.bris.ac.uk/rd/publicat/dec/

▶ *National Guidelines Clearing House*
The USA guidelines site, with a search engine and hypertext links
http://www.guidelines.gov/

Box 4.2.   Useful guidelines

▶ New Zealand blood pressure guidelines can be found on Oxford's Centre for Evidence-Based Medicine web site (http://cebm.jr2.ox.ac.uk/docs/prognosis.html) or Jackson *et al* (1993).

▶ Fahey and Peters (1996) highlight the variations in current guidelines for managing raised blood pressure by comparing five sets of guidelines.

▶ The Centre for Health Services Research in Newcastle, UK, has developed graded evidence-based guidelines specifically related to major conditions treated within primary care, e.g. asthma and angina in adults (Eccles *et al* 1996). This group continues to publish guidelines in peer-reviewed journals.

▶ *Clinical Guidelines: Report of a Local Initiative* (Haines and Hurwitz 1994).

▶ Guidelines on guidelines (Swales 1993).

▶ The Public Health Resource Unit at Oxford is running a Guidelines Database Project through which it has developed an electronic database of critically appraised clinical practice guidelines (accessed by web site address in Box 4.1).

▶ The Dutch College of General Practitioners has developed and published guidelines for a number of years. They can be contacted at nhgmail@nhg.knmg.nl and www.knmg.nl.

▶ The Royal College of General Practitioners in the UK has a guideline group and guidelines initiative officer, and its back pain guidelines are available on the College web site.

▶ The Scottish Intercollegiate Guidelines Network publish on its web site at http://www.show.scot.nhs.uk/sign/clinical.htm.

▶ National Guidelines Clearing House is the USA guidelines site with a search engine and hypertext links: http://www.guidelines.gov/.

Evidence-based guidelines: a multidisciplinary perspective

As the skill mix develops in primary care, there is a potential for GPs and managers to try to ensure 'quality and standards' by setting unrealistic protocols for professionals taking on new roles. There is little justification for attempting to bind colleagues down with unrealistic lists of dos and don'ts with no evidence base to justify their inclusion. Guidelines and protocols are only useful if they are used, and they will not be if they are impractical or too inflexible.

The current drive to establish evidence-based health care should engage *all* health-care professionals. However, the majority of existing information on clinical effectiveness and evidence-based health care is related to activities undertaken by the medical professions and very few concern the work of nurses and other health-care professionals (Appleby *et al* 1995). Much of the current guideline activity in the UK on medical interventions has been medically led. The effect of guidelines on the practice of other health-care professionals and the best methods to develop, disseminate and implement guidelines in these other disciplines remains uncertain. Yet, clinical practice guidelines may offer a means of bridging the theory–practice gap which has been highlighted for many years, e.g. in nursing (Cullum 1995). Chapter 7 covers this subject in greater depth.

Nurses and therapists have taken the lead in the development of multidisciplinary guidelines in a few areas (Cullum 1995), an example being a systematic review of research underpinning nursing management of leg ulcers in the community. The review was used to aid the development and implementation of multiprofessional guidelines in this area. There is currently a systematic review underway of the effectiveness of guidelines in professions allied to medicine (Thomas *et al* 1999, 1998). The assumption cannot be made that effective dissemination and implementation strategies for medicine will transfer to nurses and other workers because they have a different educational and management structure. Hicks and Hennessy (1997) suggest also that the emphasis on experimentation and randomised controlled trials, with relative marginalisation of alternative, more qualitative forms of research, may seriously limit the paramedical research database because of its inappropriateness for many problems. Therefore, there may need to be a more eclectic approach to evidence-based care.

Conclusion

Guidelines are likely to be increasingly part of daily clinical work. It is important that the motives for their use are to enhance patient care, as well as to ensure that the best use is made of available resources. It is vital, therefore, that guidelines are built around the best available evidence, and that where evidence is lacking, relevant research is undertaken. Guidelines need to focus on areas where they are likely to result in the greatest health gains, at least initially, and it is crucial that they are adaptable to meet local needs and circumstances. For guideline development to be of benefit to more than the worthy souls involved in that process, considerable thought and effort also needs to be expended on dissemination and implementation strategies to ensure they are of practical use and benefit to professionals and thus patients. Chapter 5 looks at the problem of dissemination and implementation, using guidelines as the main example, which is a crucial aspect of evidence-based health care.

References

Anon (1994). Implementing clinical practice guidelines: can guidelines be used to improve clinical practice? *Effective Health Care* **Bulletin 8**.

Appleby J, Walshe K, Ham C (1995). *Acting on the Evidence: A Review of Clinical Effectiveness, Sources of Information, Dissemination and Implementation*. NAHAT Research Paper No. 17. Birmingham: NAHAT.

Benech I, Wilson AE, Dowell AC (1996). Evidence-based primary care: past, present and future. *Journal of Evaluation in Clinical Practice* **2**: 249–263.

Berg M (1997). Problems and promises of the protocol. *Social Science and Medicine* **44**: 1081–1088.

Cullum N (1995). In: M Deighan and S Hitch (Eds) *Clinical Effectiveness from Guidelines to Cost-Effective Practice*. Brentwood: Earlybrave.

Eccles M, Clapp Z, Grimshaw J *et al* (1996). North of England evidence based guidelines development project: methods of guideline development. *British Medical Journal* **312**: 760–762.

Eve R, Golton I, Hodgkin P, *et al* (1996). Beyond guidelines: promoting clinical change in the real world. *Journal of Management in Medicine* **10**: 16–25.

Fahey TP, Peters TJ (1996). What constitutes controlled hypertension? Patient based comparison of hypertension guidelines. *British Medical Journal* **313**: 93–96.

Field M, Lohr K (1990). *Clinical Practice Guidelines: Directions for a New Program*. Washington: National Academy Press.

Grimshaw J, Eccles M, Russell I (1995). Developing clinically valid practice guidelines. *Journal of Evaluation in Clinical Practice* **1**: 37–48.

Grimshaw JM, Russell IT (1993). Achieving health gain through clinical guidelines. I: Developing scientifically valid guidelines. *Quality in Health Care* **2**: 243–248.

Grol R (1993). Development of guidelines for general practice care. *British Journal of General Practice* **43**: 143–151.

Haines A, Hurwitz B (1992). *Clinical Guidelines: Report of a Local Initiative*. Royal College of General Practitioners Occasional Paper 58. London: RCGP.

Hibble A, Kanka D, Pencheon D *et al* (1998). Guidelines in general practice: the new Tower of Babel? *British Medical Journal* **317**: 862–863.

Hicks C, Hennessey D (1997). Mixed messages in nursing research: their contribution to the persisting hiatus between evidence and practice. *Journal of Advanced Nursing* **25**: 595–601.

Hurwitz B (1994). Clinical guidelines: proliferation and medico legal significance. *Quality in Health Care* **3**: 37–44.

Hurwitz B (1998). *Clinical Guidelines and the Law: Negligence, Discretion and Judgement*. Oxford: Radcliffe Medical Press.

Institute of Medicine (1992). *Guidelines for Clinical Practice: From Development to Use*. Washington: National Academic Press.

Jackson R, Barham P, Bills J *et al* (1993). Management of raised blood pressure in New Zealand: a discussion document. *British Medical Journal* **307**: 107–110.

Jones J, Hunter D (1995). Consensus methods for medical and health services research. *British Medical Journal* **311**: 376–380.

Little P, Williamson I (1996). Sore throat management in general practice. *Family Practice* **13**: 317–321.

Onion CWR, Dutton CE, Walley T, *et al* (1996). Local clinical guidelines: description and evaluation of a participative method for development and implementation. *Family Practice* **13**: 28–34.

Onion CWR, Walley T (1998). Clinical guidelines: ways ahead. *Journal of Evaluation in Clinical Practice* **4**: 287–293 (see also 295–298, 299–300, 301–304, 305–307, 309–311).

Rappolt SG (1997). Clinical guidelines and the fate of medical autonomy in Ontario. *Social Science and Medicine* **44**: 977–987.

RCGP (1995). *The Development and Implementation of Clinical Guidelines*. London: Royal College of General Practitioners.

Reid NG (1988). The Delphi technique: Its contribution to the evaluation of professional practice. In: (Ellis R Ed) *Professional Competence and Quality Assurance in the Caring Professions*. New York: Chapman and Hall.

Siriwardena AN (1995). Clinical guidelines in primary care: a survey of general practitioners' attitudes and behaviour. *British Journal of General Practice* **45**: 643–647.

Stokes T, Shukla R, Schober P, *et al* (1998). A model for the development of evidence-based clinical guidelines at local level – the Leicestershire genital chlamydia guidelines project. *Journal of Evaluation in Clinical Practice* **4**: 325–338.

Swales J (1993). Guidelines on guidelines. *Journal of Hypertension* **11**: 899–903.

Thomas L, Cullum N, McColl E, *et al* (1999). Clinical guidelines in nursing, midwifery and other professions allied to medicine (Cochrane review). In: *The Cochrane Library*, Issue 1. Oxford: Update Software.

Thomas L, McColl E, Cullum N, *et al* (1998). Effect of clinical guidelines in nursing, midwifery and the therapies: a systematic review of evaluations. *Quality in Healthcare* **7:** 183–191.

Watkins C, Harvey I, Langley C, *et al* (1999). General practioners' use of guidelines in the consultation and their attitude to them. *British Journal of General Practice* **49:** 11–15.

▶5

Dissemination and Implementation Strategies

Jackie Bailey and Mark Gabbay

Getting guidelines into practice

Having produced a good quality and useful guideline, either from scratch or by identifying and modifying an existing high quality one to suit local needs, it is important to ensure that it is known about and used. In the context of guidelines, Grimshaw and Russell (1994) defined a *dissemination strategy* as an educational intervention that aims at:

> *'influencing targeted clinicians' attitudes to, and awareness, knowledge, and understanding of, a set of guidelines'.*

They identified the following dissemination strategies which have been used:

▶ publication in scientific and professional journals;

▶ postal distribution to relevant groups;

▶ incorporation within continuing medical education;

▶ educational initiatives that focus specifically on the guidelines.

In a systematic review of evaluations of clinical guidelines, Grimshaw and Russell (1994) found that many studies reported no dissemination strategy. Their review suggested that clear educational strategies were more likely to lead to the adoption of guidelines into practice:

> *'provided that dissemination of guidelines is reinforced by an implementation strategy'.*

In the context of guidelines, Grimshaw and Russell (1994) defined an *implementation strategy* as an intervention that aims at:

> *'improving targeted clinicians' compliance with guideline recommendations (that is, to turn changes in attitudes and knowledge into changes in medical practice).'*

Diverse dissemination and implementation strategies have been employed; however, limited evidence exists on the effectiveness and efficiency of these many different strategies and interpretation of the evidence is complex (Grimshaw and Thomson 1998, Bero *et al* 1998, Wensing *et al* 1998). A wide-ranging review summarising the evidence aimed at providing practical advice has recently been published (NHS Centre for Reviews and Dissemination 1999). In 1991, the central policy of the NHS became clearly allied to that of enhancing clinical effectiveness, through the incorporation of available evidence and best practice into services (the Research and Development strategy). Walshe (1998) studied the extent to which this has permeated down to clinical practice. His results (from 1996–97) indicate that a variety of implementation strategies have been adopted at health authority level; however, a substantial number had not considered it at all. Examples of good practice included GRiPP (Getting Research into Practice and Purchasing), originating in the Oxford Region in 1992, and PACE (Promoting Action on Clinical Effectiveness) organised through the King's Fund in London. The survey revealed that an organised approach was less common at trust level. It seems that the message, whilst largely accepted by planners and purchasers, is slow to penetrate through to service providers.

Below we briefly describe what strategies have been used (Oxman *et al* 1995, Mays 1994) and provide a summary of the evidence, where it exists, of their effectiveness.

Educational material

This refers to the distribution of published or printed recommendations for clinical care, including clinical practice guidelines, audiovisual materials and electronic publications.

Freemantle *et al* (1999) systematically reviewed the evidence on the effectiveness of printed educational materials in improving the behaviour of health-care professionals and patient outcomes. The review covered the distribution of published or printed recommendations for clinical care, including clinical practice guidelines and electronic publications. They found that the effects of printed educational materials, when compared with no active intervention, were at best small and of uncertain clinical significance. None of the studies included full economic analyses and thus it is unclear to what extent the effects of any of the interventions may be worth the costs involved. The authors concluded that printed materials may have a predisposing effect for change, without being sufficient in themselves to achieve a substantial impact upon practice, although there is no clear evidence for this.

Conferences

This refers to the participation of health-care providers in conferences, lectures or workshops, outside providers' practice settings.

Local consensus processes

This refers to the inclusion of participating providers in discussions to ensure that they agree the chosen clinical problem is important and the approach to managing the problem is appropriate.

Educational outreach visits or 'academic detailing'

This refers to where a trained person/expert visits a workplace and provides information and feedback on performance – providing concrete strategies to implement research findings.

The basic principles are (Soumerai and Avorn 1990):

- using interviews to determine the motivation for current practice and the possible barriers to change;

- targeting programmes to specific providers and their opinion leaders;

- defining clear objectives;

- establishing credibility and presenting both sides of the issue;

- encouraging provider participation;

- using well designed concise educational materials;

- repeating essential messages and providing alternatives;

- ideally, providing reinforcement through follow-up visits.

Eighteen studies of educational outreach were reviewed by Thomson *et al* (1999a). Although the majority of these studies show statistically significant improvement in performance with the use of this method, further research is needed into the key characteristics and cost-effectiveness of the approach.

Local opinion leaders

> '*Health providers nominated by their colleagues as "educationally influential".'*
> (Thomson *et al* 1999b)

There is some evidence of improved outcome using this method (Thomson *et al* 1999b).

Patient-mediated interventions

This refers to direct mailings to patients, patient counselling delivered by others, clinical information collected directly from patients and given to the provider, materials given to patients or placed in waiting rooms.

Audit and feedback

> '*Any summary of clinical performance of health care over a specified period of time.'* (Thomson *et al* 1999c)

Mugford *et al* (1991) reviewed studies of interventions of feedback of information, defined as the use of 'comparative information from statistical systems'. They distinguished between passive and active feedback; the former was the provision of unsolicited information, the latter engaged the interest of the clinician. They concluded that information feedback was most likely to influence clinical practice if the information was presented close to the time of decision making and the clinicians had previously agreed to review their practice.

Reminders and decision support systems

This refers to manual or computerised reminders that prompt the health-care provider to perform a specified action. From a review of the use of computer decision support systems (Johnston *et al* 1994), there is evidence that they can improve physician performance.

Marketing

This refers to the use of personal interviewing, group discussion or a survey of targeted providers to identify barriers to change and subsequent design of an intervention that addresses identified barriers.

To meet the need for evidence in this area, the Cochrane Collaboration of Effective Professional Practice (CCEPP) was established to generate systematic reviews of this developing collection of research (Freemantle *et al* 1995).

A recent study found that a variety of attributes influenced whether or not a guideline was used in practice (Grol *et al* 1998). Important influencing attributes include whether a recommendation is controversial or incompatible with current values, whether it is vague and not precisely defined, and whether it would involve changing existing working routines. The authors concluded that specific attributes of guidelines determine whether they are used in practice and that those developing guidelines need to understand and take into account these factors when making recommendations. A qualitative study (Langley *et al* 1998) exploring practitioners' perspectives identified three main significant themes summarising their views about guidelines:

- the characteristics of the guidelines, such as their intrinsic qualities, function and application, and GPs' involvement in development and appraisal;

- GP personal and individual variables, including access to IT and the ability to use it, time, means of coping with uncertainty and making decisions;

- external influences, such as patient views.

These are issues that need to be considered when seeking ways to enhance implementation.

In summary, the available evidence suggests that those strategies which operate directly upon the consultation between the professional and the patient are more likely to be effective (Freemantle *et al* 1995). These strategies include restructuring medical records, patient-specific reminders during the consultation and patient-mediated interventions. Evaluated strategies which operate outside the consultation include patient-specific feedback, aggregated feedback on compliance with guidelines, financial incentives, explicit marketing and professional peer review. Johnston *et al* (1994) argued that computerised decision support systems may be an effective method to employ, as not having the right information at the right time is an important cause of sub-optimal performance. There is some evidence that a combined implementation approach is most effective if it includes components of education, audit and management of change (Kitson *et al* 1996).

Management of change

Other evidence on professional behaviour change provides insights into effective guideline implementation. To promote change in clinical care, you must consider the general environment in which change occurs, the characteristics of the change and its consequences, and the process of change in individuals and organisations (Stocking 1992). Armstrong *et al* (1996) studied an example of this in primary care in their qualitative study of factors responsible for initiating and maintaining changes in prescribing behaviour among GPs.

The general environment

The general environment includes the local, professional, national and international environment. For change to occur, the general institutional and ideological environment must be favourable. Elements which can contribute to a favourable climate for change include:

- the availability of research evidence supporting change (e.g. where there is a large amount of high quality research supporting change);

- national consensus statements and other expert views (e.g. Royal College guidelines);

- promotion of ideas through the mass media;

- advertising to health-care professionals;

- demand from patients and patient groups (e.g. campaigning groups such as the National Childbirth Trust in the UK).

Characteristics and consequences of change

Rogers (1983) has described the following characteristics of change:

- *Relative advantage*: if a new practice is more effective than the prevailing method of care, it is more likely to be taken up. However, advantage to one group may be seen as a disadvantage to other groups. So the desired change must be perceived to have more advantages than disadvantages, both to the individual and the organisation.

- *Compatibility*: changes which fit with existing beliefs and work routines are more easily assimilated than those which challenge entrenched philosophies.

- *Complexity*: if a change requires the radical re-organisation of work and/or involves a disparate group of people, it is generally more difficult to assimilate. However, the positive side is if change is complex, it also tends to be maintained. Organisational changes tend to be more complex and this may be why they are slower to diffuse.

▶ *Observability and trialability*: those changes which can be viewed in operation or tried out in advance are more likely to be adopted.

▶ *Adaptability*: if change can be adapted to local circumstances, it is more likely to be assimilated, e.g. national guidelines are seen as external influences which can be resisted until they are adapted for local use, when they become more acceptable.

Processes of change in individuals: diffusion of innovation

The uptake of new health-care interventions has been described as following the typical S-shaped pattern of diffusion of ideas and innovation found in many areas of activity.

▶ *Innovators*: first adopters of innovation, described as 'venturesome', tend to occupy elite positions and have national and international status.

▶ *Early adopters*: described as 'respectable' – if innovation is to diffuse it must be accepted by these early adopters, who are often the opinion leaders of the group.

▶ *Early majority*: described as 'deliberate' – will only consider new ideas after peers have adopted them.

▶ *Late majority*: 'sceptical', overwhelming peer pressure needed for change.

▶ *Laggards*: small group described as 'traditional' who are resistant to pressures for change and are often socially isolated within their professional communities.

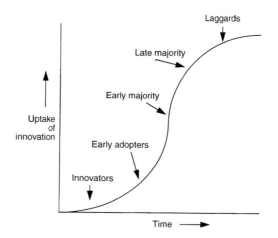

(Taken from Rogers, 1983)

Fig. 5.1. Diffusion of innovation.

As we move along the S-shaped curve from innovators to laggards, so the influence of national and international activities diminishes along with a marked decline in the influence of research evidence and a noticeable increase in the importance of immediate peers and colleagues. The effectiveness of interventions and strategies will depend on the character make-up of the group of people to whom they are targeted

(Rogers 1983). For example, for early adopters, written scientific information may be sufficient, whereas for late adopters, there may need to be additional resources, incentives, official statements and rules (Grol 1992).

Both the diffusion of innovation theory and the social influences model of behaviour change (Greer 1988, Mittman *et al* 1992) suggest that using local opinion leaders to transmit norms and model appropriate behaviour has the potential to change health-care professional practice. Peer judgements and beliefs play a major role in individuals' evaluations of new information and their resulting implications for behaviour (Mittman *et al* 1992). Opinion leaders may perform a 'sanctioning function' for the diffusion of new technologies (Greer 1988) and may enhance adaptation of general practice guidelines to suit the local environment.

Local context and organisation

The pattern of change among people is shaped not only by personal characteristics but also by the social relations of power and influence that exist in the working community. Local opinion leaders can be critical 'product champions', keeping an issue on the professional agenda and developing local coalitions in favour of change. However, this can be double-edged; if a change is heavily dependent on a particular individual who then moves on, this raises concerns about the sustainability of the change. A successful change strategy should be sensitive to the local context and seek to involve local health professionals in shaping the change agenda. In primary care, the local situation can vary from a rural to an urban practice and the practice unit can vary from single-handed to a large and diverse group of health professionals (Hutchinson *et al* 1995).

Steps to disseminate and implement guidelines in general practice

Grol (1992) has highlighted several steps needed to disseminate and implement consensus guidelines in general practice (Table 5.1). Every set of guidelines will have specific implementation barriers and a careful analysis of these should be part of the implementation strategy (Conroy and Shannon 1995).

Example of management of change initiatives

A number of initiatives have been devised to address the issue of managing change in general practice. For example, Spiegal *et al* (1992) provide a model for managing change based on a team approach. A project aimed at generating evidence-based clinical change in general practice is FACTS (Framework for Appropriate Care Throughout Sheffield) (Munro 1995). In this project, appropriate areas of clinical practice are targeted for change and the techniques employed include:

- synthesised evidence;
- endorsement by local and respected consultants;
- promotional materials for recruiting practices and prompting clinicians;
- practice-based training programmes;
- 'ready-made' audit programme;

Table 5.1. Steps to disseminate and implement guidelines in general practice and possible barriers to this (adapted from Grol 1992).

Steps	Description	Barriers to implementing new guidelines
Orientation	Attention to and becoming informed about the existence of new guidelines – feeling interested, committed	No reading or selective reading; no continuing medical education; no contact with colleagues; no needs or interests
Insight	Understanding the guidelines – awareness of (gaps in) own performance, persuasion of the need to change	Insufficient knowledge or skills; no awareness of gaps in own routines; overestimation of own performance
Acceptance	Positive attitude to the new guidelines – intention to change, confidence in success	Seeing more disadvantages than advantages; change not seen as feasible; not feeling involved or committed; expecting problems, negative consequences; negative attitude of opinion leaders in network; change requires extra time or money
Change	Actual implementation in practice, experimentation – recognition of positive outcomes, maintenance of change	Seeing no concrete alternatives; inadequate practice premises; no confidence in success; forgetting, reverting to old routines; negative outcomes of change, no reinforcement

▶ individualised advice and guidance for practices;

▶ patient leaflets.

In summary, there needs to be a development of an organisational culture supporting clinical effectiveness and the use of guidelines. The factors that influence how and why people change their behaviour must be taken into account when implementing guidelines or other research evidence. The focus for implementation strategies needs to shift from passive to active strategies. The choice of strategy should be based upon consideration of the:

▶ designated activity;

▶ targeted health-care professional groups;

▶ perceived barriers to change;

▶ available resources;

▶ management of the change processes.

There needs to be a combination of strategies so that the programme has an impact on most people, whatever their knowledge, attitudes and skills.

Discussion and conclusions

Transfer of research knowledge into practice is necessary to improve patient care and service delivery. The relationship between evidence and its transfer into practice is complex. The transfer can be facilitated by the use of guidelines and other tools, if accompanied by appropriate dissemination and implementation strategies.

The particular change that research evidence or a guideline is supporting needs analysis. What are the characteristics of the change? Is it simple and straightforward with clear benefits or will it involve complex changes for many different people? If it is the former, the change may only need widespread dissemination and a change in practice by opinion leaders. If the change is more complex, a sophisticated and multifaceted strategy may need to be employed.

Until recently, most of the emphasis on guidelines and evidence-based medicine has been in the medical domain. There is a need for a broader perspective than just GPs and other clinicians, to incorporate nurses and professions allied to medicine (see Chapter 4).

References

Armstrong D, Reyburn H, Jones R (1996). A study of general practitioners' reasons for changing their prescribing behaviour. *British Medical Journal* **312**: 949–952.

Bero L, Grilli R, Grimshaw JM, *et al* (1998). Closing the gap between research and practice: an overview of systematic reviews of interventions to promote implementation of research findings by health care professionals. *British Medical Journal* **317**: 465–468.

Conroy M, Shannon W (1995). Clinical guidelines: their implementation in general practice. *British Journal of General Practice* **45**: 371–375.

Freemantle N, Grilli R, Grimshaw J, *et al* (1995). Implementing findings of medical research: the Cochrane Collaboration on Effective Professional Practice. *Quality in Health Care* **4**: 45–47.

Freemantle N, Harvey EL, Wolf F, *et al* (1999). Printed educational materials to improve the behaviour of health care professionals and patient outcomes (Cochrane review). In: *The Cochrane Library*, Issue 1. Oxford: Update Software.

Greer AL (1988). The state of the art versus the state of the science: the diffusion of new medical technologies into practice. *International Journal of Technology Assessment in Health Care* **4**: 5–26.

Grimshaw JM, Russell IT (1994). Achieving health gain through clinical guidelines. II: Ensuring guidelines change medical practice. *Quality in Health Care* **3**: 45–52.

Grimshaw JM, Thomson MA (1998). What have new efforts to change professional practice achieved? *Journal of the Royal Society of Medicine* **91 (Suppl 35)**: 20–25.

Grol R (1992). Implementing guidelines in general practice care. *Quality in Health Care* **1**: 181–191.

Grol R, Dalhuihsen J, Thomas S, *et al* (1998). Attributes of clinical guidelines that influence use of guidelines in general practice: observational study. *British Medical Journal* **317**: 858–861.

Hutchinson A, McIntosh A, Roberts A, *et al* (1995). Evidence based health care: the challenge for general practice. In: Deighan M, Hitch S (Eds) *Clinical Effectiveness from Guidelines to Cost-effective Practice*. Essex: Earlybrave Publications Limited.

Johnston M, Langton K, Hayes B, *et al* (1994). Effects of computer-based clinical decision support systems on clinical performance and patient outcome. A critical appraisal of research. *Annals of Internal Medicine* **120**: 133–142.

Kitson A, Ahmed LB, Harvey G, *et al* (1996). From research to practice: one organisational model for promoting research-based practice. *Journal of Advanced Nursing* **23**: 430–440.

Langley C, Faulkner A, Watkins C, *et al* (1998). Use of guidelines in primary care–practitioners' perspectives. *Family Practice* **15**: 105–111.

Mays N (1994). Changing clinical behaviour: do we know how to do it? In: Harrison A (Ed) *Health Care UK 1993–1994*. Kings Fund Institute, London: pp. 102–117.

Mittman BS, Tonesk X, Jacobson PD (1992). Implementing clinical practice guidelines: social influence strategies and practitioner behaviour change. *Quality Review Bulletin* **18**: 413–422.

Mugford M, Banfield P, O'Hanlon M (1991). Effects of feedback of information on clinical practice: a review. *British Medical Journal* **303**: 398–402.

Munro J (1995). Facing the FACTS. *Health Service Journal*: Oct: 26–27.

NHS Centre for Reviews and Dissemination (1999). Getting evidence into practice. *Effective Health Care* **5**.

Oxman AD, Thomson MA, Davis DA, Haynes RB (1995). No magic bullets: a systematic review of 102 trials of interventions to improve professional practices. *Canadian Medical Association Journal* **153**: 1423–1431.

Rogers E (1983). *Diffusion of Innovations,* 3rd edn. New York: Free Press.

Soumerai SB, Avorn J (1990). Principles of educational outreach ('academic detailing') to improve clinical decision making. *Journal of American Medical Association* **263**: 549–556.

Spiegal N, Murphy E, Kinmouth A-L, *et al* (1992). Managing change in general practice: a step by step guide. *British Medical Journal* **304**: 231–234.

Stocking B (1992). Promoting change in clinical care. *Quality in Health Care* **1**: 56–60.

Thomson MA, Oxman AD, Davis DA, *et al* (1999a). Outreach visits to improve health professional practice and health care outcomes (Cochrane review). In: *The Cochrane Library*, Issue 1. Oxford: Update Software.

Thomson MA, Oxman AD, Davis DA, *et al* (1999b). Local opinion leaders to improve health professional practice and health care outcomes (Cochrane review). In: *The Cochrane Library*, Issue 1. Oxford: Update Software.

Thomson MA, Oxman AD, Davis DA, *et al* (1999c). Audit and feedback to improve health professional practice and health care outcomes (Parts I & II) (Cochrane review). In: *The Cochrane Library*, Issue 1. Oxford: Update Software.

Walshe K (1998). Evidence based healthcare, what progress in the NHS? *Journal of the Royal Society of Medicine* **91 (Suppl 35)**: 15–19.

Wensing M, van der Weijden T, Grol R (1998). Implementing guidelines and innovations in general practice: which interventions are effective? *British Journal of General Practice* **48**: 991–997.

▶ 6

Using Evidence-Based Health in Learning and Development

Mark Gabbay, Jackie Bailey, Mike Crilly and Ajay Thapar

Continuing professional development

When professionals graduate, they do not finish learning, but are involved in an ongoing process of professional education and development. Continuing professional development is an established prerequisite for most primary-care professional groups. Ideally, learning should be structured to meet personal educational needs, prompted by an honest assessment of your knowledge, skills and attitudinal biases, identified from clinical work. The individual should then develop a personal learning plan. In this way you will move from the 'dependant learner' status of traditional undergraduates, to being a 'self-directed learner' able to assess your own educational needs, and develop a personal portfolio of learning and development using a variety of educational media (Stanley *et al* 1993). Team members need to maintain their enthusiasm for learning by engaging in a variety of approaches and focusing on areas of interest. Without this continuing process of professional learning and development, practitioners can rapidly become outdated in their knowledge, lack innovation in their approach and deliver care of deteriorating quality.

Whilst it is extremely unlikely that anyone would practice without any ongoing personal education and critical evaluation of their work, it is very tempting when overwhelmed by other tasks and priorities to develop an unstructured approach to learning. This may just consist of *ad hoc* education – gleaned from reading journals (peer reviewed and not), textbooks, informal discussions with colleagues and sponsored educational meetings and events. These sources of information are often biased and may fail to reflect a balanced view of current information.

Evidence-based health (EBH) can provide a means to incorporate lifelong professional learning into busy working lives. It seeks to provide answers to questions which arise from clinical practice (practical relevance), and involves a process of subjecting what you discover to critical analysis (educational process).

Ways of learning

In this process of professional learning and development, you can employ a number of learning techniques. These may include attending or presenting talks or seminars, conducting audit or research, writing, adapting or using guidelines, or developing prescribing formularies. You are also likely to be involved in developing family-based primary care services and health promotion, screening and prevention strategies. These can also form part of an ongoing process of continuing professional development. We would argue that the quality and educational value of such activities and services will be greatly enhanced if the best use is made of available evidence.

It has been suggested that despite many GPs' approval of evidence-based approaches towards practice, few have the appropriate skills to assess the evidence and thus it is most appropriate to provide them with summaries of evidence and guidelines (McColl *et al* 1998). However, it is our belief that at least a substantial proportion of primary care staff should have a working understanding of the evidence-based approach. Our hope is that through its increasing incorporation into personal and group learning plans, this can be achieved in a relevant and stimulating way.

Audit

Many practitioners seek to learn and improve the quality of their health-care provision by undertaking clinical audits. By incorporating the principles of EBH, you can ensure that the criteria of quality that are chosen for study are evidence based, so that the standards you set out to investigate and improve have been shown by research to be relevant to enhanced clinical outcomes.

Developing agendas and priorities

It may well be that your search for knowledge and evidence uncovers gaps in published research. Whilst not all practitioners wish to carry out research, they all have a valuable part to play in asking the questions and identifying the gaps in knowledge, and thus promoting research agendas and priorities to the academic research community. The debate about researchers and academics being in ivory towers, isolated from the reality of the coal face is perhaps a cliché. However, it is essential that research and development meets the needs of practitioners, who therefore need to feed into the debate about R&D needs and priorities. It is important to build links between service providers and planners, and academic support and endeavour. Some practitioners will have research ideas and some will want to train to conduct research, but all should be able to assess it and incorporate relevant findings into their work.

Evidence and teaching

We can expect and hope that speakers and educators also make the best use of the available evidence, rather than merely giving us the benefit of their experience, valuable though that is. However, in many areas of professional work, such evidence is lacking and we rely more on the sharing of ideas. Many of us teach graduates and undergraduates of medical and related disciplines. How confident are we that what we teach can stand up to critical scrutiny? Clearly, we have much to teach about our practice and experience, but just as we expect those who teach us to ensure they make use of the best evidence available to them, so do our students. It may well be that we achieve this by encouraging the learner to seek that evidence for themselves, and then critically appraise it. Our role is to show them how to do this (or where to learn how to do it for themselves) and how to incorporate what they have learnt by adapting it to their patients and circumstances. A recent series of *British Medical Journal* articles by Greenhalgh (1997) have now been expanded and published as an excellent beginner's guide to critical reading and EBH, richly illustrated with relevant examples for primary care.

We hope that we have demonstrated how incorporating principles of EBH could benefit and focus group or individual learning and teaching programmes.

Answering clinical questions

Learning occurs most readily when it relates to real clinical situations and when what has been learnt has then to be applied. The EBH approach begins with the clinical problem that the patient brings to his doctor. This clinical problem is then converted into an answerable question, usually in the format of 'patient details–intervention–comparison–outcome'. The best evidence to answer this question is then tracked down and critically appraised. The final step is to decide whether this evidence applies to the original clinical problem and whether this evidence could or indeed should be incorporated into day-to-day clinical practice (Sackett *et al* 1997, see Chapter 3).

Questions related to diagnosis, prognosis, therapy and harm have traditionally been dealt with by EBH. During normal clinical responsibilities, many questions will naturally arise. Many remain unanswered and indeed may be difficult to answer using the EBH approach. Other questions get directed to colleagues or authoritative textbooks are referred to. Although colleagues' opinions may be useful, they may also be unreliable. Textbooks unfortunately quickly become out of date and may present unbalanced summaries of the available evidence. The purpose of acquiring skills in EBH is for the practitioner to appraise the most relevant evidence himself and hence solve practical problems that arise in caring for patients.

Shared learning

Many clinicians prefer to learn with their peers and in the UK a number of different models have developed to facilitate this. 'Young Practitioners Groups' are formed by GPs who have been in practice for up to 10 years and who meet on a regular basis to learn together and support each other. They identify learning interests and needs and may then invite outside speakers, present seminars to each other or discuss interesting journal articles. Systems of mentoring are developing whereby more experienced practitioners agree to support and guide those new to practice. Practice nurses and other team members increasingly have access to external and peer clinical supervision and support.

Learning evidence-based health in a small group

Working in a small group is one of the most effective ways to become skilled in EBH. Small groups, ideally of 8–12 people, allow participants to experience the EBH approach from start to finish. Inexperienced groups require facilitation by someone able to guide them through the initial stages (see below).

The process begins with a relevant problem. A common clinical event – such as parents bringing a child with earache to see the doctor – can be used to start things off. Provided the clinical problem selected is relevant to the group, there is usually no problem in ensuring a lively discussion of the best way to manage the patient. Such discussions often reveal disagreements and uncertainty about the best clinical management, and leads onto consideration of the evidence to support clinical decisions. The available evidence can be found by searching electronic databases such as *The Cochrane Library*, Best Evidence and MEDLINE (see Chapter 3).

If there is little previous experience with EBH it is best to choose a paper that evaluates a common treatment in a well-conducted randomised controlled clinical trial (e.g. Burke *et al* 1991). Once a group is comfortable with the basic EBH approach, studies that combine the results of several studies can also be used (e.g. Del Mar *et al* 1997). It is helpful to have a written guide on how critically to appraise evidence available for reference such as those provided in Sackett *et al* (1997), Guyatt *et al* (1993, 1994) and Oxman *et al* (1994). Chapters 2 and 3 also provide frameworks and further relevant reading lists.

Tutor's role in small groups

Learning something new is not an easy process. It is important that positive feedback is given by the tutor so that both individuals and the group are aware of the progress they are making. The role of the tutor in any small group is central to its success. The tutor is not there to provide all the answers, but rather to help people discover the answers for themselves. Instead of answering questions raised by individuals in the group, it is more appropriate for the tutor to reflect these back to the whole group for discussion ('What do other people think of this?').

The key role of the tutor is to encourage open discussion within the group and to facilitate learning by helping the individuals in the group to work together. This sometimes involves the difficult task of encouraging the quieter members of the group to contribute more and the talkative members to contribute less. The tutor needs to encourage active listening and non-judgemental discussion between all members of the group.

Difficulties in learning evidence-based health

It is normal for a group to jump from issue to issue in the early stages of learning EBH, but this settles down as individuals become more familiar with the process. If several different issues get mixed up, it can be helpful to write them down and for the group to agree how they should be tackled. It is important not to be too ambitious about the amount of material that can be covered in 1–2 hours.

Tensions can develop within a group, particularly around those who consider themselves to be 'experts' and individuals who insist on repeatedly bringing up the same issue. At times it can be helpful to split up even a small group to complete a specific task (e.g. interpreting the results of a study), before bringing the group as a whole back together again.

Many people have concerns about dealing with statistics in research papers and look to the tutor for authoritative advice. There are a variety of texts on the statistical interpretation of scientific literature (see Chapter 10, Sackett *et al* (1997) and Greenhalgh (1997)). Reassuringly for most clinicians, perhaps, a detailed knowledge of statistics is not usually required in order to appraise research for EBH.

Evidence-based health in daily practice

Outside the group setting, individual clinicians can use the EBH approach in caring for their patients. Indeed, this is the whole purpose of EBH. The starting point is to identify important knowledge gaps and uncertainties that arise when caring for individual patients. Focusing on problems that are frequently encountered is likely to benefit the greatest number of patients. The main barriers to the EBH approach are time and access to original articles. Fortunately, the development of electronic databases (such as the Cochrane Collaboration and Best Evidence) and the wider availability of computers in medicine are making it much easier to overcome these barriers. Encourage local postgraduate libraries to concentrate on those journals most likely to be of benefit. The librarians may have lists of all the journal sources in the area, e.g. other hospitals and universities. If this is not available locally, lobby for it. Local providers and primary care groups could share their resources, perhaps through the local medical library. Only a minority of journal articles are available via electronic media.

Involving patients

There is a growing interest in and commitment to user or patient involvement in health care. Many governments are encouraging public rights and responsibilities in health decisions. Increasingly, the patient voice is being legitimised in planning, and primary care groups have lay members and are likely to make increasing use of patient participation groups, community health councils and voluntary bodies. All of these may represent patient views and the latter two in particular may well be compiling reports based on evidence themselves.

Patients and service users can be involved in the practice of EBH in a variety of ways. They can influence clinical practice through patient-mediated interventions, such as patient-specific reminders. They may have a role as members of guideline development groups. They can be involved in shared decision making with health-care professionals about available treatment and management options. Chapter 9 explores these issues.

As practitioners we are used to learning from our experiences with patients, but are perhaps less used actively to involving them in our education and development process, both for ourselves and our services. However, a number of projects are aimed at sharing effectiveness data with service users as a means of promoting the implementation of research findings. The Cochrane Collaboration seeks input and feedback from consumers. A Consumer Network has been established to reflect consumer interests within the Cochrane Collaboration. The Centre for Health Information Quality (www.centreforhiq@demon.co.uk) has been established to promote quality tools, checklists and guidelines, to appraise consumer health information and to provide a database and training programmes. Patient-mediated interventions include activity designed to change the performance of providers by giving information or advice on health-care effectiveness directly to patients, or by obtaining patients' views on the current pattern of practice and passing them to the provider (Mays 1994). If patients are to be encouraged to express their preferences and participate actively in decisions about their care, they will need access to good quality information and decision aids to support informed choice. Thus, they adopt an evidence-based approach to their education to facilitate decision making.

One example of a decision aid is the interactive videodisk. The 'Shared Decision Making Program' (Kasper et al 1992) enables the patient to share directly in the decision-making process with the doctor; the resulting new information results in a new pattern of choices and better outcomes. Although it has to be recognised that individual patients and users have widely differing demands for information, and not all patients want to share decisions, their participation in decision making can reduce demands for interventions and result in better outcomes. Chapter 24 explores in more detail how patient preferences can be incorporated into a decision-tree approach.

Patient participation groups are a useful forum for discussing health priorities and proposed guidelines. The local community health council may be interested in garnering local patient views and inputing their considerable networks and knowledge of local concerns and audits concerning health care. Needs assessment, whilst an essential tool for systematic health-care planning, is outwith the scope of this book (for introductory reading refer to Harris (1998) and Stevens and Gabbay (1989)). The results of such data collections will gel well with EBH.

References

Burke P, Bain J, Robinson D, et al (1991). Acute red ear in children: controlled trial of non-antibiotic treatment in general practice. British Medical Journal 303: 558–562.

Del Mar CB, Glasziou PP, Hayem M (1997). Are antibiotics indicated as an initial treatment for children with acute otitis media? A meta-analysis. British Medical Journal 314: 1526–1529.

Greenhalgh T (1997). How to Read a Paper, the Basics of Evidence Based Medicine. London: BMJ Publishing.

Guyatt GH, Sackett DL, Cook DJ (1993). Users guide to the medical literature. How to use an article about therapy or prevention. A. Are the results valid? Journal of the American Medical Association 270: 2598–2601.

Guyatt GH, Sackett DL, Cook DJ (1994). Users guide to the medical literature. How to use an article about therapy or prevention. B. What are the results and will they help me in caring for my patients? Journal of the American Medical Association 271: 59–63.

Harris A (Ed) (1998). Needs to Know: A Guide to Needs Assessment for Primary Care. London: RSM Publications.

Kasper J, Mulley A, Wennberg J (1992). Developing shared decision-making programs to improve the quality of health care. Quality Review Bulletin 18: 182–190.

Mays N (1994). Changing clinical behaviour: do we know how to do it? In: Harrison A (Ed) Health Care UK 1993–1994. London: King's Fund Institute, pp. 102–117.

McColl A, Smith H, White P, et al (1998). General practitioners' perceptions of the route to evidence based medicine: a questionnaire survey. British Medical Journal 316: 361–365.

Oxman AD, Cook DJ, Guyatt G (1994). Users guides to the literature. VI. How to use an overview. Journal of the American Medical Association 272: 1367–1371.

Rogers E (1983) Diffusion of Innovations 3 edn: Free Press, New York.

Sackett DL, Richardson WS, Rosenberg W, et al (1997). Evidence-based medicine. Edinburgh: Churchill Livingstone.

Stanley I, Al-Sheri A, Thomas P (1993). Continuing education for general practice. 1. Experience, competence and the media of self directed learning for established general practitioners. British Journal of General Practice 43: 210–214.

Stevens A and Gabbay J (1989). Needs assessment. Health Trends 23: 20–23.

Nursing and Evidence-Based Practice: A World Away from Evidence-Based Health

Rumona Dickson and Carrie Morrison

Introduction

Nurses working in primary care are in both ideal and disadvantaged positions in relation to the implementation of evidence-based practice. On the positive side, nurses have:

- ► continuous contact and communication with their patients;
- ► the opportunity to develop effective evidence-based care plans with their patients;
- ► the opportunity to work within innovative health-care teams.

However, nurses may be disadvantaged or limited in that they have:

- ► limited autonomy in relation to making patient care decisions;
- ► limited access to research findings;
- ► limited academic preparation in their use of research evidence;
- ► limited support within their work environments to implement evidence-based practice;
- ► limited access to continuing professional development.

Current publications promote the concept that evidence-based health care should include participation from all members of the professional health-care team. That the concept was originally introduced as evidence-based *medicine* speaks volumes. Recently, Booth (1998) compiled a summary of reports that attempted to measure the proportion of health care that is evidence based. His summary includes only one section related to general practice whilst no mention is made of care delivered by anyone other than physicians. Of course, his purpose was to summarise available information and it could be reasonably argued that there is a limited amount of information on the use of evidence by nurses in their clinical practice. This previously identified gap is the basis for a UK-based project that is examining the use of research by nurses in their clinical practice (Centre for Evidence-Based Nursing 1998).

A number of current initiatives attest to the recognition of the importance of nurses participating in the evolution of evidence-based practice. In January 1998, the first edition of the journal *Evidence-Based Nursing* was published. The primary objective of this journal is to identify quality research that is important to good nursing practice whilst publishing the results of this research in abstract form accompanied by clinical commentaries (Anon 1998). The journal is a collaborative venture and is co-edited by three prominent nurse-researchers from Canada and the UK, and is a joint publication of the BMJ Publishing Group and RCN Publishing.

Internationally, we have seen the establishment of centres promoting evidence-based nursing in Australia, Canada, Hong Kong and New Zealand. In England, leading nurse-researchers have established the Centre for Evidence-Based Nursing at the University of York. The main objectives of this centre are to identify completed primary research, undertake essential research, encourage nurses to participate in research, and increase the capabilities of nurses to employ research findings (Centre for Evidence-Based Nursing 1998).

Research on the most effective mechanisms for implementing these research findings in practice provides us with important information on where we might best invest our limited human and financial resources. Extensive work done by the *Cochrane Collaboration* for Effective Practice and Organisation of Care Review Group has produced a number of systematic reviews that examine issues related to the effectiveness of implementation strategies (EPOC 1998). This work provides direction for future endeavours to implement research findings into clinical practice. Although some of the studies included in these reviews include work with nurses, the majority examine changes in physician-based practice. A summary of findings is presented in Box 7.1.

Box 7.1. Cochrane Group summary of systematic reviews of implementation strategies (Adapted from Bero *et al* (1998) with permission)

Strategies that are consistently effective:

- Use of education outreach (one-to-one professional contact in care settings)

- Reminders/prompts (manual or computerised)

- Multifaceted interventions (combinations of two or more activities, e.g. audit and feedback, reminders, local consensus processes and patient-mediated interventions)

- Interactive educational meetings (workshops that include discussion)

Strategies with mixed effects:

- Audit and feedback

- Local opinion leaders

- Local consensus processes

- Patient-mediated interventions

Strategies with little or no effect:

- Educational materials, including the distribution of printed or published recommendations

- Didactic educational meetings (lectures)

Barriers to adoption of evidence-based practice

But what does all of this activity mean for primary care nurses and the use of evidence in their clinical practice? One important factor is whether nurses believe that the care they deliver should be based on the best available evidence. If they do not hold this belief, they are unlikely to initiate changes in their clinical practice and may implement changes only when directed to do so.

However, even if nurses are convinced that evidence-based practise is a good idea, the primary factor limiting the use of evidence in their clinical practice is a lack of both actual and perceived professional autonomy. In almost all aspects of their education and their professional careers, nurses are reminded that they do not make the primary decisions related to the care they provide. Rogers and Shoemaker (1971) characterised this as placing nurses in positions of making 'contingent' decisions, i.e. the majority of the decisions made in relation to patient care are based on the decisions of others, such as physicians or practice managers. Even when nurses are the primary implementers of changes in clinical practice, they may have limited input into the design of these changes (Campbell *et al* 1998). Although these situations are changing as primary care nurses undertake greater responsibility for patient care decisions, the adoption of evidence-based practice by primary care nurses will be limited until the issue of autonomy in decision making is addressed.

A second important issue is the potentially erroneous assumption that the approach used to implement changes in physician-care practices will be appropriate for nurses. Primary care physicians are in a better position independently to develop their skills and institute the changes necessary to implement evidence-based care in their clinical practices. In fact, we do not know what combination of strategies will be the most effective in changing nursing practice.

It is our belief that there is a need to use an approach different from that for physicians when developing evidence-based practice for nurses. This hypothesis is based partly on the issue of autonomy discussed above and partly on evidence that changes in practice are more likely to occur when multiple strategies are used (Bero *et al* 1998) and when these strategies include groups of health-care workers (Ross-Degnan *et al* 1997). Given the position of nurses within the clinical practice structure, their history of working within multidisciplinary teams and the acknowledged difficulties of implementing changes within nursing (McKenna 1997), it may be more effective to develop evidence-based practice project teams. The roles of such teams would be to define research questions, identify the best evidence and develop implementation strategies (see below).

There are a number of ways to look at the issues related to evidence-based practice in primary care nursing. In this chapter, we examine the issues from three perspectives: the nurses, nursing education, and the environments in which nurses work. The initial section focuses on the requisite skills and abilities needed by nurses in order for them to employ evidence in their practice; the second section considers the roles of educational programmes in providing nurses with the skills needed to implement evidence into practice, and the final section discusses issues related to the clinical environments in which nurses work (Table 7.1).

Table 7.1. Factors facilitating evidence-based health care in nursing

Nurses need the ability to:	*Educational environment* should provide:	*Clinical environment* should encourage:
Define clinical questions	An atmosphere that actively promotes critical thinking and problem solving	Questioning of current practice
Access the research evidence	Integration of evidence in curricula	Implementation of change
Assess the research evidence	Integration of critical appraisal and research	
Implement change	methodology in curricula	

Nurse requirements

It first needs to be acknowledged that primary health-care nurses are working in dramatically changing situations in which nurses are also being asked to extend their care delivery skills and change their clinical responsibilities (Kenrick and Luker 1995). The implementation of evidence-based practice is therefore just one issue amongst many others that need to be addressed.

Ability to define clinical questions

Many primary care nurses believe that evidence-based practice is a worthwhile goal. However, to make the necessary changes, nurses must be able to identify the important patient care factors that, if altered, could result in positive patient outcomes. To do this, nurses require skills in the identification and definition of specific clinical questions. The development of these skills takes time and experience.

Ability to access the research evidence

Let us assume that a group of primary care nurses identify a clinical problem and defines a clinically important question, i.e. they decide there is a specific area of their current practice that could benefit from examination within the context of current research evidence. How do these nurses access this evidence? Whilst international initiatives have expanded the availability of research information, currently in the UK access to this information is limited.

On the positive side, there has been a recognition of the needs of primary care nurses. Publication of books specifically related to their clinical needs (e.g. Kenrick and Luker 1995) and systematic reviews (e.g. *Effective Health Care Bulletin*) are important and readily available resources. Expansion of information sources via computers and the Internet means that access to information is increasing in many areas (see Chapter 3). Of course, this assumes that nurses have the necessary knowledge and access to utilise computers and computer-based information sites. However, existing computer-based information sites are not primarily designed for nurses. In fact, of the 98 evidence-based practice Internet sites listed in the comprehensive School of Health and Related Research guide, only four are specifically targeted towards nurses (ScHARR 1999).

Nurses working in primary care settings have limited access to published research. The clinical practices in which they work are unlikely to subscribe to many clinically relevant journals and the costs of journal subscriptions restrict personal access.

Local hospitals often have small but relatively well supplied libraries. However, the resources of these libraries are not always available to nurses. For example, among three hospitals we recently contacted, whilst all had medical libraries, one restricted its use to physicians only and one to clinical staff employed at the hospital, and one library had an open system that welcomed community users. All of these facilities had limited opening hours and only one provided computer access to database searching such as MEDLINE. Whilst it is common to find that nurses are restricted or excluded from hospital libraries, the culture is changing.

Recent changes in *local university library* policies have resulted in limited access for non-university users; access is often restricted because of concerns about electronic searching and CD-ROM information systems copyright restrictions. This restrictive use includes on-site access only and no access to inter-library loan facilities (Casey 1997).

Ability to assess the research evidence

But let us say that our nurses have compiled the evidence related to their clinical question. It is likely that the knowledge they gained in their nursing education will not have provided them with the necessary skills for assessing the quality of this evidence. These are vital skills if they wish to make decisions regarding implementation within their clinical practice. Continuing or in-service education programmes are now available to help nurses develop these skills. Nevertheless, only a limited number of nurses have been able to take advantage of these programmes.

Ability to implement change

Let us assume that our nurses have either the necessary critical appraisal skills or find someone to help them undertake the appraisal. The group decides that, given the evidence, it should change current care patterns. As noted earlier, experience and evidence of the effectiveness of change strategies in primary care settings are limited. However, nurses have a history of innovation and our group would be able to design a mechanism for implementing change. The probable limiting factor for these nurses will be that, even as a group, they will not have the authority necessary to implement the changes within their clinical practice setting. Therefore, any strategies that they develop will be complicated by a need to convince those in positions of authority that the clinical changes are important, necessary and possible.

What we have outlined here is a list of hurdles that primary care nurses must overcome before they can begin to contemplate the implementation of evidence-based practice. Given the length and complexity of this list it is easy to see that a group of nurses may be more likely than an individual nurse successfully to undertake such an endeavour. However, these barriers are not insurmountable and there are numerous signs indicating that, in fact, all are being addressed within the clinical practice arenas. One such initiative has been developed by the Research and Development Support Unit for Merseyside and Cheshire. Its purpose is to help develop research capacity by increasing the involvement of health professionals. It provides support in the form of assistance in the development of research proposals, provision of methodological advice (economic, statistical and review advice on an individual and a group basis) and capacity building activities tailored to the needs of specific health groups or trusts (Research and Development Support Unit 1998).

Requirements of the educational environment

The nursing education environment has historically not included the concepts of evidence-based practice. Three particular areas within this environment will be discussed here. The first concerns the methods of instruction used, the second looks at the integration of evidence into nursing curricula, whilst the third discusses the integration of research methodology and critical appraisal skills into the curricula.

To promote problem solving

One of the key factors in implementing evidence-based practice is changing the way that health professionals address clinical problems. Currently, nursing education relies predominantly on lectures and clinical experiences. We know that didactic lectures are one of the least effective methods of promoting active learning (Alavi 1995, Bero et al 1998), whilst the quality of the clinical experiences are dependent on the individual tutors and the clinical atmosphere in which they occur (Martin 1996). There are clear indications that changing this educational model to one of problem-based learning would be beneficial to nurses, assisting both the short- and long-term development of the skills needed to define and solve clinical problems (Alavi 1995). Medical students from problem-based learning programmes are more likely to integrate new evidence into their clinical practice (Shin et al 1993). Nurses educated in similar programmes could be expected to develop these important skills.

Integration of evidence

A shift to problem-based learning is only the first step to providing nurses with the information required to use evidence in their practice. All curricula must also include the best available evidence of effectiveness. Current nursing education initiatives in the UK are helping to move this agenda forward and we now see the inclusion of evidence into certain segments of nursing curricula (Wood 1998). Examples include the use of evidence-based guidelines developed by nurses and reviews carried out by nurses in curricula (Kenrick and Luker 1995).

Integration of critical appraisal

Regardless of the strengths of current curricula, nurses need to continue to identify new research that may affect their future practice, and be able critically to assess the quality of this research. This means that courses on basic research methodologies, critical appraisal and the use of systematic reviews need to be part of basic and graduate-level programmes. These changes are occurring in some UK nursing education programmes (C Carlisle and H Waterman, personal communication). Nonetheless, the move towards evidence-based practice will be limited until the majority of nurses develop an understanding of these concepts.

Continuing professional education

The above three areas deal with basic and graduate education. The other important area for nurses currently practising is continuing professional education (Wood 1998). Within this there are two components to be addressed:

- availability and accessibility to continuing professional education for nurses;

- content of these programmes.

Limited institutional funding for continuing education and low salary levels preclude most nurses from taking part in such programmes. Means need to be found to provide affordable continuing education for all nurses. At the same time, the content and presentation of continuing education programmes need to reflect current evidence of effectiveness and include multifaceted presentation approaches which we know to be the most effective for changing practice. Therefore, to acquire and develop the skills that nurses require to improve their clinical practice, methods must be found to support non-credit learning opportunities.

Short programmes such as the Critical Appraisal Skills Programme (CASP), which are now available as open-learning resources, are designed to meet some of these needs. Conference planners should be encouraged to consider format changes that will help better meet the needs of the participating nurses. Moreover, designers of distance-education programmes should be encouraged to include aspects of evidence-based practice in their curricula.

Requirements of the clinical environment

To encourage questioning

No matter how committed any nurse or group of nurses is to the implementation of evidence in their clinical practice, their work environment will dictate whether they will be able to move their agenda forward. Clinical practices that focus on task-based nursing, or on the premise of 'we have always done it this way', are fewer than they once were, but certainly still exist. Work atmospheres like this do not allow nurses to question the delivery of their care, let alone change the way in which they deliver it. Conversely, the number of primary health-care settings where questioning of clinical practice is encouraged are increasing. In these situations, changes may, in theory, be possible.

Encourage nurses to implement change

However, frustrations arise when nurses either lack the skills to fully evaluate the clinical situation, or are not in a position (or not allowed) to implement changes to their practice. An example of these different circumstances has arisen in the treatment of leg ulcers. Leading nurse-researchers in the UK have conducted systematic reviews and provided evidence of effectiveness (NHS Centre for Reviews and Dissemination 1997). As a result, some nurses have been able to implement changes in their clinical practice that reflect this evidence. However, others have found that physicians refuse to consider the systematically reviewed evidence and do not allow changes to nursing clinical practice (Lahiff 1998).

Even in clinical environments that have the necessary components in place for facilitating the definition of clinical questions, assessing the evidence, and implementing the changes, the process is not so simple. It requires a large measure of time, determination and commitment from all health-care professionals. Experience has shown that the needs of nurses and physicians are different, and that time is needed to develop team and personal skills that allow *all* team members to take part in the changes in practice (T Lipman, personal communication).

The team approach

There is good reason to believe that a team approach to evidence-based practice may be appropriate and effective given the limitations of primary care nurses in relation to the use of research. Teams of nurses may combine their skills (e.g. defining clinical questions, critical appraisal of research, etc.) and be more confident as a result in the conclusions drawn. In addition, a well-informed and involved team is in a better position to devise appropriate implementation strategies. Such team approaches have worked in tertiary care settings (M Edwards, personal communication), in regional health authorities in Canada (Kalinka 1998), and in changing prescribing patterns in developing countries (Ross-Degnan *et al* 1997). Whether such a team approach could be effective in UK primary care settings needs to be assessed. Moreover, it needs to be ascertained whether such primary care teams would be more or less effective if physicians were included as team members.

Conclusion

Evidence-based practice is moving rapidly into the forum of primary health care. As in other clinical areas, the focus has been on the use of evidence by physicians. This has resulted in two possible outcomes: either nurses, and the needs and contributions of nurses, have been forgotten, or there has been an assumption that what works with physicians will also work with nurses. From the perspective of primary care nurses, both of these scenarios are problematic. In the first, nurses are excluded and remain in a secondary role following the directions provided by physicians or practice managers. In the second, their backgrounds, skills and decision-making autonomy are presumed to be the same as their physician counterparts. None of these assumptions is correct. Nurses come from significantly different educational backgrounds which have provided them with particular skills but have failed to provide them with the problem solving and research assessment skills that are critical to the implementation of evidence-based practice. The culture within which they work has placed them in positions where the major patient care decisions they make are contingent on decisions made by others (physicians and practice managers).

However, there are many signs that the implementation of evidence-based practice by primary care nurses is not only possible but is actually happening. Many primary health-care nurses have developed the skills necessary to formulate well-defined clinical questions and to examine their practice. Many are able to identify and assess the research evidence and to develop strategies to implement changes in clinical practice.

Educational programmes are modifying teaching techniques to facilitate an atmosphere that encourages problem-based learning whilst updating curricula to include the best available evidence. Continuing education programmes are being developed to provide opportunities for nurses to develop both their clinical and research skills.

The clinical environment in which nurses practice is also changing significantly. Many primary health-care teams approach the delivery of care in a multidisciplinary manner that attempts to utilise best the skills of all the team members in order to improve the quality of care provided to patients. Future monitoring and research evaluation, related to the role of primary health-care nurses in evidence-based practise, is required to maximise the impact of these nurses in relation to positive patient outcomes and good quality care.

References

Alavi C (Ed) (1995). *Problem-Based Learning in a Health Science Curriculum*. London: Routledge.

Anon (1998). Purpose and procedure. *Evidence-Based Nursing* 1: 2–3.

Bero L, Grilli R *et al* (1998). Closing the gap between research and practice: an overview of systematic reviews of interventions to promote the implementation of research findings. In: Haines A and Donald A (Eds) *Getting Research Findings into Practice*. London: BMJ Publishing pp 27–35.

Booth A (1998). What proportion of health care is evidence based? *Resource Guide* http://www.shef.ac.uk/~scharr/ir/percent.html

Campbell N, Thain J, Deans HG, *et al* (1998). Secondary prevention clinics for coronary heart disease: randomised trial of effect on health. *British Medical Journal* **316**: 1434–1437.

Casey N (1997). Library access: campaigning for better information [editorial]. *Nursing Standard* **12**: 1.

Centre for Evidence-Based Nursing (1998). Background and objectives of the Centre. http://www.york.ac.uk/depts/hstd/entrres/evidence/ev-intro.htm

Effective Health Care Bulletin (1997). *Compression Therapy for Venous Leg Ulcers*. York: NHS Centre for Reviews and Dissemination.

EPOC (1998). Effective Practice and Organisation of Care Review Group Scope. http://www.abdn.ac.uk/public_health/hsru/epoc

Kalinka S (1998). *SEARCH (Swift, Efficient, Application of Research in Community Health)*. Ottawa: International Society of Technology Assessment in Health Care.

Kenrick M and Luker K (Eds) (1995). *Clinical Nursing Practice in the Community*. Oxford: Blackwell Science Ltd.

Lahiff M (1998). Nursing research: The why and the why not? In: Smith P (Ed) *Nursing Research: Setting New Agendas*. London: Arnold.

Martin G (1996). An approach to the facilitation and assessment of critical thinking in nurse education. *Nurse Education Today* **16**: 3–9.

McKenna H (1997). *Nursing Theories and Models*. London: Routledge.

NHS Centre for Reviews and Dissemination. Compression therapy for venous leg ulcers. *Effective Health Care* **3(4)**.

Research and Development Support Unit (1998). *Report of First Six Months of Operation*. Liverpool: University of Liverpool.

Rogers E and Shoemaker FF (1971). *Communication of Innovations: A Cross-Cultural Approach*. London: Collier-MacMillan Ltd.

Ross-Degnan D, Laing R *et al* (1997). Improving pharmaceutical use in primary care in developing countries: a critical review of experience and lack of experience. *International Conference on Improving Use of Medicines*, Chiang Mai, Thailand.

ScHARR (1999). Netting the Evidence. A ScHARR Introduction to Evidence-Based Practice on the Internet. School for Health and Related Research. World Wide Web: http://www.shef.ac.uk/~scharr/ir/netting/html

Shin J, Haynes R *et al* (1993). Effect of problem-based, self-directed undergraduate education on life-long learning. *Canadian Medical Association Journal* **149**: 794–795.

Wood I (1998). The effects of continuing professional education on the clinical practice of nurses: a review of the literature. *International Journal of Nursing Studies* **35**: 125–131.

►8

Evidence-Based Health, Patient Consent and Consumerism

Lucy Frith

Introduction

One of the consequences of evidence-based health (EBH) is that medical information is now more easily available to patients. This, it is claimed, will enable patients to be better informed about their treatments and hence the consent they give will be made on the basis of a more extensive knowledge of the relevant information. Increasing the amount and availability of medical information is part of the trend that encourages patient participation and empowerment in health care. The way that patient empowerment is fostered, at least in government policy, is by the consideration of patient as consumer, i.e. a client of the health service.

In this chapter I want to consider the way that EBH can be used to help patients make more informed choices. Encouraging patients to be better informed is an ethically desirable end. However, ethical problems can arise if this information giving operates within a consumerist model of health care and patient empowerment.

There are three important reasons why patients cannot be seen as consumers of health care and therefore why information giving driven by consumerist policies is not an adequate way of ensuring that patients make fully informed and appropriate choices.

- ► The complexity of medical information means that it may not be possible for lay people to be able to understand and make medical choices unaided.

- ► Consumers are usually healthy and in full possession of their faculties, whereas patients may be suffering from various levels of physical and mental distress and unable to make complex decisions.

- ► Consumer spending activities are rarely directly curtailed for the good of themselves or others. If something is legally allowed to be sold then, if we can afford it, we have a right to buy it. In health care, however, there sometimes have to be restrictions placed on the patient's choice either for his own good or the good of others.

The purpose of this discussion is not to argue that EBH is not useful in giving patients more information, nor that patients should not have greater access to information. The purpose is to stress that simply to see the provision of information as an unqualified good without considering the way it is used and the context in which it is given is naive.

Patient consent

In essence EBH is concerned with increasing the amount of medical evidence available so that the relevant parties can make more informed decisions. In this way it is thought that EBH can be an important tool in informing the consent patients give to medical procedures. Two features of the EBH approach have particular implications for patient consent:

- improvement in the availability of medical information due to technological advances, such as the Internet and MEDLINE;
- move towards presenting medical information so that it is more easily understandable and accessible to the non-specialist.

Availability of information

In order for patients to participate fully in their health-care decisions they need to be informed about all the aspects and alternatives to the procedure to which they are being asked to consent. The EBH movement has been concerned with making medical evidence more accessible and therefore can be a useful tool for enabling patients to be better informed about their treatment. This argument is based on a straightforward claim that as there is more information available in more accessible forms, then patients will be better informed.

The explosion in information technology has not just affected the medical profession: it is now easier for patients to find medical information for themselves. With computer technology such as CD-ROMs and the Internet, patients can do their own research. Most doctors now have a tale about a patient who read something on the Internet and presents armed with his own diagnosis and management strategy.

Accessibility of information

Not only is medical information more accessible with computer technology, it is also easier to understand due to the use of abstracts, systematic reviews and a concern to write for the non-specialist (See http://ihs.ac.uk/casp/statistics/html, a guide to statistical and research terms for the uninitiated). The *APC Journal Club*, for example, started in 1991 with the aim of disseminating research findings. The editorial team scans the medical journals and identifies articles of clinical relevance, the research findings are scrutinised and conclusions thought to be invalid or inapplicable are rejected. The selected articles are then presented on one page and accompanied by an expert commentary to integrate them with other practice and draw out the practical implications. Hence, medical information is now presented in a much more accessible form for the non-specialist clinician or student, and patients can take advantage of this.

For example, an article in *The Guardian*, 27th October 1998, gave readers web site addresses and CD-ROM details for finding systematic reviews of research trials.

This greater availability of information makes it is easier for patients to make fully autonomous decisions about their health care. There are two vital elements to enabling patients to make autonomous decisions:

▶ giving them enough information on which to base their decision;

▶ allowing them to make the decision themselves without undue coercion or pressure.

This chapter focuses on the first element.

If someone is not given all the relevant facts about a course of action they cannot make an autonomous decision: they will not be able to weigh up all the pros and cons for themselves.

If I offer to lend you my car so you can get to the hospital more quickly in an emergency but neglect to tell you that the brakes are not working properly, then you might agree to take the car without being aware of the full implications of your decision. However, if I tell you about the brakes, you can weigh up if the benefit of getting to the hospital quickly is worth risking the possibility of the brakes failing.

Hence, information giving is an important element in enabling patients to make autonomous decisions.

The increase in the availability of information outside the formal medical encounter and the concern to make this information as 'user friendly' as possible are positive steps to enabling patients to make more informed decisions. However, the debate cannot stop there. Simply making more medical information available does not solve all the problems of ensuring that patients give fully informed consent. In practice, information giving and respecting patient autonomy have tended to be fostered within a consumerist framework. I will argue that if information giving is seen solely as a mechanism for enabling patients to exercise their rights as consumers, then this can create ethical difficulties.

Autonomy, empowerment and consumerism

The increase in the availability of medical information has occurred alongside the general trend of encouraging patients to be more active participants in their own health care: to become consumers of health care rather than passive recipients. By fostering consumerism it is thought that patients will be able to act as more autonomous agents in the health-care system and that rights enshrined in the Patients' Charter to protect them will ensure a more satisfactory service. Consumerism has become the dominant means by which it is thought that the NHS can ensure both patient autonomy is respected and a decent service provided.

This trend comes from a variety of perspectives and political persuasions but it was the last government's reforms of the NHS which were instrumental in fostering consumerism in health care. These reforms involved the creation of an internal market which was designed to simulate a market economy within the health service by encouraging competition. This competition would cut costs, improve quality and make the health service more responsive to the users' needs. Within this simulated market the users of the health service were to be seen as consumers of health care and not patients. The term 'consumer' implies a more active and autonomous role than 'patient'.

> 'Consumers are viewed as adopting a more active social role associated with the notion of rights, power and empowerment.' (Melville 1997)

The focus for consumerist rhetoric is fostering patient autonomy. One of the aims of creating the internal market was to give consumers increased bargaining power and therefore more choice over their health care. Consumers would influence providers by the decisions they made and the health service would respond to the consumer rather than the providers of the service. As Margaret Thatcher said in the government white paper *Working for Patients*:

> 'We aim to extend patient choice ... All the proposals in the white paper put the needs of the patient first ... The patient's needs will always be paramount.' (Department of Health 1989)

This extension of patient choice was largely to be done by attempting to give patients greater freedom to choose the health care they wanted, in ethical language encouraging the exercising of patient autonomy.

This concern for patient autonomy is laudable, but I will argue that simply giving patients medical information and then expecting them to use it independently as consumers would use information, is not an adequate way of ensuring that patients make fully informed and appropriate choices about their health care. The duties of the health professionals go beyond information provision and extend to trying to ensure that patients understand it and use it well. This is because the medical profession has a positive duty of beneficence to their patients which distinguishes health care from commercial organisations which only have a negative duty not to cause undue harm.

As consumers of products we expect that the product will be fit for the purpose for which it is sold. For example, crisp manufacturers have a duty not to cause us undue harm, i.e. their crisps should not contain toxic substances. However, we do not expect them to stop selling crisps because they are not very good for us and we should be encouraged to snack on fruit rather than fatty foods with little nutritional value; i.e. we do not expect the manufacturers to act beneficently towards us. Health care, however, is another matter. The provision of health care and professionals' duties do not just extend to ensuring that people have unfettered choice or that people are protected from undue harm. Rather they have positive duties to do good for their patients. Simply allowing people to exercise free choice may not be doing the best for them and doctors, while aiming at all times to maximise patient autonomy, have to balance this against their duties to act beneficently.

Concerns from wider availability of medical information

With the development of EBH patients will have access to medial information outside the formal medical encounter and while this can be very useful in helping patients understand their condition and treatment, there are some potential pitfalls that need to be recognised. The most important of these is that patients need doctors to help them understand and interpret medical information. Unlike buying a cooker where an understanding of the relevant information to make an informed purchase is relatively straightforward, the skills needed to understand medical information take years of training to develop.

A review of a decision-making guide for patients on CD, *Urinary Disorders and Male Health*, that would be used by patients in the waiting room, highlights the difficulty in presenting information that is easily understandable to the layman.

> '*It assumes that its audience is conversant with medical terminology and freely uses words such as hyperplasia, transitional cells, and carcinoma in situ.*' (Gibbs 1998)[1]

Despite the difficulties in presenting information in an easily understandable format, it is not impossible and many projects are concerned with writing patient information leaflets in a comprehensible and informative way (Buckland and Gann 1997).

However, even if patient information leaflets or information found on the Internet are easily understandable, patients still need to discuss the information with a practitioner to contextualize it. Each case is different and the general information about a condition needs to be applied to the individual patient. This is important as particular pieces of health information might be particularly distressing. For instance, patients consulting *Urinary Disorders and Male Health* might see the word carcinoma and panic, thinking that was the likely cause of their urinary problems. Simply providing medical information is not enough to ensure that patients give informed consent. Patients need help in the form of support and interpreting of data so they can make proper use of any information they find.

A further problem with medical information received outside the formal medical encounter is that the information patients get from the media and the Internet could be of variable quality. This is a particular problem for the Internet as there is no inherent quality control (Jadad and Gagliardi 1998). Patients will not be equipped to decide which web sites are worth visiting and which information is trustworthy.

> '*As the number of health related sites continues to rise, so does the concern about possible "information overload", with high quality sites becoming lost in the mass of "hits" retrieved by search engines.*' (Grant and Henshaw 1998)

For instance, The American Federal Trade Commission found 400 web sites that made fraudulent or dangerous claims about treatment.

---

[1] This is not to say these aids are not valuable. As Gibbs (1998) says, the CD will be useful to general practitioners and junior doctors so that they will be able to answer 'all those difficult questions that patients ask after seeing the consultant or, more commonly, after seeing a television programme the night before.'

These problems are not, of course, inherent in the use of the Internet. It is possible that a quality mark could be developed that would indicate that a site conformed to some sort of standard, such as Health on the Net.[1] There are various rating tools (Grant and Henshaw 1998), such as the *Britannica Internet Guide*, that aim to give browsers some idea of the quality of the sites. With these kinds of checks and rating tools the Internet could be an invaluable source of good, up-to-date information.

In summary, due to the complex nature of medical information, simply providing patients with this information does not ensure that they are able to give fully informed consent. Information giving is an invaluable start to the process, giving the patient an idea of the pertinent questions to ask and the issues at stake. Ultimately, however, the doctor has to help the patient act autonomously by facilitating their decision making and supporting the patient throughout this process: it is this beneficent concern that is lacking in the consumerism model of information giving.

Reasoning and decision-making abilities

Patients, unlike consumers, are often not functioning optimally: they are ill and by definition perhaps not able to process information to the best of their ability. Therefore, the problem of getting fully informed consent is often not necessarily one of lack of information but how, where and when the information is given. Does the patient fully understand what he is being told? Are there opportunities to discuss the information at a later date after it has been absorbed? Is the patient encouraged to ask questions? To ensure that patients understand the information they are given, three areas need to be addressed:

▶ communication skills of the individual health carer need to be adequate to the task;

▶ institutional procedures need to allow the carer ample time to impart the information properly;

▶ a system of checks needs to make sure the relevant information has been given and that information is given regularly and not just at the onset of treatment.

Before the issue of how information is imparted is addressed, there has to be some agreement over what is the relevant information to give the patient. Clearly, if the doctor has to tell the patient about every single aspect of the treatment, he will have no time to administer it. Also, it is sometimes argued that to give all the information to the patient could harm him and not be in his best interests. Although the paternalistic withholding of information is largely discredited, there still has to be some selectivity over what is disclosed both for practical and ethical reasons.

The case of *Chatterton v. Gerson* [1981] illustrates the legal approach to the question of how much information should be disclosed.

---

[1] Health on the Net.URL. http://www.hon.ch/ Global/about_HON.html. There is also Healthfinder developed by the US Department of Health and Human Services, that directs the public to reliable sources of health information, http://www.healthfinder.org/.

> Miss Chatterton took a case against her doctor, arguing that she had not given informed consent to a surgical procedure because she had not been given information on all the possible risks involved in the treatment. Her action failed as the judge said that a consent to surgery was valid providing that the patient was 'informed in broad terms of the nature of the procedure which is intended' (Brazier 1992). Miss Chatterton then took a negligence action and this failed too. The judge found that although the doctor should have told her about the most common risks inherent in the procedure, he did not have to tell her every single risk there might be. The decision of how much to tell her should be made by taking into account 'the personality of the patient, the likelihood of misfortune and what in the way of warning is for the particular patient's welfare' (Brazier 1992).

This case illustrates that there is no legal definition of precisely how much information should be given to the patient. In English law, generally, the reasonable professional standard of information giving is adopted. Thus, it is largely left to the professional to decide how much information should be given to the patient.

However, the courts have not always accepted the reasonable professional standard of information giving, and one of the judges in the case of *Sideway v. Bethlem Royal Hospital Governors* [1985] stated that, in certain cases:

> 'disclosure of a particular risk was so obviously necessary to an informed choice on the part of the patient that no reasonably prudent medical man would fail to make it.'

This judgement encapsulates the idea that doctors should act reasonably as well as acting in accordance with a responsible body of medical opinion.

Hence, the law leaves the question of how much information to divulge up to the judgement of the individual doctor, stipulating that those decisions have to balance the patient's welfare and the patient's autonomy by giving enough information for the patient to make an informed choice. It is the inclusion of a consideration of the patient's welfare that distinguishes both the legal and ethical position from the consumerist model of information giving. Under the consumerist model, the patient would be given all the information, which would respect his autonomy. However, the doctor has a duty of beneficence to the patient and in this context he should ensure that the patient is not harmed by the information. Thus, the doctor, in my view, must aim both to respect the patient's autonomy and act beneficently towards the patient.

The following case study illustrates how not balancing beneficence and autonomy can lead to difficulties.

> A complaint was made by a woman who had been admitted to hospital, in great distress, with blood clots on the lung and had been put on a drip of heparin. Later in the course of treatment her arm swelled up but she was not told why the swelling had occurred. Although it was treated successfully, the woman complained because she thought the swelling had occurred as a result of the nurse not cleaning her wound properly.

When she was admitted, the doctor acted beneficently, administering the drip and telling her very little about the treatment, simply saying that everything would be alright. However, no more information was given when her condition stabilised. The issue here is not whether the woman would have refused consent if she had been given more information at the onset of treatment, as it is unlikely that she would have refused life-saving treatment. Rather, it illustrates the problems caused by viewing consent solely as an authorisation to proceed with a treatment. If consent had been seen as an ongoing process with information being given gradually throughout the treatment, then when her condition had stabilised the doctor would have then given her more information and discussed her treatment with her in more detail, thus increasing her autonomy. She would have been told what was happening when the swelling occurred, i.e. that it was a normal side-effect of a drip, and this would have alleviated her distress.

In conclusion, many of the most thorny problems of informed consent in medical practice concern questions of what is the relevant information to give patients and the means by which it is disseminated, rather than a lack of available information. If information giving operates within a consumerist model then the onus will simply be on information provision. Such a solution does not provide the best service for patients. Health professionals have a responsibility to act beneficently towards their patients and ensure that they understand the information and have support and care while receiving it.

Restricting autonomy to promote beneficence

In carrying out their duty of beneficence there may be occasions when health professionals feel that they should not respect a patient's autonomy: if it is not in the patient's best interests or if it is not in the interests of the greater good. Clinical staff have a duty to ensure that their patients make the most appropriate decisions for themselves, but they also have a duty to the wider community, either their hospital trust or the NHS depending on how widely the responsibility is cast, to ensure that individual's decisions do not harm the greater good. I shall consider these two areas in turn.

Individual good

In the majority of medical encounters the patient is guided by the professional, options are presented or one course of action is strongly recommended and an agreement is reached. However, what should happen in cases where the professional and the patient disagree?

A patient goes to his GP with flu and asks for a prescription. When pressed, he says he wants antibiotics because he wants to get well quickly in time for an important event.

A strictly consumerist response to this would be to give the patient the treatment he wants. This would respect his freedom of choice and respect his autonomy. However, the goal of patient care is to help patients fulfil their desired ends and achieve the best outcome. Mill (1976) when discussing the legitimate reasons for restricting someone's liberty, states:

> 'If either a public officer or anyone else saw a person attempting to cross a bridge which had been ascertained to be unsafe, and there was no time to warn him of the danger, they might seize him and turn him back, without any real infringement of his liberty; for liberty consists in doing what he desires, and he does not desire to fall into the river.'

The patient desires to get well quickly and preserve his health and antibiotics do not facilitate this end. Thus, the doctor should explain why antibiotics should not be given and attempt to reach an agreement with the patient. However, if an agreement cannot be reached, the doctor is justified in still refusing to prescribe the antibiotics, as it could be argued that the patient is not perceiving his own best interests accurately and his desire to get well conflicts with his desire to have antibiotics.

Two aspects of patient choice need to be distinguished here:

- free choice within a particular set of options;

- free choice over the range of options.

One of the main aims of EBH is to ensure that the options the NHS provides are the most effective and the clinician should present the patient with a range of the most effective treatment options. Choices between the particular options, if they have equivalent effectiveness, should be left to the patient. The limiting of options on the grounds that they are unsafe or inappropriate is not an unwarranted restriction of patients' choices. Choices must be extended within definable boundaries, i.e. promoting a good outcome for the patient. It is the extension of the right *kind* of options that is important, not just simply increasing the overall number of available options.

General good

Just as the clinician has a duty of beneficence to an individual patient, it can also be argued that he has a duty of beneficence to the wider community, e.g. his trust. A health professional should aim to promote the welfare of the trust and be mindful of the effects of his patients' choices might have on the collective.

The Child B case was an example where the treatment choice of one individual patient was seen to harm the greater good of the health authority.

Child B, who was suffering from leukaemia, was refused a second bone marrow transplant by Cambridge Health Authority. Her father challenged the decision in the High Court; it then went to the Appeal Court where the Health Authority's (HA) decision was upheld. The interesting aspects of this case are that the HA was considering the implications for its patients as a whole and focused on the cost of the treatment versus the expected outcome. The HA told the Appeal Court that it had refused treatment on the grounds that, in its view, this would not be a cost-effective use of resources. The treatment cost of £75 000 was not justified by the predicted success rate which was very low. If they spent the money elsewhere they might procure more benefit.

Assuming for the sake of the argument that the treatment was in Child B's best interests, it is possible to see that the duty of the doctor to promote beneficence for his patient and the duty of beneficence to the HA could come into conflict. This conflict in duties is not easily solved and it is one that tests health authorities and hospital trusts when making resource allocation decisions (Frith (in press)). However, there clearly needs to be some kind of balance between the needs of the individual patient and the general good. Within a consumerist model, such a balance could never be struck as the focus would always be on the individual patient to get as much out of the system as he could, neglecting to recognise the obligations he has to other users of the health service. As Sorell (1997) states:

> 'Consumerism is usually unconcerned with responsibilities of users or consumers to one another, and it tends to ignore all but the relations affecting economic competition between providers. In the NHS context, however, users have responsibilities to one another ... Users have responsibilities not to overburden the NHS, for example.'

I would argue that as health care is a basic human good, the provision of which should not be limited by someone's economic status, we have obligations to pay for the health service even if we are lucky enough never to use it, and obligations not to overburden it with unwarranted demands. Clinicians also have obligations to consider their patients' choices and balance them against the welfare of other patients. This is not to say that the good of the individual should be of secondary importance to the greater good but, in certain circumstances, that has to be a factor in weighing up what is the right course of action.

Conclusion

Increasing the amount and improving the availability of medical information for patients is important both ethically and legally. Patients should be given as much information about their proposed treatment as possible and fully informed consent, while possibly only an ideal, should still be strived for. Consumerism encourages the giving of information to patients on the grounds that it respects their autonomy and enables them to be 'good' consumers of health care. I have argued that the duties of health professionals go further than simply ensuring that information is available for patients if they want it. The health professions have a duty of beneficence towards patients and this involves making sure patients understand the information, supporting them while it is given and helping them make appropriate health-care choices. It is this duty that distinguishes health care from commercial enterprises and, hopefully, ensures that patients are able to make the best choices for themselves about their medical care.

References

Brazier M (1992). *Medicine, Patients and the Law*. Harmondsworth: Penguin Books.

Buckland S and Gann B (1997). *Disseminating Treatment Outcomes Information to Consumers*. London: King's Fund Publishing.

Department of Health (1989). *Working for Patients*. London: HMSO.

Frith L (in press). Evidence based medicine and priority setting. *Health Care Analysis*.

Gibbs T (1998). A review of urinary disorders and male health. *British Medical Journal* **317**: 1258.

Grant M and Henshaw S (1998). Internet quality criteria. *Health Expectations* **1**: 69–71.

Jadad AR and Gagliardi A (1998). Rating health information on the Internet: navigating to knowledge or to Babel. *Journal of the American Medical Association* **279**: 611–614.

Melville M (1997). Consumerism: do patients have power in health care? *British Journal of Nursing* **6**: 337–340.

Mill JS (1976). In: Himmelfarb G (Ed) *On Liberty*. Harmondsworth: Penguin Books.

Sorell T (1997). Morality, consumerism and the internal market in health care. *Journal of Medical Ethics* **23**: 71–76.

▶9

Patient Involvement in Evidence-Based Health in Relation to Clinical Guidelines

Anna van Wersch and Martin Eccles

Introduction

Health care is changing. According to Cheah (1998) the 1990s will be remembered as the decade when quality assurance, evidence-based health (EBH) and clinical quality improvement were the key issues in health care. Patient dissatisfaction with health care, however, has remained a consistent finding over many decades. The criticisms cited in research include: poor and contradictory information; cold, authoritarian and jargon-based communication; and inconsistent diagnosis and treatment protocols. Irvine (1997) asserts that unless these criticisms are dealt with, public trust in the medical profession could be seriously damaged.

Medical practice was supposed to be too complicated for care to be standardised or described. New research evidence in medicine was largely ignored by clinicians, partly because of their lack of time for keeping up to date, and partly because of resistance to changing learned practices. The recent growth of clinical guidelines is a positive development within health care (Eccles *et al* 1996a,b, Field and Lohr 1992). In order for these guidelines to be valid, an explicit link should be made between recommendations and scientific evidence (see Chapter 4; Grimshaw *et al* 1995). Advantages envisaged from the use of valid guidelines are (Heffner 1998):

▶ decreasing physician practice variation;

▶ slower rise of health-care costs;

▶ monitoring of inappropriate care;

▶ assisting clinicians to stay abreast of new clinical information;

▶ setting research priorities;

▶ promoting better health-care outcomes.

However, at the core of the health-care system are the patients. Patients are no longer seen as passive recipients of health care, but as consumers who act as 'rational' actors in the context of the medical encounter (see Chapter 8; Lupton 1997). According to Meryn (1998), patients today are health consumers who want to be active participants in medical decision making. Weed (1997) argues that patients should be able to manage their own health and illness in the same way as they can manage their own transport. He furthermore states that patients, rather than doctors, should become the primary decision makers in medicine, but that this requires up-to-date, clear, non-contradictory, understandable and easily accessible information:

> *'In a demystified health, care system modern information tools should be used routinely by all patients, in conjunction with providers who are trained to help at various steps in the system where patients cannot function on their own (such as feeling their own spleen or replacing their own hip).'*

Reading the literature on EBH, you wonder what the patients' role and involvement is in this new approach.

▶ Do patients have access to EBH, and if so in what form?

▶ What role, if any, do patients play in the development, implementation and evaluation of valid evidence-based clinical guidelines?

▶ Do they have a role to play when there is a lack of research evidence?

▶ Should patients participate in development groups?

▶ Are their needs, expectations and satisfaction accounted for, and if not, why?

▶ Why are guidelines for clinicians' use only? Why put so much work into providing evidence-based information for doctors and not also use it for patients?

This chapter looks at patient involvement in EBH in relation to clinical guidelines in two parts: patient involvement in developing clinical guidelines; and a patient version of the guidelines.

Patients' role in guideline development

Guideline development groups

In addition to the explicit use of the best available scientific evidence to assure the validity of clinical guidelines, Grimshaw *et al* (1995) recommend that national or regional guideline development groups should include representatives of key disciplines. If you accept that effective health care also requires the participation of rational, informed patients in partnership with professionals, then you would expect them to be included in these groups. However, this is relatively unusual. Benbow (1996) states:

> *'It is difficult to imagine how a plan of care could be developed without the involvement of the patient, but unfortunately it does still happen.'*

Hadorn and Baker (1994), who tackle the methodological and procedural issues of guideline development, and describe in detail the constitution of the panel and the conducting of meetings, mention nowhere the involvement of patients. Eccles *et al* (1996a) did invite two patients to be group members, but described them as 'non-participating observers' of technical discussions to which they can hardly offer any input.

The perceived status difference between health professionals and patients might inhibit any constructive contribution by patients, who may also feel themselves to be an uncomfortable 'minority'. Bond and Grimshaw (1995) acknowledged this as an inhibiting factor among health professionals in their case study from community pharmacy:

> 'There are difficulties inherent in multidisciplinary guideline development, relating to professional hierarchies and mutual ignorance of different professionals' skills and modus operandi.'

Williamson (1989) stresses the importance of the 'marriage' between doctors and patients in doctor–patient working groups, in order to explore similarities and differences in perspectives, values and interests. In her plea for incorporating patients in collaboration groups, she distinguishes three types of patient representatives and outlines the contributions and skills each can be expected to bring:

▶ fellow patients: who would mainly present their own views;

▶ a member of a patient group: who would present the group's views;

▶ patient advocates: who would present knowledge of patients' views.

Guideline literature rarely identifies the background of patient representatives (if any) on the development or working group and/or how they were chosen. Furthermore, it is not clear what is expected of them. The main reason for patient participation is to help achieve a consensus between health professionals' and patients' views (Davies and Hopkins 1997, Girgis and Sanson-Fisher 1995). That these perceptions differ has been shown in several studies (Jennings and Muhlenkamp 1981, Jung et al 1997, Ogden et al 1997, Roberts et al 1994).

Patients' perspectives

Research into patients' health-care perceptions can be incorporated into guideline development. A variety of methodologies may be appropriate, including randomised controlled trials. However, most research follows an observational design, which may also provide evidence, depending on whether it was the most suitable method.

Several researchers stress the importance of including research on patients' views in the process of guideline development, as an adjunct to clinical-based evidence on effectiveness. Gottlieb et al (1992) have constructed a quality improvement model to assist the development of clinical algorithms and guidelines. The process of the model is divided into four steps, the second being guideline development based on an understanding of patient needs, scientific evidence and clinical experience. Spiers (1996) argues that the evidence needed for evidence-based health care should not only come from clinical studies but also from patients and users. The experience and knowledge of patients in the diagnosis and treatment process should be shared with professionals, patients and potential patients. Huttin (1997) debates that for those grey areas where clinical guideline development is difficult because of a lack of evidence, clinical reasoning should be based on factors other than just clinical science such as experience and patient preferences.

There are clear arguments therefore for considering patient satisfaction data and consumer views on the provision of care when developing clinical guidelines.

Patients' needs and satisfaction

Koning *et al* (1995) concluded their literature review with:

> 'To date, guidelines and consensus reports on quality care for asthma and chronic obstructive pulmonary disease (COPD) are mainly based on research and opinions of care providers. Patients' viewpoints on good medical care have rarely been studied.'

Their survey of 121 patients about the care they received identified several unfulfilled needs: Patients would have liked more information on diagnostic tests, prognosis and long-term use of medication. In addition, they wanted more written information about the nature of the disease, and one-third would have liked more participation in decisions about their treatment.

Williamson (1989) interviewed 177 mothers of children under 5 to measure patient satisfaction with GP services. One of the suggestions for improvement was the development of written guidelines on childhood ailments.

Patients' preferences and expectations

Differences in patients' preferences may lead to differences in the preferred therapy. Owens (1998) argues that guideline developers should identify those decisions in which patient preferences are important and for these decisions to be clearly noted in the written guideline.

Examples from research include:

- Ravdin *et al*'s (1998) survey of breast cancer patients' knowledge and expectations of adjuvant therapy found that women overestimate the value of adjuvant therapy and will accept remarkably low degrees of net benefit. They argued that improvements in doctor–patient communication might be important to truly informed decision making, and that flexibility for individual patients' preferences should not be superseded by rigid treatment guidelines.

- Eisenberg (1997) discusses the incorporation of patients' preferences and expectations about alternative therapies into guidelines. He proposes a step-by-step strategy whereby conventionally trained medical providers and their patients can proactively discuss the use or avoidance of alternative therapies.

- 'Preference-based' methods explicitly incorporate the views of patients in respect of their outcome preferences (Huttin 1997). Balance sheets are an example of tools useful in the decision-making process. They provide the patient and health professional with an overview of the possible outcomes of the different treatment options. Leard *et al* (1997) presented individual patients with a comparison of the potential risks and benefits of colorectal screening options for average-risk patients, and found that patients do have preferences and that these are very diverse. Their work acknowledges the omission of patient preferences in the development of national guidelines:

'These recommendations [of the guidelines] take into consideration efficacy, effectiveness, risks, and occasionally cost, but not patient preferences.'

Patients' role in the implementation and evaluation of guidelines

The most difficult stage in the development of guidelines is ensuring their actual implementation (see Chapters 4 and 5). Levin *et al* (1997) stress that it is a priority for the implementation of guidelines that professionals *and* patients are educated according to the contents of the guidelines in order to encourage compliance.

Reminders

These have been established as a strategy to enhance professionals' guideline use. However, they have also been directed at patients (Murray *et al* 1992) to encourage their compliance and involvement.

Research

The extent of guideline adherence can be assessed using patient dossiers or clinical outcomes. Examples of research into these approaches include:

- Grilli *et al* (1990, 1991) evaluated the implementation of guidelines for breast, colorectal and ovarian cancer in Italy through a survey of 770 physicians, exploring their knowledge and attitude, and a review of the medical records of 1482 patients. They found, with reference to guideline recommendations, that the quality of care was far from optimal, especially in relation to diagnosis and staging. Furthermore, the awareness of the guidelines was unsatisfactorily low and seemed to be related to individual physicians' interest.

- Guidelines related to long-term oxygen treatment had been in place more than 5 years when Restrick *et al* (1993) audited its prescription and use among 176 patients of GPs. They reported that the guidelines were largely followed and that patients complied with the treatment.

- Button *et al* (1998) evaluated primary health-care team clinical guidelines for the promotion and management of incontinence care by means of a postal patient questionnaire. They concluded that the clinical guidelines did not have any impact on the clinical outcomes measured.

- Guidelines for the management of breast cancer-related lymphoedema were evaluated by looking at patient outcome variables (Kirshbaum 1996). Patients were assessed with two quality-of-life questionnaires, diaries they filled in and semi-structured interviews in order to elicit data on practitioner compliance and practical issues of implementing change using clinical guidelines. The results showed high levels of compliance from the practitioners as well as the patients.

Summary

If you accept the assessment that patients in the 1990s and beyond should be encouraged to be rational, active, independent partners in health care, they surely have an important role in guideline development, implementation and evaluation. This would ensure their clear involvement in the move to incorporate the evidence-based philosophy into primary care. Furthermore, they might have a role to play in participating – either directly or indirectly – in guideline development groups, in order to reach consensus between the views of health professionals and patients. In that case it is important to identify what is expected of patient contributions and to define what sort of patient (fellow patient, member of a patient group or a patient advocate) would be most suitable for that role. You should also incorporate the best available evidence about patient satisfaction, preferences, expectations and needs when considering service provision and commissioning, as well as clinical decision making.

Patients' guidelines

In this section we will argue the need for a patient version of clinical guidelines, as a means of giving patients access to the best evidence available, which is both relevant and appropriate to their needs. This can be justified under the following headings:

▶ patients' demands for information;

▶ the positive effects of different forms of information on patients' well-being;

▶ problems with the reliability of current information;

▶ the role of information in shared decision making.

Information

Most complaints from patients deal with problems of communication and not with clinical competence (Richards 1990). Most satisfaction research within health care identifies complaint about the provision of information. Patients want more and better information about their problem and its prognosis, more openness about the side effects of treatment, relief of pain and emotional distress, and advice on what they can do for themselves (Meryn 1998).

Provision of information

Positive effects of written information on patients' experiences, social–psychological problems and satisfaction have been found in many studies (Fawzy 1995, Last and van Veldhuizen 1996, van Wersch et al 1997a, b). Studies have also looked at the influence of audio tapes (Davison and Degner 1997, McHugh et al 1995, Ong et al 1995) and videotapes (Flood et al 1996, Rainey 1985, Shapira et al 1997) on patient satisfaction and quality of life. These different methods of information provision have their advantages and disadvantages. The main disadvantage mentioned by Smith and Timoney (1997) is that the information is inevitably pitched at a level which, whilst too complex for some, will be insufficiently detailed for others. Furthermore, updating of such tapes and leaflets tends to lag significantly behind developments.

Reliability of information

Written information

Problems with written information are commonly found within the literature. A few have already come up in the first section of this chapter (Koning *et al* 1995, Williamson 1989).

Smith *et al* (1998) evaluated the readability and accuracy of 168 different patient information leaflets on asthma and concluded that 20% contained inaccurate or misleading statements, and that all but one was at least 6 years old. They recommend that health professionals ensure that the information they are providing is accurate and up to date.

According to Smith and Timoney (1997):

'It is impossible to predict how much outdated information is given to patients.'

Information on the web

Much of health information is nowadays available on the Internet. In 1997 over 10 000 health-related web sites were found, and over a third of Internet users accessed the web to retrieve health and medical information (Coulter 1998). Researchers warn that even though the web makes it very easy for people to disseminate information, by allowing anonymous authors to conceal commercial or other conflicts of interest, it does not help readers to discriminate between genuine insight and deliberate invention (Silberg *et al* 1997, Wyatt 1997).

According to Haines and Donald (1998), the changing relation between patient and doctor is partly due to patients being able to arm themselves with information from the Internet, facilitating their development into information brokers and interpreters. However, Impicciatore *et al* (1997) found in their systematic survey of advice on managing fever in children at home that only four of the 41 web pages adhered closely to the main recommendations in the guidelines on managing fever in children. They suggest an urgent need to check health-care information on the Internet and oriented at the public for accuracy, completeness and consistency.

Shared decision making

It has been increasingly recognised that provision of patient information has an important role to play in the process of shared decision making between patient and doctor (Entwistle *et al* 1996, Field and Lohr 1992, Hack *et al* 1994, Johnson *et al* 1996, Walker *et al* 1996, Wijma *et al* 1992). Studies show that the majority of patients are positive about the value of information in their treatment decision (Barry *et al* 1995, Shepperd *et al* 1995).

Without patient information, only the medical staff have the knowledge that is required to make decisions about a treatment (Crawford *et al* 1997). It has been shown that giving patients information verbally is not enough as the recall and understanding of what has been said is very low (Dunn *et al* 1993, Michie *et al* 1997).

Davison *et al* (1995) found that men diagnosed with prostate cancer preferred a passive decision-making role rather than an active one. However, new studies are required to determine if this preference will change to a more active role with increasing and relevant information provision. The men who did not prefer an active role still wanted more information about disease advancement, likelihood of cure and types of treatment available.

As health care and the patient's role within the system evolves, there is growing interest in providing information to support patients' participation in choosing treatments and deciding on strategies for managing their health problems (Coulter 1998).

Kaplan *et al* (1996) showed in a study of 7730 patients and their doctors that patients tend to leave doctors who fail to involve them in decisions. However, this was not the case for all patients. Further research is required about which, if any, patient characteristics such as age, education, gender or other factors such as the type of illness, are related to patient responses in this regard.

Following the publication of the guidelines on Do-Not-Resuscitate (DNR) orders, Lofmark and Nilstun (1997) investigated the extent of patient involvement in decisions about their DNR status; and considered how the ethical conflict involved in informing patients about their status could be described and analysed. They found that two-thirds of the health professionals had made a decision about DNR without discussing it with the patient. Consultation was apparently confined to those considered to be 'competent patients'. The authors argued that patients should be routinely informed about their DNR status, as to deny them this could be harmful. They recommended prospective research to find out if patients want to be informed, and how and when this should be done.

Evidence-based health and patient guidelines

This leads us to the question: Do patients have access to EBH and, if yes, in what form?

Fahey (1998) argued that applying evidence from clinical trials and systematic reviews to individual patients in primary care is complex and challenging. Oliver *et al* (1996) showed the differences in the views of ultrasonographers and patients when patients were provided with leaflets based on the best available evidence about the effectiveness of routine ultrasonography in early pregnancy. Ultrasonogaphers were concerned that the leaflets would raise women's anxiety, reduce uptake of scans and disrupt hospital organisation. The patients were shocked by aspects of the information but thought it appropriate to include both advantages and disadvantages. van Wersch *et al* (1997a,b) found similar differences between health professionals and patients in their study evaluating the use of a care protocol for cancer patients. The patients were provided with a very detailed jargon-free description of all aspects of the care, including a full account of operation techniques. In the pre-test phase, health professionals were pessimistic about the effects of this form of information provision. They believed that patients would not read or understand it and would become unnecessarily anxious. The post-test study, however, showed that most patients had read it, could understand it and there were no negative psychological effects. The health professionals' views had changed, and they found that patients asked fewer and more interesting questions than before the implementation of the protocol. Similarly, Bokamp and Pfeiffer (1984) provided their patients with detailed information about events surrounding an operation and concluded:

> 'Contrary to widely-held opinion, almost all patients were highly interested in detailed information and demonstrated considerable knowledge of their complaints, the surgical method and the risks involved.'

Much effort has been put into developing leaflets and other information packages, but as Coulter (1998) says, good intentions are not enough to guarantee quality and usefulness in the information provided. Especially if patients are going to be active participants in decisions about their care, it is important that the information is based on evidence and presented in a form that is acceptable and useful. So far, more attention has been given to presentation and readability than to content. Coulter goes as far to say that because lots of information material was developed for the lowest possible reading age, much of it is of 'infantile' quality. She states that there is:

> 'no excuse for palming patients off with unscientific clinical opinion which does not conform to the standards required for evidence-based medicine.'

Haines and Donald (1998) stress the role patients themselves can play in demanding care of a high standard:

> 'Patients may influence practitioners' behaviour towards clinically effective practice by requesting interventions that have proved to be effective.'

Terry (1994) examined the effects of a patient guidebook developed to summarise risk-based clinical prevention screening guidelines. Significant gaps and misconceptions were found concerning patients' knowledge of the guidelines for colon examinations, blood pressure and Pap tests. Providing patients with their own version of the guidelines would be perhaps the most effective and accurate way of providing information, enabling shared decision making and reducing anxiety and uncertainty. It would also reflect enhanced patient autonomy within the evolving relationship between doctors and patients. It would guarantee up-to-date, clear, non-contradictory information, made understandable for the lay person. The information needs to be at an appropriate reading level, but sufficiently sophisticated in its content to provide patients and their carers with sufficient, accurate and relevant information to enable them to make informed choices. Thus, it could be used as an information tool per se, as a medium in the shared-decision process, or as a plan for managing patients' own care process. When clinicians and patients follow the same guidelines, differences in views should be reduced and compliance enhanced.

Another worthwhile development would be to make such patient guidelines available on the Internet. This would benefit from a system of guarantee from the clinicians' organisations – perhaps a form of hallmark which patients can recognise as denoting quality assurance.

The main problem remains how to construct these guidelines (at one reading level or various levels?); and how this information is going to be delivered in a timely way so that patient decision making will be improved.

Conclusion

This chapter has tried to show ways in which patients should and could be active participants in clinical guideline development and evaluation, as well as users of EBH through patient versions of these guidelines. Whilst detailed, robust research is currently limited, observational studies support our assertions. Furthermore, there is increasing consensus that patient participation is important. Many guidelines remain to be developed, and more research is needed into how this should be done and what the most appropriate format(s) is.

Patient involvement in EBH is implicit if EBH is to be effective and ethical. This involvement should include patient participation in guideline development to ensure that health services take account of the views of their users. Furthermore, patients should have access to EBH through the use of patient guidelines, which are almost unavoidable in the current changing health-care environment. As Irvine (1997) states:

> 'People know more about health matters because they have independent access to clinical information and because their interest has been stimulated by media attention. More patients want an open relation with their doctors, they want to be well informed and involved in decisions about their care.'

Our role as health professionals is to ensure that the information we impart is relevant, understandable, and accurate, and that our communication skills enable us to share it with patients.

References

Barry MJ, Fowler FJ, Mulley AG, et al (1995). Patient reactions to a program designed to facilitate patient participation in treatment decisions for benign prostatic hyperplasmis. Medical Care 33: 771–782.

Benbow M (1996). Pressure sore guidelines: patient/carer involvement and education. British Journal of Nursing 5: 182–187.

Bokamp H and Pfeiffer WM (1984). Preoperative education consultation from the viewpoint of the patient. Zeitschrift Orthop 122: 623–627.

Bond CM and Grimshaw JM (1995). Multi-disciplinary guideline development: a case study from community pharmacy. Health Bulletin 53: 26–33.

Button D, Roe B, Webb C, et al (1998). Consensus guidelines for the promotion and management of continence by primary health care teams: development, implementation and evaluation. NHS Executive Nursing Directorate. Journal of Advanced Nursing 27: 91–99.

Cheah TS (1998). The impact of clinical guidelines and clinical pathways on medical practice: effectiveness and medico-legal aspects. Annual Academica Medica Singapore 27: 533–539.

Coulter A (1998). Evidence based patient information is important, so there needs to be a national strategy to ensure it. British Medical Journal 317: 225–226.

Crawford ED, Bennett CL, Stone NN et al (1997). Comparison of perspectives on prostate cancer: analyses of survey data. Urology 50: 366–372.

Davies E and Hopkins A (1997). Good practice in the management of adults with malignant cerebral glioma: clinical guidelines. Working group, Royal College of Physicians. British Journal of Neurosurgery 11: 318–330.

Davison BJ, Degner LF, Morgan TR (1995). Information and decision-making preferences of men with prostate cancer. *Oncological Nursing Forum* **22**: 1401–1408.

Davison BJ and Degner LF (1997). Empowerment of men newly diagnosed with prostate cancer. *Cancer Nursing* **20**: 187–196.

Dunn SM, Butow PN, Tattersall ML *et al* (1993). General information tapes inhibit recall of cancer diagnosis. *Journal of Clinical Oncology* **11**: 2279–2285.

Eccles M, Clapp Z, Grimshaw J *et al* (1996a). Developing valid guidelines: methodological and procedural issues from the North of England Evidence Based Guideline Development Project. *Quality in Health Care* **5**: 44–50.

Eccles M, Clapp Z, Grimshaw J *et al* (1996b). North of England Evidence Based Guidelines Development Project: methods of guideline development. *British Medical Journal* **312**: 760–762.

Eisenberg DM (1997). Advising patients who seek alternative medical therapies. *Annals of Internal Medicine* **127**: 61–69.

Entwistle VA, Sheldon TA, Sowden AJ, *et al* (1996). Supporting consumer involvement in decision making: what constitutes quality in consumer health information? *International Journal of Quality in Health Care* **8**: 425–437.

Fahey T (1998). Applying the results of clinical trials to patients to general practice: perceived problems, strengths, assumptions, and challenges for the future. *British Journal of General Practice* **48**: 1173–1178.

Fawzy FI (1995). A short-term psychoeducational intervention for patients newly diagnosed with cancer. *Support Care Cancer* **3**: 235–238.

Field MJ and Lohr KN (Eds) (1992). *Guidelines for Clinical Practice*. Institute of Medicine. Washington: National Academy Press.

Flood AB, Wennberg JE, Nease RF Jr, *et al* (1996). The importance of patient preference in the decision to screen for prostate cancer. Prostate Patient Outcome Research Team. *Journal of General Internal Medicine* **11**: 342–349.

Girgis A and Sanson-Fisher RW (1995). Breaking bad news: consensus guidelines for medical practitioners. *Journal of Clinical Oncology* **13**: 2449–2456.

Gottlieb L, Sokol H, Oates AB, *et al* (1992). Algorithm-based clinical quality improvement. *HMO Practice* **6**: 5–12.

Grilli R, Apalone G, Liberati A, Nicolucci A (1990). Impact of the National Task Force on the quality of assistance to neoplasm patients: results and implications of a study on implementation of educational intervention. *Epidemiological Prevention* **12**: 50–61.

Grilli R, Apolone G, Marsoni S, *et al* (1991). The impact of patient management guidelines on the care of breast, colorectal, and ovarian cancer patients in Italy. *Medical Care* **29**: 50–61.

Grimshaw J, Eccles M, Russell IT (1995) Developing clinically valid guidelines. *Journal of Evaluating Clinical Practice* **1**: 37–48.

Hack TF, Degner LF, Dyck DG (1994). Relationship between preferences for decisional control and illness information among women with breast cancer: a quantitative and qualitative analysis. *Social Science and Medicine* **39**: 279–289.

Hadorn DC and Baker D (1994). Development of the AHCPR-Sponsored Heart Failure Guideline: Methodological and procedural issues. *Journal of Quality Improvement* **20**: 539–547.

Haines A and Donald A (1998). Making better use of research findings. *British Medical Journal* **317**: 72–75.

Heffner JE (1998). Does evidence-based medicine help the development of clinical practice guidelines? *Chest* **113**: 172–178.

Huttin C (1997). The use of clinical guidelines to improve medical practice: main issues in the United States. *International Journal for Quality in Health Care* **9**: 207–214.

Impicciatore P, Pandolfini C, Casella N, *et al* (1997). Reliability of health information for the public on the World Wide Web: systematic survey of advice on managing fever in children at home. *British Medical Journal* **314**: 1875–1879.

Irvine D (1997). The performance of doctors. I: Professionalism and self regulation in a changing world. *British Medical Journal* **314**: 1540–1542.

Jennings BM and Muhlenkamp AF (1981). Systematic misperception: oncology patients' self-reported affective states and their care-givers' perceptions. *Cancer Nursing* **12**: 485–489.

Johnson JD, Roberts CS, Cox CE, *et al* (1996). Breast cancer patients' personality style, age and treatment decision making. *Journal of Surgical Oncology* **63**: 183–186.

Jung HP, Wensink M and Grol R (1997). What makes a good general practitioner: do patients and doctors have different views? *British Journal of General Practice* **47**: 805–809.

Kaplan SH, Greenfield S, Gandek B, *et al* (1996). Characteristics of physicians with participatory decision-making styles. *Annals of Internal Medicine* **124**: 497–504.

Kirshbaum M (1996). The development, implementation and evaluation of guidelines for the management of breast cancer related lymphoedema. *European Journal of Cancer Care* **5**: 246–251.

Koning CJM, Maille AR, Stevens I, et al (1995). Patients' opinions on respiratory care: Do doctors fulfill their needs? *Journal of Asthma* **32**: 355–363.

Last BF and van Veldhuizen AM (1996). Information about diagnosis and prognosis relating to anxiety and depression in children with cancer aged 8–16 years. *European Journal of Cancer* **32A**: 290–294.

Leard LE, Savides TJ, Graniats TG (1997). Patient preferences for colorectal cancer screening. *Journal of Family Practice* **45**: 211–218.

Levin N, Eknoyan G, Pipp M et al (1997). National Kidney Foundation: Dialysis Outcome Quality Initiative – development of methodology for clinical practice guidelines. *Nephrology Dialysis and Transplantation* **12**: 2060–2063.

Lofmark R and Nilstun T (1997). Do-not-resuscitate orders – should the patient be informed? *Journal of Internal Medicine* **241**: 421–425.

Lupton D (1997). Consumerism, reflexivity, and the medical encounter. *Social Science and Medicine* **45**: 373–381.

McHugh P, Lewis S, Ford S et al (1995). The efficacy of audiotapes in promoting psychological well-being in cancer patients: a randomised, controlled trial. *British Journal of Cancer* **71**: 388–392.

Meryn S (1998). Improving doctor–patient communication. *British Medical Journal* **316**: 1922–1930.

Michie S, McDonals V, Marteau TM (1997). Genetic counselling: information given, recall and satisfaction. *Patient Education and Counselling* **32**: 101–106.

Murray KO, Gottlieb LK, Schoenbaum SC (1992). Implementing clinical guidelines: a quality management approach to reminder systems. *Quality Review Bulletin* **18**: 423–433.

Ogden J, Andrane J, Eisner M et al (1997). To treat? To befriend? To prevent? Patients' and GPs' views of the doctor's role. *Scandinavian Journal of Primary Care* **15**: 114–117.

Oliver S, Rajan L, Turner H et al (1996). Informed choice for users of health services: views on ultrasonography leaflets of women in early pregnancy, midwives, and ultrasonographers. *British Medical Journal* **313**: 1251–1253.

Ong LM, de Haes JC, Kruyver IP, et al (1995). Providing patients with an audio recording of the outpatient oncological consultation; experiences of patients and physicians. *Nederlands Tijdschrift voor de Genneskunde (Dutch Medical Journal)* **139**: 77–80.

Owens DK (1998). Spine update. Patient preferences and the development of practical guidelines. *Spine* **23**: 1073–1079.

Rainey LC (1985). Effects of preparatory patient education for radiation oncology patients. *Cancer* **56**: 1056–1061.

Ravdin PM, Siminoff IA, Harvey JA (1998). Survey of breast cancer patients concerning their knowledge and expectations of adjuvant therapy. *Journal of Clinical Oncology* **16**: 515–521.

Restrick LJ, Paul EA, Braid GM, et al (1993). Assessment and follow up of patients prescribed long term oxygen treatment. *Thorax* **48**: 708–713.

Richards T (1990). Chasms in communication. *British Medical Journal* **301**: 1407–1408.

Roberts CS, Cox CE, Reintgens DS, et al (1994). Influence of physician communication on newly diagnosed breast cancer patients' psychological adjustment and decision-making. *Cancer* **74**: 336–341.

Shapira MM, Meade C, Nattinger AB (1997). Enhanced decision-making: the use of a videotape decision-aid for patients with prostate cancer. *Journal of Biocommunication* **23**: 8–12.

Shepperd S, Coulter A, Farmer A (1995). Using interactive videos in general practice to inform patients about treatment choices: a pilot study. *Family Practice* **12**: 443–447.

Silberg WM, Lundberg GD, Musacchio RA (1997). Assessing, controlling and assuring the quality of medical information on the internet. *Journal of the American Medical Association* **727**: 1244–1245.

Smith H, Gooding S, Brown R, et al (1998). Evaluation of readability and accuracy of information leaflets in general practice for patients with asthma. *British Medical Journal* **317**: 264–265.

Smith D and Timoney A (1997). Patient information systems. *British Journal of Urology* **80**: 27–30.

Spiers J (1996). Evidence-based health care and patient choice. But will it work for me doctor? In: Dunning M, Needham G, Weston S (Eds) *But Will It Work, Doctor?* London: On The Black Limited, pp.10–14.

Terry PE (1994). The effects of a materials-based intervention on knowledge of risk-based clinical prevention screening guidelines. *Journal of Occupational Medicine* **36**: 365–371.

van Wersch A, Bonnema J, Prinsen B, et al (1997a). Continuity of information for breast cancer patients: the development, use and evaluation of a multidisciplinary care-protocol. *Patient Education and Counselling* **30**: 175–186.

van Wersch A, de Boer MF, van der Does E et al (1997b). Continuity of information in cancer care: evaluation of a logbook. *Patient Education and Counselling* **31**: 223–236.

Walker BL, Nail LM, Larsen L, et al (1996). Concerns, affect, and cognitive disruption following completion of radiation treatment for localised breast or prostate cancer. *Oncological Nursing Forum* **23**: 1181–1187.

Weed LL (1997). New connections between medical knowledge and patient care. *British Medical Journal* **315**: 231–235.

Wijma K, Varenhorst E, Hjertberg H *et al* (1992). A study on prostate cancer. The patient can decide himself: medical or surgical treatment. *Lakartidningen* **89**: 1659–1661.

Williamson V (1989). Patients' satisfaction with general practitioner services: a survey by a community health council. *Journal of the Royal College of General Practitioners* **39**: 452–455.

Wyatt JC (1997). Commentary: measuring quality and impact of the world wide web. *British Medicial Journal* **314**: 1879.

▶10

Fundamental Statistics for Evidence-Based Health in Primary Care

Alan Gibbs

Introduction

It is useful to have at least a basic understanding of statistics when assessing evidence reporting quantitative research. This chapter is designed to lead readers through basic concepts, and some useful methods to enable clinicians to apply results to their daily work and reading. It also explains the statistical aspects of the basis of evidence, and how quantitative research may be assessed for its strengths and weaknesses. It is not intended to provide detailed information, or equip readers to carry out their own statistical calculations. There are many other texts available for such purposes, some of which are mentioned in the text.

Definitions and basic concepts

Randomised controlled trials

Since in most discussions of the strength of the evidence for the use of a particular therapy, the results from randomised controlled trials (RCTs) tend to be treated as important, it is useful to review briefly the conduct of these trials and the statistical analyses of the results from them. An introduction to clinical trials can be found in Altman (1991), and a more extensive coverage in Pocock (1983).

A group of patients who are thought appropriate to be entered into the trial are divided into two groups by a random mechanism, ideally involving random numbers. An outcome measure is determined before the start of the trial. The two treatments to be compared are applied to the two groups. In order that the comparison between the two treatments should be fair, and that any assessment of the outcome measure should be unbiased, it is desirable, as far as possible, that the treatment and assessment should be carried out on a blind basis, i.e. that those involved in administering the treatment and assessing the outcome, as well as the patients in the trial, should be unaware of the allocation of the treatment to individual patients. Since the comparison of two treatments can include the situation when one of the treatments is in fact no active treatment, it is desirable that a placebo procedure or drug should be used in order to maintain the blindness of those carrying out the trial and assessing the outcome, as well as the patients in the trial.

Statistical tests

The traditional statistical approach to analysing the results of such a trial is to assume provisionally that the two treatments have the same effect. In statistical terms, this is called the null hypothesis, where null means none or nothing. This does not mean that you should get exactly the same outcomes in the two groups experiencing the treatments: the outcomes will vary according to the individual characteristics of the patients but if the assumption of equality of treatment effect is correct, the outcomes of individuals in the two groups can be treated as samples from a single underlying population. The probability of the observed or greater difference between the two samples can then be calculated using the appropriate statistical techniques. The particular approach used will depend on the nature of the outcome measure chosen, the size of the groups involved and any assumptions that can reasonably be made.

Statistical significance

The initial assumption of no treatment effect (the null hypothesis) is now considered in the light of the probability calculated in the above manner. If the probability is large, then this implies that the observed or greater difference in the outcomes in the two samples is likely to occur if the two treatments are equal in their effect. On the other hand, if the calculated probability is small, then there are two possible alternatives to consider:

1. the assumption of equal treatment effect is correct, but a difference in the outcomes in the two groups has occurred because of individual variability between patients; or
2. the treatments have different effects on outcome which give rise to the observed differences in the samples.

It is reasonable to say that the smaller the calculated probability is, the less likely we are to accept alternative (1) and the more likely we are to accept alternative (2). Traditionally, the approach has been to set a particular probability value before the start of the trial and to take this as the dividing line between accepting alternatives 1 and 2. The specific probability chosen is referred to as the significance level. Conventionally, it is often chosen to be 0.05, and calculated probabilities less than this are said to be 'significant at the 0.05 probability level' or more briefly 'significant'. The value of 0.05 is quite arbitrary, and recently there has been a tendency to calculate the probability and leave the implications of this to the reader. This has been helped by the development of computer programs that will carry out the calculations involved which are sometimes difficult. Whatever the approach used, it is certainly rational to conclude the smaller the probability, the stronger the evidence against the null hypothesis of equal treatment effect. A more detailed discussion of this approach, called hypothesis testing, can be found in Altman (1991).

Advantages of the statistical approach

It is important to realise that since this approach is based on probability it does not guarantee that the right decision is made. However, it does provide an objective numerical technique based on the data from the trial for making decisions, which have a high probability of being correct in the long run.

A confidence interval approach

A disadvantage of the hypothesis testing approach is that it does not provide a measure of by how much a given treatment is superior to another. This can be made by calculating a confidence interval for some appropriate measure of difference in outcome between the two treatments. The choice of measure will depend on the nature of the outcome initially chosen.

A confidence interval is a range of values that has a specific probability of including a particular characteristic of the outcome. For example, in a comparison of antibiotics in acute bronchitis in general practice (Cooper *et al* 1978), the percentage having a successful response at 7 days was 86% for 21 patients treated with septrin, and 74% for 19 patients treated with amoxycillin. A hypothesis test approach using Fisher's exact test would give a probability (P) of 0.44 which is clearly greater than the conventional level of 0.05. This would not be strong evidence against the null hypothesis of equal effectiveness of the two drugs. A confidence interval approach to the same data would be to calculate a 95% confidence interval for the difference in the percentage of successful outcomes for the two treatments. Using the formula given in Gardner and Altman (1989), an approximate 95% confidence interval for the difference in the percentage of successful outcomes would be –17% to +41%.

The above interval includes the value 0, indicating that the difference in the effect could be 0. However, the width of the 95% confidence interval indicates that the result of the trial is consistent with a wide range of differences in the percentages with a successful conclusion. This range of possible values for the difference is usually felt to be more informative than a statistical test giving a calculated probability of 0.44, or a statement that the result is not significant at the 0.05 probability level.

Meaning of a confidence interval

The wide range of possible values is a consequence of the smallness of the size of the trial: it can be reduced by increasing the numbers in the two groups. It should be borne in mind that there is no guarantee that the confidence interval will include the true difference, however large the associated probability. What can be said is that in the long run 95% confidence intervals will contain the true difference 95% of the time.

Confidence intervals and hypothesis tests

There is a direct correspondence between a confidence interval and an hypothesis test. If the hypothesis test is not significant at the 0.05 (5%) level, then the 95% confidence interval will contain the null value of no difference, and *vice versa*, as here. If the hypothesis test is significant at the 0.05 (5%) level, i.e. if the calculated probability is < 0.05, then the 95% confidence interval will not contain the null value of no difference, and *vice versa*. In fact, the above relationship may not hold exactly in practice because slightly different approximations may have been used in the two procedures. In addition, it may not always be possible to calculate exact confidence intervals. Gardner and Altman (1989) give formulae and worked examples for the calculation of confidence intervals in a wide range of situations, as well as a useful discussion of confidence intervals and their relationship with hypothesis tests.

Strength of evidence

The area in which evidence-based health (EBH) has had the greatest effect is in defining different kinds of evidence and ordering them according to their strength. Formal details can be found on the world wide web at http://cebm.jr2.ox.uk/docs/levels.html. These have been developed in the main with regard to therapy but have been extended to other areas, including diagnosis and prognosis.

   The most recent development (17.09.98) of levels of evidence from the Cochrane Centre for Evidence-Based Medicine in Oxford relative to therapy are given in Box 10.1.

Box 10.1.   Centre for Evidence-Based Medicine levels of evidence

Recommendation grade

A   1a Systematic reviews with homogeneity of individual RCTs

    1b A single RCT with a narrow confidence interval

    1c 'All or none' outcomes

B   2a Systematic review with homogeneity of cohort studies

    2b A single cohort study or a RCT of poor quality

    2c Outcome research. This corresponds to systematic samples of patients where the relationship of outcome to treatment has been studied

C   3a Systematic review with homogeneity of case-control studies

    3b An individual case-control study

    4   Case series (and poor quality cohort and case-control studies).

An ordering of recommendation is implied above, in that A is preferred to B and so on, and within a particular grade there is an ordering of evidence in that 1a is preferable to 1b and so on.

   An '*all or none*' outcome is a situation involving a treatment when all the patients died before the treatment became available, but now some survive on it, or when some of the patients died before the treatment became available, but now none die on it.

   It is further suggested that a – (minus) sign can be added to the recommendation if, for example, a RCT gives rise to a wide confidence interval which might not be statistically significant but might include a clinically important benefit.

   This can be illustrated in the following example (Fig. 10.1): suppose studies compare a treatment with a placebo control group and the results are summarised by calculating a 95% confidence interval for the difference in some appropriate outcome measure. For comparison A the confidence interval is for the difference in outcome measure which includes a difference in benefit of 0 but not the measure of benefit previously determined as clinically important. Clearly, the treatment cannot be recommended. For comparison B the confidence interval is for difference in benefit which includes a clinically important value but not the 0 value of no benefit difference. This suggests that the treatment is effective. For comparison C the confidence interval of difference in benefit includes a clinically important value and the 0 value of no benefit difference. In this comparison the treatment may be more effective than the control but the result is inconclusive.

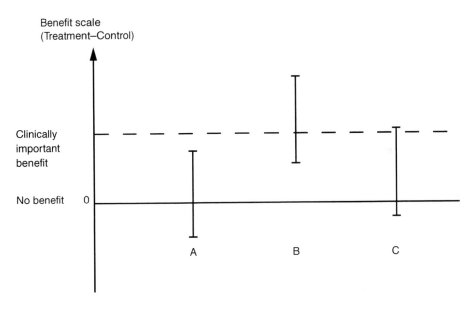

Fig. 10.1. 95% Confidence intervals for treatment benefit.

Homo- or hetero-geneity?

Homogeneity is mentioned in three of the levels above (1a, 2a, 3a). It means there is no evidence of underlying differences between the measures of benefit chosen in the different studies being considered. A conventional approach would be to use a statistical approach to test for homogeneity in outcome and to decide to reject homogeneity if the differences are statistically significant at the conventional level of 0.05. However, it must be borne in mind that the usual test for homogeneity lacks power (in a statistical sense, that is, it has a low probability of achieving a significant result if real differences exist), and so it might be more appropriate to use a significance level of 0.10 or 0.20.

Studies of poor quality

Reference is made in some levels to studies of poor quality. An example of a RCT of poor quality would be one in which < 80% of subjects were followed up. Of course there are many other ways in which RCTs can be of poor quality.

Cohort studies can be of poor quality if:

▶ comparison groups were not clearly defined;

▶ exposures and/or outcomes were not measured in the same objective and preferably blinded way for both groups;

▶ known confounders were not identified and/or controlled for in the same way for both groups;

▶ subjects were not followed up either adequately or for a long enough period.

Case-control studies can be of poor quality if they suffer from the first three of these faults.

Other hierarchies of evidence

An alternative simpler ordering of evidence, which is a modification of that produced by the Centre for Evidence-Based Medicine (Box 10.2), is adopted by *Bandolier* (Anon 1995a), – a journal of evidence-based health care produced by the Pain Relief Unit, The Churchill Hospital, Oxford. The journal is also available on the world wide web at: www.jr2.ox.ac.uk/bandolier

---

Box 10.2. *Bandolier* system of ordering evidence

1. Strong evidence from at least 1 systematic review of multiple well-designed RCTs

2. Strong evidence from at least 1 properly designed RCT of appropriate size

3. Evidence from well-designed trials without randomisation, single group pre/post, cohort, time series or matched case-controlled studies

4. Evidence from well-designed non-experimental studies from more than one centre or research group

5. Opinions of respected authorities, based on clinical evidence, descriptive studies or reports of expert committees.

Other hierarchies exist but appear to have common features with those described above, with evidence from RCTs at the top, and non-experimental studies and opinions of respected authorities at the bottom.

Randomised controlled trials

What constitutes a well-designed RCT can be deduced from the CONSORT statement (Altman 1996). This is a statement of how such trials should be reported as agreed by the editors of several respected medical journals. Desirable features should include:

▶ a prospectively defined hypothesis, together with any subgroup analysis planned, and any co-variates thought necessary to be included, being indicated;

▶ the planned study population with any inclusion or exclusion criteria;

- the outcome measures used, the minimum difference thought important, together with details of how the planned sample size was determined;

- the unit and method of randomisation, techniques of concealment of treatment allocation;

- techniques used to ensure blinding of those conducting and assessing the trial;

- results given in adequate detail together with a point estimate and a confidence interval for the effect of the intervention on the outcome measures, together with an indication of whether analysis was on an intention-to-treat basis.

The above list is not exhaustive but it indicates some of the key points. A further point that could be added is an outcome measure of clinical importance.

Progress of patients in the trial
The CONSORT statement also suggested that a flow chart should be produced which included:

- the number of patients eligible for randomisation;

- the number actually randomised;

- the numbers allocated to the different treatments but not actually receiving the allocated treatment;

- the numbers withdrawn because of treatment failure, and for other reasons, in the allocated groups;

- the numbers lost to follow-up in the allocated groups;

- the numbers completing the trial in the allocated groups.

This flow chart would enable readers to make a judgement on the degree of selectivity of patients into the trial, and the efficiency with which the trial was carried out.

Systematic reviews
For the highest level of evidence the results from several trials should be combined in a systematic review. A high quality systematic review should have the following characteristics:

- the methods used to search for information are indicated, and the search is reasonably comprehensive;

- the criteria which determined which studies would be included are given, and they are fairly used;

- the criteria for determining the validity of the study are given, and applied fairly and consistently to the studies;

- the techniques for combining the findings of the studies are indicated and correctly applied.

Conflicting conclusions

Hopayian and Mugford (1999) discuss the interesting situation that arose where two systematic reviews (Watts and Silagy 1995, and Koes *et al* 1995) drew different conclusions when looking at epidural steroid injections for sciatica. The difference in the conclusions arose for two main reasons. One of the reviews (Koes *et al* 1995) made a much more detailed assessment of the quality of the papers considered, and Watts and Silagy (1995) looked only at possible sources of bias in the assessment of outcome difference between the treatment and control groups.

Both reviews considered three aspects:

▶ quality of the random allocation;

▶ extent to which every patient randomised was included in the primary analysis;

▶ extent to which the assessors were blinded.

The review by Koes *et al* (1995) included the following points in addition:

▶ sample size;

▶ relevance of the outcome measures;

▶ evidence of co-interventions.

This suggests that the review by Koes *et al* (1995) was more satisfactory. On the other hand, the statistical techniques used by the Watts and Silagy (1995) review were more appropriate. They calculated a pooled odds ratio for the numbers achieving 75% pain relief, based on the studies judged to be satisfactory. This gave a significant odds ratio. Koes *et al* (1995) simply divided the studies into those that were statistically significant and those that were not, which is an inappropriate method of summary. It takes no account of the size of individual differences or the different sample sizes. The Koes *et al* (1995) review found that half the studies were statistically significant and half were not, and concluded that the effectiveness of epidural steroid injections had not been established.

This emphasises that systematic reviews should themselves be subjected to the same rigorous critical analysis as the original papers.

Meta-analysis

Systematic reviews may lead on to meta-analysis, which is usually taken to mean combining results from different studies to get a more precise estimate of a treatment effect than could be obtained from a single trial.

Although this argument appears persuasive, it assumes that differences in trial results are simply due to chance, when in fact they may be due to differences in underlying or study populations, treatments, outcome measures, trial design, etc.

Publication bias

One of the arguments against calculating overall effects is the question of publication bias. It is a well accepted fact that studies with a statistically significant result are more likely to be published than studies that are not significant (Egger and Davey Smith 1998). It has also been suggested that studies involving small numbers are less likely to be published because of possible unreliability and lack of power. The implication of these two effects is that small, non-significant studies will tend not to be published and this will lead to an overestimate of treatment effect and the precision of the estimate will also appear to be greater than it actually is.

A graphical check for the existence of publication bias can be seen in the *'funnel plot'*. If a measure of treatment effect, typically the odds ratio on a log scale, is plotted against trial size, then if the assumptions behind meta-analysis are correct the pattern of results should follow a 'funnel' pattern (Fig. 10.2), with wide variability for small trials, diminishing as trial size increases. If, however, there are few results in the area marked A (Fig. 10.2), corresponding to small, non-significant trials, then publication bias may be suspected. In fact, a formal statistical test for publication bias has been developed (Egger *et al* 1997).

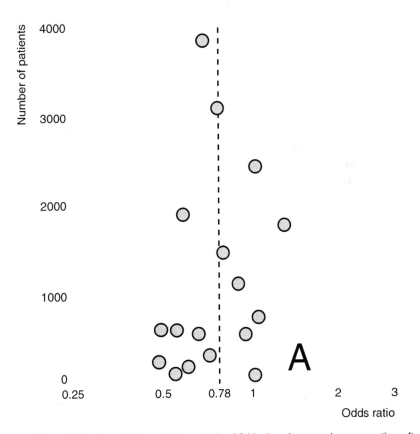

Fig. 10.2. Funnel plot of mortality results from trials of ß-blockers in secondary prevention after myocardial infarction. The odds ratios are plotted against study sample size.

Perhaps a less well known problem is duplicate publication, where the same study is published more than once. Since this is more likely to happen with trials showing a statistically significant outcome, this means that the size of the treatment effect and its precision will be overestimated.

An attempt to avoid publication bias has been made with the establishment of a controlled trial register by the Cochrane Collaboration. This will record the existence of trials even if the results are not published.

If meta-analyses are exclusively based on small studies, then the interpretation of their conclusions should be treated with scepticism because of the possible problems of publication bias and poor quality. Ideally, their results should be confirmed by large-scale, high-quality RCTs, though this will not always be possible. One of the questions raised in meta-analysis is whether unpublished studies should be included or not in the overall analysis. Their inclusion increases the number of subjects involved, but also means that the quality of the studies cannot be checked. For reasons of commercial confidentiality there may be a tendency for some commercially-funded research to remain unpublished, so a high proportion of unpublished material may be of this kind. The suggestion has been made that the results should be analysed with and without the unpublished data as a form of sensitivity analysis, and if conclusions differ between the two analyses, then the results should be treated with caution (Koes *et al* 1995).

Meta-analysis on original data

It is important to note that meta-analyses can be divided into those that are based on the summarised published data alone, and analyses based on individual records. Of course, this latter type of analysis is only possible if the data are still available, and those responsible for collecting the data are willing to provide them to those carrying out the meta-analyses. If the original data are available and extensive enough, then it might be possible to carry out a re-analysis so that, for example, outcomes could be examined on an intention-to-treat basis if this was not done originally, or a different outcome measure selected. When the original data are available, it can be re-analysed in respect of underlying risk; it also allows errors to be corrected and for more appropriate statistical analyses to be carried out (Davey Smith and Egger 1998).

Presenting the results of research

For published research to be of value to the primary care team member it is important that results should be expressed in a form that the primary care team member can make use of. It has also been shown that the form in which information is conveyed can have a major effect on the action taken (Hux and Naylor 1995, Cranney and Walley 1996).

Measurement of treatment effectiveness

It is widely accepted that differences between treatment and placebo or between different treatments can only be judged to be real if the differences are statistically significant at some conventionally accepted significance level (e.g. 0.05). This, of course, gives no indication of the magnitude of the difference in outcome and has led to a demand for results to be given in terms of the magnitude of the outcome difference between treatments or between treatments and control, with a 95% confidence interval as an indication of variability.

Outcomes can be measured in many different ways, but probably a widely accepted approach is to look at the proportion satisfying some objective criteria, chosen before the start of the study. For example, in a meta-analysis of the treatment of migraine with oral sumatriptan (Anon 1999), the measure chosen is the proportion of patients having no or mild pain 2 hours after the start of treatment. The result for individuals in the trial is whether they satisfied this criteria or not. The results from this trial can be summarised in many ways, probably the most obvious being the difference between treatment and control in the proportion of patients having the desired outcome of pain reduction (Table 10.1).

Table 10.1. Overall results for the treatment of migraine with oral sumatriptan.

Outcome (mild or no pain 2 hours after start)	Treatment	Control
Success	1067	256
Failure	787	780
Total	1854	1036

Table 10.2. Summarised measures of success for the migraine data.

Odds ratio	=	4.13*
Relative risk	=	2.33*
Absolute risk reduction	=	0.328
Relative risk reduction	=	0.436

*The odds ratio and relative risk are for the association of treatment and success. If the same statistics were calculated for the association between treatment and failure, the reciprocal of these values would appear.

The results given in Table 10.1 can be expressed in many different ways (see Table 10.2), none of which is particularly helpful to the GP.

In this study the proportion with the desired outcome in the treatment group was:

$$\frac{1067}{1854} = 0.576$$

and in the control group was:

$$\frac{256}{1036} = 0.247.$$

Using any statistical test the difference between the two will be significant at any reasonable significance level. Statistical significance is strong evidence that treatment and placebo differ in their effect, but it does not tell us how great or how small the difference is. The best estimate of the difference is:

$$0.567 - 0.247 = 0.328$$

which is known as the absolute risk reduction (ARR), with an approximate 95% confidence interval of 0.291–0.366. This is clearly consistent with the result of the above statistical test as the interval does not include the 0 value of no difference. This indicates that the long-term percentage having a desired outcome when treated with the drug will be between 29 and 37% compared with the outcome on placebo.

Number needed to treat

It has been suggested that results can be more usefully expressed by inverting the ARR, which gives the number needed to treat (NNT) with the drug to get a single successful outcome compared with that achieved on placebo. In the above example:

$$NNT = 1/0.328 = 3.04.$$

The 95% confidence interval can similarly be inverted to give a 95% confidence interval for the number needed to treat of 2.73 (= 1/0.366) and 3.44 (=1/0.291). Obviously, the lower confidence limit for the proportion corresponds to the upper confidence limit for the number needed to treat, and *vice versa*.

For successful treatments, the NNT can vary from 1, which corresponds to the unrealistic situation when the treatment has a successful outcome for all patients and the placebo is totally ineffective, to infinity, where the proportion of successful outcomes is the same for both treatment and placebo. A negative NNT implies that the treatment is less effective than the placebo.

For a statistically significantly effective treatment, the end points of the 95% confidence interval of the NNT will always be positive. If one of the end points of the 95% confidence interval is negative, then this implies that the difference between the treatment and placebo is not statistically significant. If both of the end points are negative, then this means that the treatment is significantly different from and worse than the control. A negative endpoint is often not given but is replaced by the words 'no benefit'.

An alternative approach is discussed by Altman (1998) who points out that a negative NNT to benefit one individual (NNT) actually corresponds to a NNT to harm one individual (NNH) and thus a negative value for the end point of the confidence interval of NNT can be expressed as a positive value for NNH. To emphasise the fact that the interval includes no difference, the value infinity (∞) for the number needed to treat is included in the interval.

Size of number needed to treat

Clearly, NNTs as close to 1 as possible are desirable, but what values are acceptable will depend on the severity of the disease, the prevalence of side effects, and the alternative treatments available. One of the smallest NNTs (1.09) was that produced in a meta-analysis of triple therapy (bismuth, tetracycline and metronidazole) with either ranitidine or omeprazole *versus* a combined control group consisting of patients treated with histamine-receptor antagonists or omeprazole alone for the eradication of *Helicobacter pylori* (Anon 1995b).

A 95% confidence interval for NNT that is as small as possible is also desirable, as this indicates reduced uncertainty in the estimate of the NNT. However, this will in part depend on the overall size of studies on which the NNT calculation is based.

Empirically, NNTs for successful treatments are hopefully small, certainly in single figures. If prophylaxis is considered, then the NNT as defined above will be negative, since you are looking for a reduction of undesirable outcomes in the treatment group compared to the control group. Also, since undesirable outcomes are hopefully relatively infrequent even in the control group, the absolute value for the NNT will usually be large.

L'Abbé plots

A simple visual method for graphically summarising the results from a meta-analysis is to draw a L'Abbé plot (L'Abbé *et al* 1987). For each separate study in a meta-analysis, a point is plotted on a graph with co-ordinates corresponding to the proportion of successful outcomes in the control and treatment groups on the horizontal and vertical axes, respectively. A further modification is to replace the point by a circle whose area is in line with the size of the study in question; although this has the disadvantage that some results may be obscured, it highlights larger studies (Fig. 10.3). The line at the 45° angle represents equality between treatment and control. Points in the upper level triangular area represent studies that favour the treatment, whereas results in the lower right triangular area favour the control. Variability in the percentage success in the treatment and control is clearly indicated. Whether any study differs markedly from the rest, or whether some of the studies favour the control, can easily be seen. The variability seen between the proportion of successes with placebo is often quite sobering.

Applying meta-analysis to subgroups

A major problem of meta-analysis in general practice is that it is geared to discovering average effects based on large numbers of subjects, whereas the interest of the GP is the individual patient, and whether a particular treatment is right for him/her.

This can lead to a focus on subgroup analysis which may be misleading. Subgroup analyses are often carried out when the overall analysis is not statistically significant, and it may be that the data have been divided in several different ways so that there are potentially many ways of defining subgroups. This, of course, increases the probability of a statistically significant result when real differences do not exist (which may have been the motivation for the subgroup analysis in the first place!). This means that the most important question to ask is whether the subgroup analysis was planned before

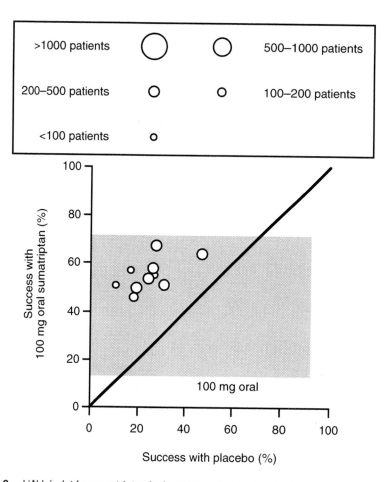

Fig. 10.3. L'Abbé plot for sumatriptan in the treatment of acute migraine.

the study started, or whether it was suggested by examination of the data. If the latter, then subgroup analysis should be treated as an hypothesis-generating, rather than an hypothesis-testing, exercise. Even in the former case, a subgroup analysis is inevitably based on smaller numbers than those in the total study group, and is therefore likely to be more subject to the play of chance.

Problems with subgroup analysis

In an examination of the data from the ISIS-1 randomised trial of the treatment of patients with suspected acute myocardial infarction, there was a significant reduction overall (P<0.05) in the odds of death during treatment (Collins *et al* 1987). However, if the data were re-analysed for subgroups defined by the patients' star sign, then for those with the star sign Scorpio there was an even larger reduction in the odds of death, with a slightly more significant result (P<0.04). In addition, those not born under the sign of Scorpio did not show a significant reduction in the odds of death (P>0.05). You can probably assume that anyone carrying out this type of analysis has looked at the results for all 12 star signs, but will have reported only the most 'significant' result. Carrying out 12 analyses obviously increases the chance of a significant result.

Now it is possible that the sign of the zodiac, which is of course related to birth period, may be an important factor in defining response to treatment, but it seems more likely that this is a chance finding. In any event, it would be prudent to see if this is confirmed by other studies.

Guidelines for subgroup analysis

The following guidelines have been suggested for determining whether apparent differences in subgroup response are real or not (Oxman and Guyatt 1992).

▶ Is the magnitude of the difference clinically important?

▶ Was the difference statistically significant?

▶ Did the hypotheses precede rather than follow the analysis?

▶ Was the subgroup analysis one of a small number of hypotheses tested?

▶ Was the difference suggested by comparisons within rather than between studies?

▶ Was the difference consistent across studies?

▶ Is there indirect evidence that supports the suggested difference?

Evidence-based diagnosis

An interesting 'case study' of using EBH to diagnose a non-smoking patient with a chronic unproductive cough of more than 20 years duration has recently been published (Glasziou 1998). Using a rather complex search strategy it was claimed that four articles dealing with the diagnosis of chronic cough, including information on the frequency of different aetiologies, were located using MEDLINE. However, subsequent letters (Bates 1998, Zucala *et al* 1998) suggested that a large number of irrelevant references would also be generated, and that two of the references concerned would not in fact have been located because of the time limit of the previous 5 years chosen in the search strategy. This highlights one of the practical problems of searching for information of either being swamped by irrelevant data or missing important references.

Evidence-based treatment

A serious attempt to illustrate the perceived problem of applying EBH to the individual patient with a particular condition has been discussed (Fahey 1998). In the paper it is suggested that it is possible to carry out RCTs in general practice, and that the results for trials not carried out in general practice can also be relied on, because the outcome is more likely to be determined by patient characteristics than trial setting. In addition, as medical journals apply the CONSORT principles to the reporting of clinical trials, it will be easier to judge the representativeness or otherwise of the trial study population. A clinical scenario of two patients with sinusitis of different levels of severity was suggested. MEDLINE was used to locate a RCT of confirmed acute sinusitis treated by antibiotics (Lindbaek *et al* 1996). Using a scale of severity also provided by the trial report, and the frequency and severity of possible side effects of treatment, a quantitative ratio of expected benefit to harm was calculated for the two patients. This clearly indicated whether treatment was beneficial or otherwise in the two cases, and thus whether treatment with antibiotics should be used or not. This implies that there must be a common scale on which the benefits and disadvantages of treatment can be measured. The need to produce this means that any assumptions about benefit and harm are made explicit.

The application of a treatment regimen tested in a RCT to individual patients, with a clear attempt to quantify benefit/harm expected, was impressive. However, the author admitted that while the paper was being written another study of sinusitis which suggested that antibiotics had little effect on acute sinusitis, was published (van Buchem *et al* 1997; see also Chaper 19). Letters to the journal concerned claimed that the diagnosis of acute sinusitis in general practice was difficult (Sweeney *et al* 1998), and that trying to put into practice the techniques suggested in the paper in the time usually available for consultation would be quite impracticable (Kernick 1998).

Development of guidelines

The above example suggests that applying the principles of EBH by an individual GP during consultation may be difficult (see also Chapter 17). A more practical alternative may be the development of evidence-based guidelines in common conditions, such as those produced in *Effective Health Care* by the NHS Centre for Reviews and Dissemination in York (see Chaper 4). It will be important for GPs to be involved in the production of these guidelines, so that they are seen as relevant and practical, and that they should be updated at regular intervals. In this way, more and more aspects of general practice may become evidence based.

References

Altman DG (1991). *Practical Statistics for Medical Research*. London: Chapman and Hall, Chapter 15.

Altman DG (1996). Better reporting of randomised controlled trials : the CONSORT statement. *British Medical Journal* **313**: 570–571.

Altman DG (1998). Confidence intervals for the number needed to treat. *British Medical Journal* **317**: 1309–1312.

Anon (1995a). Evidence-based everything. *Bandolier* **12**: 1.

Anon (1995b). *H Pylori*: Numbers needed to treat. *Bandolier* **12**: 2–5.

Anon (1999). Making sense of migraine treatments. *Bandolier* **6**: 1–4.

Bates D (1998). Results of search strategy should be given to readers. *British Medical Journal* **317**: 138.

Collins R, Gray R, Godwin J, *et al* (1987). Avoidance of large biases and large random errors in the assessment of moderate treatment effects; the need for systematic overviews. *Statistics in Medicine* **6**: 245–250.

Cooper J, McGillion FB, West B (1978). A comparison of cotrimoxazole and amoxycillin in acute bronchitis. *Practitioner* **220**: 798–802.

Cranney M, Walley T (1996). Same information, different decisions: the influence of evidence on the management of hypertension in the elderly. *British Journal of General Practice* **46**: 661–663.

Davey Smith G, Egger M (1998). Meta-analysis: unresolved issues and future developments. *British Medical Journal* **316**: 221–225.

Egger M, Davey Smith G (1998). Meta-analysis: bias in location and selection of studies. *British Medical Journal* **316**: 61–66.

Egger M, Davey Smith G, Schneider M, *et al* (1997). Meta-analysis: bias in meta-analysis detected by a simple graphical test. *British Medical Journal* **315**: 629–634.

Fahey T (1998). Applying the results of clinical trials to patients in general practice: perceived problems, strengths, assumptions and challenges for the future. *British Journal of General Practice* **48**: 1173–1178.

Gardner MJ, Altman DG (1989). *Statistics with Confidence.* London: BMJ Publishing.

Glasziou P (1998). Twenty year cough in a non smoker. *British Medical Journal* **316**: 1660–1661.

Hopayian K, Mugford M (1999). Conflicting conclusions from two systematic reviews of epidural steroid injections for sciatica: which evidence should general practitioners heed? *British Journal of General Practice* **49**: 57–61.

Hux JE, Naylor CD (1995). Communicating the benefits of chronic preventive therapy: does the format of efficacy data determine patient's acceptance of treatment? *Medical Decision Making* **15**: 152–157.

Kernick D (1998). From theory to reality. *British Journal of General Practice* **48**: 1433.

Koes BW, Scholten RJPM, Mens JMA, *et al* (1995). Efficacy of epidural steroid injections for low back pain and sciatica: a systematic review of randomised clinical trials. *Pain* **63**: 279–288.

L'Abbé KA, Detsky AS, O'Rourke K (1987). Meta-analysis in clinical research. *Annals of Internal Medicine* **107**: 224–233.

Lindbaek M, Hjortdahl P, Johnsen UL-H (1996). Randomised, double blind, placebo controlled trial of penicillin V and amoxycillin in treatment of acute sinus infections in adults. *British Medical Journal* **313**: 325–329.

Oxman AD, Guyatt GH (1992). The consumer's guide to subgroup analysis. *Annals of Internal Medicine* **116**: 78–84.

Pocock SJ (1983). *Clinical Trials: A Practical Approach.* Chichester: Wiley.

Sweeney K, Evans P, Pereira Gray D, *et al* (1998). Applying the results of clinical trials to patients. *British Journal of General Practice* **48**: 1612–1613.

The Cochrane Collaboration (1997). *The Cochrane Library.* Oxford: Update Software.

van Buchem FL, Knottnerus JA, Schrijnemaekers V, *et al* (1997). Primary-care based randomised placebo-controlled trial of antibiotic treatment in acute maxillary sinusitis. *Lancet* **349**: 683–687.

Watts RW, Silagy CA (1995). A meta-analysis on the efficacy of epidural corticosteroids in the treatment of sciatica. *Anaesthesia and Intensive Care* **23**: 564–569.

Zuccala G, Pedone C, Carbonin P (1998). Evidence based medicine is not magic. *British Medical Journal* **317**: 1387.

SECTION 2

EVIDENCE-BASED PRIMARY CARE COMMISSIONING AND PRESCRIBING

This section is particularly aimed at evidence as it pertains to commissioning, including some worked examples. As primary care groups in the UK increase their sphere of influence in decisions about the use of resources, and the services provided for patients, they are likely increasingly to want to draw upon the best available evidence to help them in their task.

This section begins with an overview of evidence and commissioning, including the evidence about the effectiveness of the UK process, and how evidence of effectiveness may be used by commissioners. This is followed by a chapter outlining the approach, using the example of commissioning stroke services.

The following pair of chapters present an overview of health economic evidence plus a detailed worked example, exploring how you may use a paper giving health economic information. Many professionals are concerned about the practical challenges of applying evidence to individual patients. This is explored by focusing on barriers to evidence-based prescribing, and potential solutions. It has become increasingly popular to involve pharmacists in primary care prescribing reviews, and we have included a chapter exploring the evidence about the effectiveness of this approach.

Finally, as an introduction to the final section, there is a chapter summarising real questions and real answers from practice. Some practices have started using evidence-based approaches in their work. This chapter illustrates the variety of questions and the process of finding answers from evidence, including the time taken and the results.

▶11

Evidence-Based Commissioning in Primary Care

Stephen Gillam

Introduction

The advent of the NHS internal market in 1990 heralded changes of lasting significance for general practice. The implicit power of the 'gatekeeper' had long been recognised but fundholding extended this influence in a visible and contentious way. While its benefits remain disputed, there is no doubt that fundholding shifted the balance of power within the medical profession and the NHS as a whole. But with these new powers have come new responsibilities. Primary care groups (PCGs) extend the commissioning franchise to all primary care professionals and carry important implications for their basic and postgraduate training.

Just as evidence-based clinical practice applies the judicious use of the best evidence available when making decisions for individual patients, evidence-based commissioning implies the consistent use of evidence when planning populations' health services. Increasingly, GPs need skills in 'knowledge management', a term that embraces the abilities to scan, sift and appraise new evidence before distributing, storing and applying it (Boxes 11.1–11.3).

After a brief historical detour, I will summarise the evidence related to primary care-centred commissioning. The next section focuses specifically on the challenge of basing commissioning decisions on evidence. Finally, I will discuss the implications of this work for the development of PCGs.

Box 11.1. Searching skills for commissioning decision teams (see Chapters 3 and 4 for examples of sources)

Commissioners should have:
- ▶ a knowledge, and preferably some experience, of searching sources of information other than their local postgraduate library;

- ▶ a working knowledge of at least two databases of relevance to their work;

- ▶ an understanding and ability to use the electronic search interfaces they refer to, including 'MESH', explode and Boolean operators;

- ▶ ability to conduct a search, using more than one database or approach.

Box 11.2. Appraisal skills for commissioning decision teams

Commissioners should be able to:

▶ appraise the type of research papers they commonly use, such as systematic reviews, meta-analyses, randomised trials, cohort studies, case-control studies and other surveys, according to a criteria-based framework;

▶ present such appraisal, outlining the strengths and weaknesses of the literature they have identified;

▶ write a review of an appraised search.

In this way, commissioners can share their findings with others in a way that can efficiently aid evidence-based decisions.

Box 11.3. System for storing and retrieving evidence

▶ A computer-based reference management system (more versatile than a card-based system).

▶ Commissioning decision team should be able to:
— input records into it;
— download electronic search results onto it;
— search in it.

Commissioning in evolution

The 1991 NHS reforms introduced two different types of purchaser: the district health authorities, which were responsible for purchasing the full range of services for relatively large populations (approximately 500 000), and GP fundholders, who had budgets to purchase a selected range of services for relatively small practice populations (approximately 10 000). From these two basic models, several different approaches emerged involving GPs in needs assessment, service evaluation, and planning, but without necessarily delegating budgetary control (Mays and Dixon 1996). Recent government measures have encouraged convergence between the two main models (NHS Executive 1997a).

In opposition to budget holding, the National Association of General Practitioners championed the role of multipractice collectives. General practitioner commissioning groups (GPCGs) went 'live' in April 1998. They cover populations of not less than 50 000, with pooled prescribing budgets, working in co-operation with health authorities to commission hospital and community health services (HCHS) (NHS Executive 1997b). HCHS budgets are indicative only, but the commissioning groups can decide how to spend savings from their prescribing budgets. These arrangements are being piloted over a 2-year period in localities with previously low GP involvement in commissioning or purchasing.

The total purchasing pilots (TPPs) provided an opportunity for volunteer fundholding practices to receive delegated budgets from their local health authorities to purchase potentially all hospital and community health services for their patients (Total Purchasing National Evaluation Team 1997). Pertinent findings from the national evaluation of TPPs are discussed in the final section.

The government funded an evaluation of GPCGs but is not waiting for its findings. The white paper *The New NHS – Modern, Dependable* (NHS Executive 1998) inaugurated the next evolutionary variant: primary care groups (PCGs). PCGs have a budget covering GP prescribing and practice infrastructure. Only as PCGs develop will they take responsibility for an increasing share of HCHS and general medical services (GMS) budgets. PCGs will grow out of the existing range of commissioning schemes around 'natural communities' of between 47 000 and 260 000 patients.

Commissioning-based evidence

Doctor as patient's agent

A commonly stated advantage of involving GPs in the commissioning process is that they are closer to patients and therefore can help to ensure that plans take account of patients' needs and preferences (NHS Executive 1994). The assumption that GPs' views and priorities are congruent with their patients' needs has not been tested.

Leverage

Priorities tend to change when GPs play a leading role in commissioning because they place greater emphasis on certain services than does the health authority. For example, the Audit Commission (1996) found that many fundholders used their leverage to change the provision of district nursing services, to improve the provision of hospital discharge information, or to secure faster turn around times for pathology tests. Non-fundholders involved in commissioning groups reported similar concerns but with less confidence that they could effect changes (Graffy and Williams 1994).

General practitioner's role

Direct involvement in decisions about resource allocation places the GP in the role of rationer, a task with which many GPs feel uncomfortable because it conflicts with their preferred role as patient's advocate (Robinson and Hayter 1995, Ayres 1996). Patients may be less willing to accept the advice that they do not need treatment or referral if they believe the GP's decision is influenced by budgetary considerations. This could undermine the doctor–patient relationship with possible adverse consequences on the effectiveness of clinical care (Cornell 1996).

It is clear that many GPs do not want to accept direct responsibility for delegated budgets. Many had ideological objections to fundholding (Robinson and Hayter 1995, Primary Care Support Force 1996). Some argue that time spent on budget management has a detrimental effect on their ability to provide good clinical care. Others claim they do not have the requisite skills in financial management. Experience of non-fundholding commissioning groups suggests that it is possible to involve primary care staff in setting priorities without delegating budgetary control (Black *et al* 1994), but there are still questions about whether they will remain committed in the longer term. Budget holding offers greater incentives for GPs than commissioning alone.

To date there have been few published examples of nurses and other primary care staff playing a leading role in the development of fundholding or commissioning. *The New NHS–Modern, Dependable* white paper seeks to change that (NHS Executive 1998).

Needs assessment

Much of the impetus for developing commissioning groups came from doctors themselves (Smith *et al* 1997). General practitioner-led commissioning has been based on single practices or clusters of practices (Smith and Shapiro 1997). However, much health data, e.g. that used to assess health needs, are based on electoral wards, i.e. geographical boundaries rather than practice boundaries. Practice boundaries do not necessarily fit into 'natural' communities, nor are they co-terminous with local authority boundaries used by social services and other agencies. Co-ordination of information sources can be especially difficult in urban areas where practice selection effects operate more powerfully.

Appropriate population size

In absolute terms the appropriate population size for commissioning depends on what services are to be commissioned. The notion of 'epidemiological stability' suggests that community nursing and many other 'attached' community health services, elective surgery and other facilities covered by standard fundholding are logically purchased at practice level, while most other secondary care services, including A&E and maternity services, may better be purchased under block contracts by organisations covering populations of around 100 000–300 000, leaving tertiary and more highly specialised services to be covered at a 'regional' level (roughly 1 000 000) (Murray 1993).

Financial risk and resource allocation

Financial risk resulting from unpredicted demand is greater when the population pool is small. The experience of health maintenance organizations in the USA suggests that purchasing for populations of <50 000 involves punitive transaction costs and unmanageable risk (Sheffler 1989), but this view has been challenged (Weiner and Ferris 1990). Models have been devised for spreading the risk over 3–5 years, but these have not yet been tested (Bachmann and Bevan 1996). Attempts to devise a resource allocation formula for fundholding which would be robust at the practice level proved unsuccessful (Sheldon *et al* 1994).

Quality of care

Most research on fundholding concentrated on access to secondary care or on changes in prescribing patterns and costs (Goodwin 1996). The scheme appeared to make only limited impact on referral rates (Surrender *et al* 1995) and emergency admissions (Toth *et al* 1997). There is some evidence of an effect on prescribing costs but this is hotly contested (Gosden and Torgerson 1997). These measures of utilisation tell us very little about the quality of care. On the whole, studies have failed to measure the impact on patients' health and it is therefore impossible to draw firm conclusions on the relative efficiency of the scheme in terms of costs and benefits (Gosden *et al* 1997).

Shifting the balance

The current policy concern to shift the balance of care from secondary to primary settings is led in part by a desire to contain rising health-care costs. There are few signs that giving secondary care budgets to GPs has achieved the desired shift (Coulter 1996). Fundholders have made considerable investments in their practices, but as yet these have not led to reductions in the demand for secondary services.

The realisation that current arrangements may not have gone far enough has increased interest in merging budgets for primary and secondary care. The 1997 NHS (Primary Care) Act allows scope for experimentation with unified budgets for GMS and HCHS, although piloting of these arrangements has been deferred. In theory unified budgets could provide more powerful incentives to shift the balance of care and to ensure that investment in primary care is matched by reductions in expenditure on specialist services. The risks are considerable (Coulter and Mays 1997). The creative tension of contestability introduced by the purchaser–provider split will be diluted if GPs purchase and provide from the same budget and there is greater potential for conflicts of interest. On the other hand, unified budgets can be used to plan cost-effective services that break down barriers between providers. The growth of community-based intermediate care provides an example (Steiner 1997).

Evidence-based commissioning

Clinical effectiveness

The Audit Commission (1996) found that most fundholders were not making full use of the increasing body of knowledge about clinical effectiveness to change the way they commission. Of the fundholders surveyed, only a third said that their purchasing plans had been influenced by literature on evidence-based health. Most fundholders have been reluctant to challenge the standards of clinical care provided in hospitals (Douglas *et al* 1997). Needs and demands are not the same thing and it is possible that GP-led commissioning will encourage responsiveness at the expense of appropriateness and cost-effectiveness. PCGs are more likely to include representatives with an interest in audit or education and should be better at processing and sharing this knowledge.

Primary care groups can expect to be held to account for the quality of their decision making. Health authorities have been notoriously haphazard in scrutinising new evidence but most now have strategies in place to promote clinically effective practice (Walshe 1998). PCGs will need to be alert to new electronic sources of information. Clinical governance leads will need to ensure the more systematic distribution of relevant material between and within practices.

Nature of evidence

Too reductionist an emphasis on randomised control led trials can downgrade those services, e.g. talking therapies, that will ever elude such approaches to evaluation. Disinvestment in, for example, school nursing may have costly long-term consequences. The importance of qualitative research (and the ability to appraise it) is increasingly acknowledged. Having no evidence for the effectiveness of an intervention should not be confused with having evidence for its ineffectiveness. The key is to seek evidence appropriate to the questions asked.

Expertise

Effective purchasing requires a wide range of skills, including needs assessment, contracting, performance monitoring, accounting and budget management. Beyond an understanding of the processes of commissioning, some specialist knowledge is required to make strategically coherent purchasing decisions. This knowledge may not always be vested in general practice (Howells 1996). For example, people with learning disabilities have special needs of which their GPs may not always be aware (Royal College of General Practitioners 1996).

Health authorities tend to rely on the generalist skills of public health physicians for advice on purchasing specialist services, but they may not necessarily be more expert in particular specialties than GPs involved in fundholding. What public health specialists do have, in contrast to most GPs, is training in information retrieval, epidemiology and research methods, skills which are central to the assessment of health needs. Effective purchasing relies on knowing how and when to obtain expert advice, as well as having the time to research needs and service options (Audit Commission 1996). An understanding of how to evolve true partnerships is essential to furthering public health aims. The first generation of PCG boards are likely to 'learn by doing'. In time, training opportunities should emerge that are PCG led, multidisciplinary, use existing resources (in health authorities and trusts) and are based on assessment of existing skills (Wilson et al 1998).

Towards the new NHS

Learning from the total purchasing pilots

The TTPs varied greatly in size, organisation and ambition (Total Purchasing National Evaluation Team 1997). With no detailed blueprint for total purchasing, TPPs interpreted the concept in different ways and developed at different rates. The level of achievement between pilots therefore varied widely. Achievement was more likely to be reported in primary than in secondary care. Reported achievements in reducing length of stay and emergency admissions were corroborated by analysis of hospital episode statistics. Single practice and small multi-practice projects were more likely than large multi-projects to achieve their objectives in the first year. Achievements were also associated with higher direct management cost per head and the ability to undertake independent contracting. Large multi-practice pilots required considerable organisational development before progress could be made.

The TPP evaluation suggests that budget holding and independent contracting is important if PCGs are to manage demand for hospital services. The perception that PCGs lack power to effect change could be a major barrier against wider participation in these groups. It will be important to assess the extent to which PCGs are able to exert influence in order to achieve beneficial changes in the delivery of local services (Gillam and Coulter 1998).

Clinical governance

Engendering collective responsibility among all practitioners for staying within budget or adhering to prescribing and referral protocols will prove difficult. The reduction in individual autonomy and a greater emphasis on cost effectiveness remains antipathetic to many doctors. They are ambivalent about taking responsibility for rationing. The extent to which they will share a commitment to the needs of the locality as opposed to those of their own practice will crucially affect the development of PCGs. Groups will include practices at different levels of development with a variety of practice styles; as a result some types of practices could be marginalised. Practices with low referral rates or efficient prescribing policies may be unwilling to share risk with practices perceived as less developed. On the other hand, closer working between more and less developed practices has most potential to raise the quality of primary care in a locality. Performance indicator packages are at an early stage of development. Technical obstacles such as the difficulties of controlling for case-mix are not easily resolved. Few outcome measures have been validated. The data most easily obtainable are often least easily interpreted. Both high and low referral rates, for example, may be markers of inadequate practice.

Equity

Fundholding tended to attract well organised practices from better-off parts of the country, with inner city practices particularly under-represented (Audit Commission 1995). It remains to be seen whether GPs and practice staff working in 'difficult' areas will have the time or the inclination to get involved in PCGs and whether the scheme will help to improve services in disadvantaged areas. Smaller practices and single-handed GPs may get left out.

Transaction costs

Transaction costs are likely to be substantially lower when budgetary control remains with the health authority because the need for numerous contracts with small-scale purchasers is avoided, but these efficiency gains must be balanced against reduced incentives for practices to control demand by restricting referrals or investing in practice-based facilities as a substitute for more expensive secondary services.

Management support

Not enough is known about the level of administrative support necessary to underpin commissioning at the different levels. Experience with TPPs thus far does not suggest they reduce bureaucracy, but purchasing processes could become more streamlined as the practices gain experience (Total Purchasing National Evaluation Team 1997). Ever more stringent cuts in management costs will be counter-productive if access to relevant information and evidence is thereby impaired.

Public accountability

Primary care groups may struggle to secure user involvement. While patients might find it easy to identify with their own general practice, aggregates of practices or localities seem less relevant to them. This question of identity links to the wider question of accountability. Accountability arrangements for fundholders tended to focus on financial management, with little emphasis on accountability to patients or the local public. It will be important to examine ways in which PCGs can make themselves accountable to the people on whose behalf they are securing access to services.

Conclusion

The ability to create effective commissioning organisations should not be underestimated. The necessary organisational development of PCGs will require time and resources, particularly as some of the practices participating will have little experience of commissioning.

References

Audit Commission (1995). Briefing on General Practitioner Fundholding. London: HMSO.

Audit Commission (1996). What the Doctor Ordered: A Study of General Practitioner Fundholders in England and Wales. London: HMSO.

Ayres P (1996). Rationing health care: views from general practice. Social Science and Medicine 42: 1021–1025.

Bachmann MO and Bevan G (1996). Determining the size of a total purchasing site to manage the finance from risks of rare costly referrals: computer simulation model. British Medical Journal 313: 1054–1056.

Black DG, Birchall AD, Trimble IMG (1994). Non-fundholding in Nottingham: a vision of the future. British Medical Journal 309: 930–932.

Cornell J (1996). Has general practice fundholding been good for patients? Public Health 110: 5–6.

Coulter A (1996). Why should health services be primary care-led? Journal of Health Services Research and Policy 1: 122–124.

Coulter A and Mays N (1997). Deregulating primary care. British Medical Journal 314: 510–513.

Douglas HR, Humphrey C, Lloyd M, et al (1997). Promoting clinically effective practice: attitudes of fundholding general practitioners to the role of commissioning. Journal of Management in Medicine 11: 26–34.

Gillam S and Coulter A (1998). Evaluating primary care groups. British Journal of General Practice 48: 1640–1641.

Goodwin N (1996). General practitioner fundholding: a review of the evidence. In: Harrison A (Ed) *Health Care UK 1995/6*. London: King's Fund.

Gosden T and Torgerson D (1997). The effect of fundholding on prescribing and referral costs: a review of the evidence. *Health Policy* **40**: 103–114.

Gosden T, Torgerson D, Maynard A (1997). What is to be done about fundholding? *British Medical Journal* **315**: 170–171.

Graffy JP and Williams J (1994). Purchasing for all: an alternative to fundholding. *British Medical Journal* **308**: 391–394.

Howells G (1996). Situations vacant: doctors required to provide care for people with learning disability. *British Journal of General Practice* **46**: 59–60.

Mays N and Dixon J (1996). *Purchaser Plurality in UK Health Care*. London: King's Fund.

Murray D (1993). *Patterns in NHS Commissioning? A Review and Discussion of Alternative Models of Integrated Locally Sensitive Commissioning*. London: London School of Hygiene and Tropical Medicine.

NHS Executive (1994). *Developing NHS Purchasing and General Practitioner Fundholding: Towards a Primary Care-Led NHS*. EL(94)79. Leeds: Department of Health.

NHS Executive (1997a). *Changing the Internal Market*. EL(97)33. Leeds: Department of Health.

NHS Executive (1997b). *General Practitioner Commissioning Groups*. EL(97)37. Leeds: Department of Health.

NHS Executive (1998). *The New NHS – Modern, Dependable*. Leeds: Department of Health.

Primary Care Support Force (1996). *What Works Well? What Needs to Happen?: General Practitioners in Commissioning*. London: Primary Care Support Force.

Robinson R and Hayter P (1995). *Why do General Practitioners Choose not to Apply for Fundholding?* Southampton: Institute for Health Policy Studies.

Royal College of General Practitioners (1996). *The Nature of General Medical Practice. Report from General Practice 27*. London: Royal College of General Practitioners.

Sheffler R (1989). Adverse selection: the Achilles heel of the NHS reforms. *Lancet* No. 8644: 950–952.

Sheldon T, Seith P, Borowirz M, *et al* (1994). Attempt at deriving a formula for setting general practitioner fundholding budgets. *British Medical Journal* **309**: 1059–1064.

Smith J and Shapiro J (1997). *Holding on While Letting Go: Evaluation of Locality Commissioning in County Durham and Newcastle/North Tyneside*. University of Birmingham: Health Services Management Centre.

Smith J, Bamford M, Ham C, *et al*. *Beyond Fundholding: A Mosaic of Primary Care Led Commissioning and Provision in the West Midlands*. University of Birmingham and Keele University.

Steiner A (1997). *Intermediate Care: A Conceptual Framework and Review of the Literature*. London: King's Fund.

Surender R, Bradlow J, Coulter A, *et al* (1995). Prospective study of trends in referral patterns in fundholding and non-fundholding practices in the Oxford region 1990–4. *British Medical Journal* **311**: 1205–1208.

Total Purchasing National Evaluation Team (1997). *Total Purchasing: A Profile of National Pilot Projects*. London: King's Fund.

Toth B, Harvey I, Peters T (1997). Did the introduction of general practice fundholding change patterns of emergency admission to hospital? *Journal of Health Services Research and Policy* **2**: 71–74.

Walshe K (1998). Evidence-based healthcare: what progress in the NHS? *Journal of the Royal Society of Medicine* **91 (suppl 35)**: 15–19.

Weiner J and Ferris D (1990). *General Practitioner Budget Holding in the UK: Lessons from America*. London: King's Fund.

Wilson T, Butler F, Wright J (1998). *Defining the Education and Training Needs of PCGs*. Oxford: PCG Resource Unit.

▶12

Commissioning Stroke Services

David Chappel

This practical chapter differs from others in this book because it is about decision making for a population rather than for an individual patient. This leads to a number of differences in approach. Although health authority commissioners worked up the example described here, fundholders faced similar issues and primary care groups (PCGs) will shortly do so.

The question

What is the best way to organise stroke services for our population?

The question arose because the condition is common and serious (it was a target in *Health of the Nation* and *Our Healthier Nation*) rather than because there was a perceived problem with services, i.e. a proactive rather than reactive approach. Such an approach is not easily amenable to the formulation of a clear-cut question. Indeed, it would be a mistake to focus too quickly on answerable questions before thinking through the breadth of the problem. I have used a similar question as a 'trick' question in training staff on search strategies. I asked them when they arrived to 'see how many references you can find (on MEDLINE) on the topic 'effective treatments for stroke'. The point about the need to refine questions and use a strategy was quickly apparent.

A district stroke group, comprising staff from the health authority, primary care, trusts and social services, discussed the breadth of the problem. They defined four broad areas:

▶ *Prevention*: This includes primary prevention (i.e. interventions to prevent stroke) and secondary prevention (interventions to prevent further strokes following a first stroke or transient ischaemic attack) since many of the activities are similar in both areas.

▶ *Treatment*: This includes the diagnosis and initial treatment for patients with stroke in the acute stage, including acute nursing care and the prevention of complications.

▶ *Rehabilitation*: This includes early and long-term rehabilitation (and its organisation), particularly therapies such as physiotherapy, occupational therapy and speech therapy.

▶ *Long-term support*: This includes the work of carers, the voluntary sector (e.g. support groups) and the private sector (e.g. accommodation), as well as the work of the statutory sector (local authority and NHS).

This process ensures that prioritisation is not simply based on the presence or absence of evidence (which is predominantly available for treatment and primary prevention), but takes a broad view of the important issues. The formation of a group to work on this topic is also important for other reasons. Implementation of any findings will need to involve many professionals so their co-operation is needed throughout, and the group will form a useful network to help with the search for evidence (later additions to the group included the voluntary sector). However, each member of the group will bring his own specific interests and prejudices and this bias must always be borne in mind.

The search

One thing you can be sure of is that someone else has worked on a question like this before. Virtually all health authorities (and increasingly PCGs from 1999 onwards) are likely to have thought about it, even if not at the level that you want. This means that someone can save you time, if you can identify them. The problem is that the review you want may not have been formally published but may just be a locally used report – so-called 'grey literature'. Chapter 3 outlines how this type of literature may be searched in more detail.

Contact with 'experts'

No-one is an expert in all aspects of stroke care but there are many people who may be able to point to others who have done the work. It was through this 'networking', both within and outside the stroke group that the most useful references were found.

Through public health contacts I was already aware of the Oxford Region's GRiPP (Getting Research into Practice and Purchasing) project (Blais 1994), and was able to obtain a copy of its stroke literature review. I was also aware that the Department of Health had a review of evidence (Wade 1994) that was in the local medical school library. A local consultant in stroke medicine put me on the track of a Stroke Association document (Wolfe *et al* 1996) and a recently published book (Warlow *et al* 1996). A senior lecturer in public health medicine had a copy of a document from another region (MacLeod *et al* 1993), and reminded me to start from *The Cochrane Library* (The Cochrane Collaboration 1999) before going much further and that there was an *Effective Health Care Bulletin* on stroke rehabilitation (though it was already a bit out of date) (NHS Centre for Reviews and Dissemination 1994).

The Cochrane Library looks promising as there is an active Stroke Collaborative Review Group. Disappointingly, a search through the titles showed that many topics have not progressed beyond protocols, and those that have cover only a small part of overall stroke care. However, where a topic has been covered, the authoritative nature of Cochrane reviews are helpful in controversial areas; e.g.

> *'there is insufficient evidence to recommend the use of thrombolytic drugs to treat acute ischaemic stroke at the moment . . .'* (Wardlaw *et al* 1998)

Without these contacts most of the documents could still have been found through local consultants, contacting the Royal Colleges and the appropriate research charities (such as the Stroke Association). A new GP group, interested in stroke and evidence-based practice, has recently been established (Action for Stroke Group, PO Box 9939, London W6 9WZ). A potential network to contact may include:

- physiotherapy departments;

- community nursing;

- local academic departments of primary care, public health, nursing, physiotherapy, neurology and care of the elderly;

- relevant charities;

- Royal Colleges of nursing, physicians, GPs etc.

Using the Internet

Chapter 3 covers searching the Internet. In this case searching the Internet for information on 'effective treatments for stroke' is likely to be as futile as it would be for a MEDLINE search.

There are, however, a number of other ways in which the Internet is useful. First, it gives the chance to ask the advice of many more people – 'electronic networking'. This is where mailbases are particularly useful. (The Mailbase Consortium provides electronic discussion lists for the UK higher education community. Available from: URL: http://www.mailbase.ac.uk.) In this case I used three:

- Public Health (public-health@mailbase.ac.uk);

- Evidence-Based Health (evidence-based-health@mailbase.ac.uk);

- Northern Public Health Medicine (northern-phm@ncl.ac.uk).

Others may be contacted via the list owner or joined. These should not be used as a first-line search method, as others on the lists would expect you to have done some groundwork first. However, new or obscure reviews can be picked up this way and contact made with people addressing similar issues.

No new reviews were uncovered although the ones described were mentioned again. One system used by public health doctors is EPINET. This was originally designed for exchanging communicable disease information but as it is based in every health authority, it is sometimes used by consultants in public health medicine to ask for advice on other topics. I did not use EPINET and it may become obsolete as new links develop through the NHSnet.

For those that wish to browse, it is best to start with a suitable Internet gateway and the public health (available from URL: http://fester.his.path.cam.ac.uk/phealth/phweb.html), evidence-based health (available from: URL:http://www.shef.ac.uk/~scharr/ir/netting.html) or medical ones (available from: URL: http://omni.ac.uk/) are good starting points. These can link, for example, to Health Technology Assessment and Development and Evaluation Committee sites in some regions and provided me with some (now rather dated) information on CT scanning (South and West Regional Development and Evaluation Committee 1994, Ferguson and McCabe 1997). They also provided links to the Agency for Health Care Policy and Research (US Department of Health 1995) in the USA (available from: URL: http://www.ahcpr.gov/). A stroke-specific site has been created with drug company funding (available from: URL: http://www.strokeforum.com/).

Using specialist libraries

There are many librarians with great expertise and ingenuity who can help. The local university or medical school is a good starting point. I was lucky to have a Clinical Effectiveness Resource Centre at the Health Authority who found the AHCPR document. Regional Health Authority (now NHSE outpost) libraries or those of large organisations such as the King's Fund, Royal Society of Medicine or British Medical Association are often useful sources of information (not used here).

Searching for grey literature

There are now some useful databases of grey literature. The King's Fund has an excellent library and database for 'grey literature' (not used here). The local librarian should be able to help access some of the grey literature databases held by the British Library (available from: URL: http://www.bl.uk/), such as *British Reports Translations and Theses* and *System for Information for Grey Literature in Europe*, but I did not use these and do not think they are likely to have yielded anything to change recommendations. Chapter 3 covers this form of searching in more detail.

Appraising what you have found

Much of the grey literature will come with unsolicited appraisal ('you ought to look at X's excellent report, and I suppose you might glance at Y's'). This can be useful in getting some 'peer review' of grey literature, although it needs to be used with care. The amount of time available will determine how much effort can be put into appraising literature. There are good guidelines for reviewing reviews (see Chapter 2), but it is inevitable with 'secondary' literature that much will have to be taken on trust.

One advantage of this search was the relatively large number of documents that could be compared, focusing effort into areas of disagreement. Each review had its strengths and weaknesses: none was ideal for my purpose. The GRiPP review was as near to a systematic review as was possible, though the Stroke Association document covered a greater breadth of areas and was more up to date. The Department of Health document had good coverage of epidemiology, and the textbook gave immense detail (although it was very difficult to evaluate how evidence based some of it was). *The Cochrane Library* provided the strongest evidence, but only for very small areas when the breadth of stroke services is considered.

Keeping abreast of new developments

The information derived from previous reviews of the topics will gradually (occasionally rapidly) go out of date. Three papers were identified during the search that contained important new information (Stroke Units Trialists Collaboration 1997, International Stroke Trial Collaborative Group 1997, CAST 1997). The local consultant easily spotted them as they were in mainstream journals. It would be impossible to keep a broad review such as this fully updated and so some sort of regular search and appraisal are necessary.

'Consensus statements' and 'guidance' from respected authorities are rarely evidence based but they often point to areas where the evidence base is changing (e.g. on thrombolysis), giving the impetus to further searches. All Department of Health circulars are now on the Internet (available from: URL: http://tap.ccta.gov.uk/doh/coin4.nsf). The planned National Institute for Clinical Effectiveness may provide some help in the future with keeping abreast of 'best evidence' (Department of Health 1998).

The answer

The question has been kept broad so the answer is not simple. The findings of this search were summarised in a 70-page 'technical document' (available from the author (Gateshead and South Tyneside Health Authority and Newcastle University 1997)). The aim was to derive an agreed evidence base for developing (what has now turned out to be) the Health Improvement Plan. Some areas (e.g. hospital stroke units) had strong evidence from which to work and others (e.g. long-term support) had little.

However, a list of 43 potential recommendations was drawn up and circulated to the group to prioritise. Four areas came out 'top':

- hypertension in primary care;

- multidisciplinary teams in secondary care;

- availability of routine information on stroke;

- long-term support.

These are areas that need further refinement. Although 'evidence' was the starting point, there are many other factors to balance in deciding what to do, such as practicality and perceived importance. Although a balancing of emphasis and priorities is required with individual patient decisions, decisions on service delivery resulting in changes in other people's practice makes this even more likely.

The first priority area was hypertension in primary care. The District Stroke Group, together with the District Multidisciplinary Audit Group, set up a subgroup to implement local guidelines. Hypertension is a sufficiently focused area to define a tight question with which to search, using approaches outlined elsewhere in this book (see Section 3). Indeed, there are already systematic reviews in this field, e.g. Ebrahim (1998). The Hypertension Group took the advice of a previous district group who had looked at vascular risk:

'scoring systems were not yet feasible in primary care in this district as practices did not yet have the information systems in place.'

They therefore favoured the British Hypertension Society Guidelines (Sever *et al* 1993) over the more evidence-based New Zealand guidelines (Jackson and Sackett 1996). Once again the formation of a group allows exchange of information on other

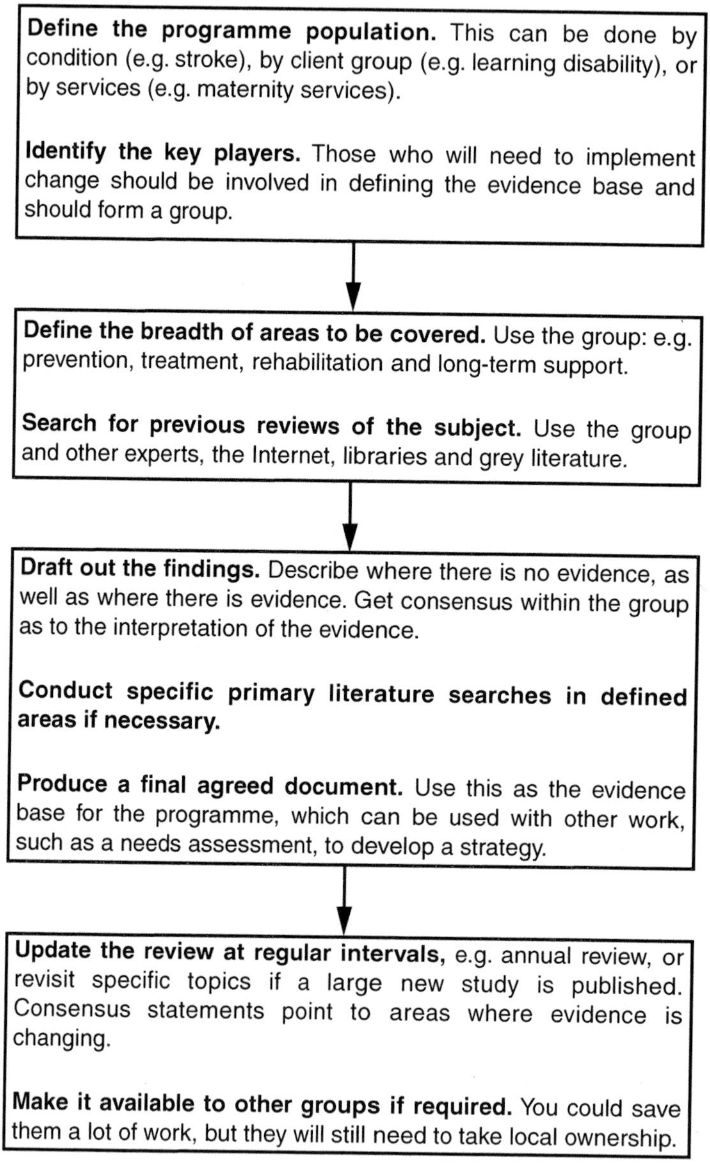

Define the programme population. This can be done by condition (e.g. stroke), by client group (e.g. learning disability), or by services (e.g. maternity services).

Identify the key players. Those who will need to implement change should be involved in defining the evidence base and should form a group.

↓

Define the breadth of areas to be covered. Use the group: e.g. prevention, treatment, rehabilitation and long-term support.

Search for previous reviews of the subject. Use the group and other experts, the Internet, libraries and grey literature.

↓

Draft out the findings. Describe where there is no evidence, as well as where there is evidence. Get consensus within the group as to the interpretation of the evidence.

Conduct specific primary literature searches in defined areas if necessary.

Produce a final agreed document. Use this as the evidence base for the programme, which can be used with other work, such as a needs assessment, to develop a strategy.

↓

Update the review at regular intervals, e.g. annual review, or revisit specific topics if a large new study is published. Consensus statements point to areas where evidence is changing.

Make it available to other groups if required. You could save them a lot of work, but they will still need to take local ownership.

Fig. 12.1. Searching for evidence for a programme of care.

work that could be used to save time. Other priority areas are being developed in a similar way.

This work is part of a research programme into commissioning of services. In time I hope to have more information on the usefulness of this approach (summarised in Fig. 12.1) and whether the 'technical document' leads to more 'evidence-based' commissioning of services.

References

Blais M-J (For the Oxford Regional Getting Research into Practice [GRiP] project) (1994). *Using the Evidence: Northamptonshire Project on Stroke: Literature Review*. Northampton: Northamptonshire Health Authority.

CAST (Chinese Acute Stroke Trial Collaborative Group) (1997). CAST: a randomised placebo controlled trial of aspirin use in 20,000 patients with acute ischaemic stroke. *Lancet* **349**: 1641–1649.

Department of Health (1998). *A First Class Service: Quality in the New NHS*. London: HMSO.

Ebrahim S (1998). Detection, adherence and control of hypertension for the prevention of stroke: a systematic review. *Health* Technology Assessment **2**.

Ferguson A and McCabe C (1997). *The Clinical and Cost-Effectiveness of Computed Tomography in the Management of Transient Ischaemic Attack and Stroke. Guidance Note for Purchasers 97/01*. Sheffield: Trent Institute for Health Services Research.

Gateshead and South Tyneside Health Authority and Newcastle University (1997). Stroke: Technical Document for a Stroke Strategy for Gateshead and South Tyneside. Newcastle: Gateshead and South Tyneside Health Authority and Newcastle University.

International Stroke Trial Collaborative Group (1997). The International Stroke Trial (IST): a randomised trial of aspirin, subcutaneous heparin, both, or neither among 19,435 patients with acute ischaemic stroke. *Lancet* **349**: 1569–1581.

Jackson RT, Sackett DL (1996). Guidelines for managing raised blood pressure. *British Medical Journal* **313**: 64–65. (see also URL http://www.nzgg.org.nz/library/gl_complete/bloodpressure/index.htm).

Macleod CA, Jenner DA, Hildreth J (1993). *Health Gain Investment Programme: Technical Review Document: Coronary Heart Disease and Stroke*. Sheffield: Trent Health.

NHS Centre for Reviews and Dissemination (1994). *Stroke Rehabilitation. Effective Health Care Bulletin Number 2*. York, NHS Centre for Reviews and Dissemination.

Sever P, Beevers G, Bulpitt C *et al* (1993). Management guidelines in essential hypertension: report of the second working party of the British Hypertension Society. *British Medical Journal* **306**: 983–987. (This has recently been updated.)

South and West Regional Development and Evaluation Committee (1994). *The Routine Use of CT Scans in the Management of Stroke*. Southampton: Wessex Institute for Health Research and Development.

Stroke Units Trialist's Collaboration (1997). Collaborative systematic review of the randomised trials of organised inpatient (stroke unit) care after stroke. *British Medical Journal* **314**: 1151–1159.

The Cochrane Collaboration (1999). *The Cochrane Library* [database on disk and CD-ROM]. Issue 2. Oxford: Update Software (Updated quarterly).

US Department of Health and Human Services Public Health Service. Agency for Health Care Policy and Research (1995). Post-stroke rehabilitation: assessment, referral, and patient management. *Clinical Practice Guidelines Quick Reference Guide for Clinicians* **May i–iii**: 1–32 (AHCPR Publication No. 95-0663).

Wade D (1994). Stroke (acute cerebrovascular disease). In: Stevens A and Raftery J (Eds) *Health Care Needs Assessments*, vol. 1. Oxford: Radcliffe Medical Press.

Wardlaw J, Yamaguchi T, del Zoppo G (1998). Thrombolytic therapy versus control in acute ischaemic stroke (Cochrane Review). In: *The Cochrane Library*, Issue 3. Oxford: Update Software.

Warlow CP, Dennis MS, van Gijn J *et al* (1996). Stroke: a practical guide to management. Oxford: Blackwell.

Wolfe C, Rudd T, Beech R (1996). *Stroke Services and Research: A Strategy for the Future*. London: Stroke Association.

▶13

Economics-Based Medical Practice: Using Evidence to Capture and Release Resources

Toby Gosden and Matthew Sutton

'Measuring "costs" along the way ... is only an intermediate step to a comparison of benefits and is of no significance in itself.' (Dowie 1997)

Introduction

Economics-based medical practice involves an extension of evidence-based health (EBH) to take account of the potential impact of delivering services to one group of patients on other patients. Economic evaluations are concerned with estimating the lost benefit, sacrifice or 'opportunity cost' as a result of using scarce resources in one use rather than another. As the above quote reveals and as we emphasise in this chapter, the presentation of the monetary costs of interventions is *not* the primary aim of economic evaluations.

In the past, health economic evidence has not been in the forefront of the minds of advocates of EBH. Indeed, recently published EBH texts rarely mention cost effectiveness or efficiency (Ridsdale 1998). Even if EBH texts do have chapters on health economics, they usually limit the discussion to a critical appraisal of economic evaluations which, whilst important, does not brief the practitioner on how to interpret the results and use the data.

The resources available to the NHS are constrained, and any increases in the total NHS budget require a commensurate decrease in expenditure elsewhere within the public purse. As the demand for health care continues to rise, there is an urgency to make the best use of the limited resources. Increasingly, cash-limited budgets are being devolved closer to practice level to encourage more efficient use of resources. The 1998 Primary Care (NHS) Act provided the flexibility to change existing contractual arrangements to increase the responsiveness of primary care to local needs and circumstances. Primary Care Act pilot sites (PCAPS) can choose either to continue to provide the same level of service that they did prior to PCAPS (termed personal medical services (PMS)) or they can increase the level of service (PMS+). Thus, in order to reshape, realign and/or increase existing services to meet local needs, pilot sites are faced with a number of decisions which inevitably involve capturing and releasing resources. More recently, the emergence of primary care groups may bring an increased emphasis on cash-limited budgets to deliver the clinical governance agenda. Therefore, increasingly practitioners will be providing care within budgets. Health economics provides a framework within which to evaluate the changes and trade-offs that may be made.

There are a number of reasons why health economics, and indeed EBH, may be particularly difficult to practice in primary rather than secondary care.

- Many of the patients seen in primary care are the 'worried well' and many of the problems presented are difficult to define and therefore deciding which intervention (apart from medication) is needed is not straightforward.

- Even if interventions were easily identifiable, there is a limited amount of economic information on primary care treatments.

- Predicting the level of patient demand is particularly difficult even with good quality epidemiology data.

- Those practising in primary care, such as nurses and GPs, may not have the time proactively to prioritise services.

- A GP's performance is based on the number of patients in his/her care and the volume of services provided and not the cost-effective use of resources. In order to cover practice expenses, GPs must earn certain levels of income; thus, the inflexibility of the general medical services (GMS) remuneration framework discourages any evidence-based move away from income-earning activities.

Various publications describe the purpose of and prescribe a methodology for economic evaluation of health-care interventions (Drummond and Jefferson 1996, Weinstein et al 1996, Drummond et al 1997, Gold et al 1996). The main types of economic analysis that can be found in the literature include:

- cost minimisation;

- cost effectiveness;

- cost consequence;

- cost utility;

- cost benefit.

The main difference between these different types is the way in which the consequences are measured (Box 13.1).

While there are many complexities and much controversy over application, the principles of economic evaluation are relatively straightforward. In this chapter we describe these basic principles and offer a guide to the aspects of economic evidence which set it apart from the other types of evidence used in EBH.

To this end we describe when:

- *Determining which treatment is more cost effective:*
  - a simple guide to the characteristics of economic evaluations and the information which EBH practitioners need to glean from them;
  - some important considerations interpreting the results of economic evaluations and assessing the appropriateness of published results for the local setting.

Box 13.1. Types of economic evaluation

A *cost-minimisation design* compares two alternative treatments for which their respective effectiveness is known to be equal, so that the evaluation question is to determine which entails the minimum cost.

The outcomes in a *cost-effectiveness analysis (CEA)* are natural and physical units of health, such as blood pressure or cholesterol levels.

A *cost-consequence analysis* evaluates the consequences, e.g. number of referrals or prescriptions, of alternative treatments or interventions for their respective costs.

A *cost-utility analysis (CUA)* takes into account the utilities that patients attach to certain health states. A typical CUA would calculate a cost per QALY, which acknowledges reductions in morbidity (quality) and mortality (quantity) associated with a treatment.

A *cost-benefit analysis (CBA)* attempts to place a monetary value on the benefits of treatment and incorporates any savings from releasing resources from competing alternatives. For example, by eliciting how much patients would hypothetically be willing to pay to see a consultant in their local surgery rather than travel to the hospital, an average 'valuation' of the benefit of outreach clinics can be estimated. The ratio of this benefit and the cost of providing the specialist outreach clinic are compared to the benefits and costs of travelling to hospital outpatient clinics.

⫸ *Utilising economic data to inform service development:*
— a three-step approach to evidence-based decision making which will allow practitioners to incorporate economic considerations into their practice.

We believe practitioners need to know how to *interpret* economic evaluations for their local setting rather than needing to understand the details of costing methodology and following its recommendations to the letter.

What is different about economic evaluations?

Economic evaluations extend the remit of health-care evaluations. They take account of the resources used in producing health-care interventions as well as measuring outcomes (Dowie 1997). Those resources might include nurse time, prescribed drugs, patient time, room space, GP time, etc. As such, economic studies look at the relationship between inputs and outputs in the production of health care. In studying such relationships, health economists are faced with controversial issues involving which inputs and outputs to consider and how these inputs and outputs can be measured and valued.

Few of these controversies have been settled in health economics. The rationale for economic evaluations favours a societal perspective for the analysis (Johannesson 1994). This involves taking account of all the consequences of an intervention, including patient time and travel costs, as well as the impact on other parts of the health service. This perspective has led economists into contention with the advocates of EBH (Sackett *et al* 1996, Maynard 1996). While these issues are clearly important, there are nevertheless simple but important features of economic evaluation which are less contentious. It is these features of economic evaluation which we highlight in this chapter.

One of the primary distinguishing features of economic evaluation is its objective to make all health-care interventions comparable. This is because most health-care resources are funded from the public purse and any mix of interventions which is chosen implies that certain types of activity have been prioritised (Williams 1994). Therefore, albeit that these decisions are not made centrally or perhaps even consciously, implicit decisions are being made. Economic evaluation aims to obtain maximum health benefits from the health-care budget by prioritising the most valuable activities. Thus, a common way of measuring the benefits from all interventions is required to make these comparisons explicit. For many comparisons this may seem on the face of it like comparing apples and oranges. Nevertheless, much of the endeavour of health economists has been dedicated to this task and we discuss these developments in more detail in the next section.

An equally important component of economic evaluation is comparison of the resource consequences of the alternative decisions. This is often misinterpreted as a desire to reduce the amount of resources consumed by the health-care system. In fact, it is motivated by a desire to maximise the benefits of health care for the population as a whole. Pursuit of this goal requires careful interpretation of the results of economic evaluations and we dedicate most of our attention later in this chapter to this feature of economic evaluation.

Outputs: The measurement of multiple types of health benefits

Because the over-arching aim of economic evaluations is to compare *all* health-care interventions regardless of the setting, condition or target population, much of the endeavour has been to develop a health benefit measure with three important properties:

> It is cardinal in the sense that twice the level of that benefit measure has twice the value.

> It reflects societal preferences so that one unit of health benefit is of equal value to society whether it is 'produced' by, for example, replacing someone's hip or counselling them for depression.

> It incorporates all aspects of the outcomes from health-care interventions which are valued by society.

Perhaps the most debated health-benefit measure offered by health economists is the quality-adjusted life-year (QALY) (Williams 1985). The QALY aims to capture health benefits by reflecting changes in both the quantity (length) and quality of life. Years of life are weighted by the quality of those years using a 'score' between 0 and 1. This score may be obtained using the Euroqol five-item (EQ-5D) questionnaire for which public valuations have been obtained (Kind *et al* 1998). The QALY has many detractors and, although it has been designed to satisfy the first two criteria in the above list, the simplicity of the EQ-5D questionnaire means that it cannot capture all the pertinent aspects of health benefit in every setting. For this reason, some health economists have suggested its use only within the same setting or disease group (Donaldson *et al* 1988). For the purposes of this chapter, however, it is sufficient to note only that economics-based medical practice does not necessarily require acceptance of QALYs (weighted using EQ-5D scores) as an outcome measure. For the comparison of some interventions, other outcome measures may fit the three properties listed above more satisfactorily.

Inputs: Reflecting differences in resource requirements

The objective of economic evaluation can be expressed in two ways (Birch and Gafni 1992):

▶ minimising the resources used to achieve a certain level of benefit; or

▶ maximising benefits within available resources.

The standard design of clinical trials lends itself to the first way of expressing the rationale for economic evaluation (Sutton 1997). A typical example in a secondary-care setting would be a comparison of day-case with inpatient care (Russell *et al* 1977). Such an analysis is called a *cost-minimisation analysis* (Box 13.1) and its preponderance in the literature may explain why economic evaluations are perceived to be about 'cost cutting' rather than benefit maximisation (Sutton 1997).

The second formulation of the objective of economic evaluation is likely to be more appropriate for practitioners (Craig and Sutton 1998). There are examples of cost-constrained evaluations in the literature. Torgerson and Gosden (1997), for example, considered how changing the age composition of women screened for breast cancer could increase the total benefits from the National Breast Screening service. The maximisation of health outcomes within constrained resources is the problem which faces practitioners every day. As we shall see, the fact that resources are constrained has important implications for whether what appear to be 'cost effective' changes in practice are feasible.

There are two main issues when considering the resource requirements of alternative interventions:

▶ ensuring that efficient use of inputs results in the maximisation of benefits;

▶ comparing interventions which utilise multiple inputs.

Initially we explain how efficient use of inputs can maximise the health benefits to the population by considering interventions which use only a single input.

Single input

A basic form of economic evaluation which fits most easily alongside a clinical trial is a *cost-minimisation analysis*. This analysis is only applicable when the outcomes for each participating patient from two alternative treatments are as near identical as possible. If this criterion is satisfied then the alternatives can be compared relatively simply on the basis of the level of resources which each requires. If the alternatives consist of only one major resource input, then the comparison is simple; the less resource-intensive option is preferred.

It is important to note, however, why this is the case. It is assumed, for example, that the provider faces limited availability of that resource and a choice of potentially beneficial uses for that resource. It is only then that *releasing* resources by adopting the less resource-intensive option will allow benefits to be reaped from the alternative uses of those resources. Chapter 14 considers such an example of releasing resources when nurse time is freed up by moving from a comprehensive screening strategy for coronary heart disease to a minimal screening strategy. It is emphasised that it is the potential benefits from alternative uses of those resources which are crucial in determining whether the least resource-intensive intervention is preferable. The underlying rationale in favour of cost-minimising interventions is that by treating one group of patients more efficiently, resources are released to offer health benefits to *other* patients.

A relatively simple comparison illustrates the concept of *opportunity cost*. Two interventions are being compared which achieve the same level of health benefit. One of the alternatives requires more resources and therefore denies some alternative use of those resources. The opportunity costs of the more resource-intensive option are higher because more health benefits are sacrificed. In general, the opportunity costs of an intervention are measured by the potential benefits which are lost through that use of resources and should represent the *best possible* alternative use of those resources.

A *cost-effectiveness analysis* is undertaken when there is evidence that the amount of health benefit received by each participating patient is significantly different between the two alternative interventions. In this case the results of the economic evaluation are traditionally summarised in terms of a ratio between the costs of each intervention and the benefits which it produces (the cost-effectiveness ratio). Cost-effectiveness analyses are most controversial when the more resource-intensive intervention is also the one which produces the most benefit per individual treated. Let us assume once again that only one input is required. If the amount of that resource is constrained then, although more benefit will be produced *in total* by implementing the more resource-intensive option, fewer people can be treated. More benefits are spread over fewer people which implies an important equity judgement and that some form of prioritisation process will be required (Sutton 1997).

It may seem as though these sensitivities can be avoided by increasing the amount of resources used for this population. However, where are these additional resources to be *captured* from? It may be that additional funding can be obtained from the Health Authority in which case the opportunity costs fall on an unidentified group of potential patients. Failing this, however, the opportunity costs will be borne by other patients within the practice.

The decision about whether to implement the more resource-intensive option therefore becomes controversial. It either requires reducing the number of patients offered the treatment or it means capturing resources from some other health-care intervention. The decision is now between the new intervention and a combination of the original intervention *plus* additional resources from a third intervention currently in practice. It is this decision which our three-step procedure attempts to address (see below). However, before describing this procedure, we discuss additional considerations in comparing interventions which use multiple inputs.

Multiple inputs

The method of comparing alternative interventions becomes more complex if they involve more than one input. Unless one option uses more of *all* inputs, it will be necessary to compare the 'value' of the inputs used. This should be done on the basis of the opportunity costs of the different resources.

In published studies resource usage tends to be summarised by attaching monetary values to all inputs. Such an approach arises out of the desire to reflect a societal perspective in the evaluation and to obtain a generalisable set of findings. It reflects an economic view that in general the market price of inputs will reflect their value so that monetary valuations of resources will on average reflect their opportunity cost.

It is worth considering, however, what factors will influence the opportunity costs of resources. Opportunity costs reflect other options available for those resources and will therefore be context specific. The value of practice nurse time, for example, will depend on the total amount of nurse time available to the practice, the demand for nurse services and their expertise and efficiency. In some areas nurse time may be particularly valuable and interventions which produce the same level of outcome but use other resources which are relatively slack would be a better way of treating patients.

Difficulties with recruitment and retention of GPs in some areas (Taylor and Leese 1997) will also influence the relative opportunity costs of different types of staff. Changes in service delivery which release GP time will be more cost-effective in areas with relative under-provision of GPs than in those which have a relatively high number of GPs. This is because GP resources are relatively more scarce and therefore their deployment has a higher opportunity cost. Use of wage costs as indicators of the value of GP time *vis-à-vis* other staff will not reflect this.

Cost figures presented in published studies may give broad conclusions but cannot reflect local conditions. Bryan and Brown (1998) suggest that local variations in:

▶ financial costs of resources;

▶ population epidemiology;

▶ 'current practice' intervention used to evaluate the new intervention;

will all affect the robustness of findings from economic evaluations to local decision-making settings. In addition, the opportunity costs of different resources will depend on local context. We recommend that published studies are used only to obtain estimates of the amount of resources required for different interventions and their effectiveness.

A three-step approach to incorporating economics into practice

In describing the basic principles of economic evaluation we have emphasised the complex considerations which arise when incorporating economic considerations into practice. Economic evaluation simplifies this complex decision through the use of the cost-effectiveness ratio. However, given the reservations outlined above about the appropriateness of estimating opportunity costs using market valuation, we suggest that this process is done more systematically in the local context. We now outline a three-step procedure which may guide practitioners through economics-based medical practice (Box 13.2).

Box 13.2.   Three-step procedure for an economic decision-making process

Step 1: Estimate the types and amounts of resources which will need to be captured for the new intervention.

Step 2: Identify where those resources can be *released* from.

Step 3: Estimate what the overall change in health benefits will be for the population as a whole.

Step 1

The first stage in assessing whether a new intervention should be adopted is to assess the type and volume of resources that will be required. Estimates of the resources required can be obtained from the published literature. However, these estimates may need to be amended to reflect local conditions (Bryan and Brown 1998). Estimates of the amounts of each type of resource should increasingly become available as recommendations now suggest that these should be reported in published papers (Walker *et al* 1997, Briggs and Sculpher 1995, Weinstein *et al* 1996).

Step 2

The second stage of an economic decision-making process is to identify where the required resources can be released from. One technique which may be useful in this process is programme budgeting and marginal analysis (PBMA). Programme budgeting is a method for investigating how resources are currently used within a service and marginal analysis considers what expansions and contractions of services are feasible (Donaldson *et al* 1995). The exercise may be best undertaken by a small group of people from within the practice but with different perspectives on current activity.

Programme budgeting

The programme budgeting stage involves a mapping of the current mix of resources onto different types of activity, such as chronic disease clinics, immunisations, etc. This stage can be time consuming and there may be some difficulty in defining the 'blocks' of activity onto which resources are to be mapped. Nevertheless, in many applications the programme budgeting stage has been reported to be useful in highlighting areas where there is a substantial mismatch between stated priorities and actual resource use (Donaldson *et al* 1995).

Marginal analysis

A misalignment between objectives and resource use is one way of generating options for change in the marginal analysis stage of the exercise. Other options include literature reviews, local opinions on current inefficiencies within the service and national policy documents, such as recent guidance on appropriate responses to cold and flu symptoms. The ultimate aim of the exercise is to identify which activities could be contracted to provide sufficient resources for the new intervention but involving the smallest loss of benefits to the practice population. It is important to consider what impact the new intervention will have on other activities within the practice and to consider the scale of the changes that are feasible. It may be, for example, that terminating one of the clinics will release more resources than is required or that this will render some other activity non-viable.

Step 3

The final stage in the process involves evaluating whether switching resources to the new intervention will result in a net increase in health benefits for the practice population. In some cases it may be that a way of releasing resources with no loss of benefit has been identified in Step 2 so that any alternative use of those released resources will be beneficial. In other cases, however, some parts of the practice population may lose out because of the service change and it is essential that the benefits from the new intervention outweigh the benefits lost by stopping the former activity.

Conclusion

The incorporation of economics into EBH can involve three distinct considerations:

▶ what perspective will be taken?

▶ how are outcomes to be measured?

▶ what are the alternative uses of the resources captured by a new intervention?

Published economic evaluations often take a societal perspective which means including patient costs and the consequences for other parts of the health service. Decision making within general practice may not reflect these societal considerations. Measurement of health status using the Euroqol quality-of-life instrument and outcomes using QALYs has become closely associated with economic evaluation. These tools have been designed with economic evaluation in mind and have particular properties which are useful for economic evaluation. However, they may not receive widespread support as appropriate measures of outcome for general practice. Despite these challenges there is still a role for economics in EBH through its emphasis on considering alternative uses of constrained resources. Economic evaluations can offer evidence for changes in activity in the following cases:

▶ If the interventions use only one important input and the health benefits are the same for each patient (cost-minimisation analysis), then implementing the least resource-intensive option releases resources for other uses which will provide benefits to other patients.

▶ If the interventions use a mix of resources, then attention needs to be paid to what resources will be released and what resources will be captured as a result of the proposed policy change.

We have suggested that PBMA can be used to identify potential areas for investment or disinvestment. Chapter 14 illustrates our approach using a paper by Field *et al* (1995).

In this chapter we have shown that the principles of economic evaluation can be demonstrated within a context, i.e. general practice, which involves no change in the types or levels of resources used. The advantage of this focus is that it does not involve the complexities introduced by changes in the mix of inputs or shifting resources across traditional budgetary boundaries (e.g. primary/secondary interface; pharmacy/general practice).

References

Birch S, Gafni A (1992). Cost effectiveness/utility analyses. Do current decision rules lead us to where we want to be? *Journal of Health Economics* **11**: 279–296.

Briggs A, Sculpher M (1995). Sensitivity analysis in economic evaluation: a review of published studies. *Health Economics* **4**: 355–372.

Bryan S, Brown J (1998). Extrapolation of cost effectiveness information to local settings. *Journal of Health Services Research and Policy* **3**: 108–112.

Craig N, Sutton M (1998). Opportunity costs on trial: new options for encouraging implementation of results from economic evaluations. In: Haines A and Donald A (Eds) *Getting Research Findings into Practice*. London: BMJ Publishing, pp 130–148.

Donaldson C, Atkinson J, Bond J (1988). Should QALYs be programme-specific? *Journal of Health Economics* **7**: 239–257.

Donaldson C, Walker A, Craig N (1995). *Programme Budgeting and Marginal Analysis: A Handbook for Applying Economics in Health Care Purchasing*. Glasgow: Scottish Needs Assessment Programme.

Dowie J (1997). Clinical trials and economic evaluations? No there are only evaluations. *Health Economics* **6**: 87–89.

Drummond M, Jefferson T (1996). Guidelines for authors and peer reviewers of economic submissions to the *BMJ. British Medical Journal* **313**: 275–283.

Drummond M, O'Brien B, Stoddart G, et al (1997). *Methods for the Economic Evaluation of Health Care Programmes*. Oxford: Oxford Medical Publications.

Field K, Thorogood M, Silagy C, et al (1995). Strategies for reducing coronary risk factors in primary care: which is most cost effective? *British Medical Journal* **310**: 1109–1112.

Gold M, Siegel J, Russell L, et al (1996). *Cost Effectiveness in Health And Medicine*. New York: Oxford University Press.

Johannesson M (1994). The concept of cost in the economic evaluation of health care. *International Journal of Technology Assessment in Health Care* **10**: 675–682.

Kind P, Dolan P, Gudex C, *et al* (1998). Variations in population health status: Results from a United Kingdom national questionnaire survey. *British Medical Journal* **316**: 736–740.

Maynard A (1996). Letter to the Editor. *British Medical Journal* **313**: 170.

Ridsdale L (Ed) (1998). *Evidence-Based Practice in Primary Care*. Edinburgh: Churchill Livingstone.

Russell I, Devlin H, Fell M, *et al* (1977). Day-case surgery for hernias and haemorrhoids: a clinical, social and economic evaluation. *Lancet* 8016: 844–847.

Sackett D, Gray J, Haynes R, *et al* (1996). Author's reply. *British Medical Journal* **313**: 170–171.

Sutton M (1997). Personal paper: how to get the best health outcome from a given amount of money. *British Medical Journal* **315**: 47–49.

Taylor D, Leese B (1997). General practitioner turnover and migration in England 1990–1994. *British Journal of General Practice* **48**: 1070–1072.

Torgerson D, Gosden T (1997). The National Breast Screening Service: is it economically efficient? *Quarterly Journal of Medicine* **90**: 423–425.

Walker A, Major K, Young D, *et al* (1997). *Economic Costs in the NHS: A Useful Insight or Just Bad Accountancy?* Paper presented to the Health Economists' Study Group, Liverpool.

Weinstein M, Siegel J, Gold M, *et al* (1996). Recommendations of the panel on cost effectiveness in health and medicine. *Journal of the American Medical Association* **276**: 1253–1258.

Williams A (1985). Economics of coronary artery bypass grafting. *British Medical Journal* **291**: 326–329.

Williams A (1994). Economics, society and health care ethics. In: Gillon R (Ed) *Principles of Health Care Ethics*. Chichester: Wiley, pp 829–842.

▶ 14

Using Evidence from Economic Studies to Inform Service Development in General Medical Practice

Toby Gosden

Introduction

Chapter 13 outlined both why and how information from economic evaluations might be incorporated into decision making within an environment of constrained resources. It was also argued that when using economic data from *cost-minimisation analyses*, choosing which intervention costs least is relatively straightforward. However, care is required when translating the findings of *cost-effectiveness analyses* to practice level as the costs and benefits of alternative interventions can be different.

In this chapter, a published cost-effectiveness analysis of health check strategies is used to illustrate one approach to *utilising* economic evidence to *inform* service development at practice level. I offer the practitioner a three-step procedure to guide service development within their practice (see Box 13.1). This framework can be informed by both economic evaluation evidence and by local patient views and expert opinion on resource and effectiveness issues.

The service development: Practice coronary heart disease screening strategy

To illustrate this approach a hypothetical practice is considered which is part of a primary care group (PCG). The PCG has allocated each practice a practice-based cash-limited budget. The practice can alter service provision to address local needs more effectively as long as it stays within budget.

Following an audit of health checks, the practice decides that it might not be making best use of its resources. The GPs and practice nurses had been providing full health checks (full history taking and physical examination) to every new patient and to those patients who had not visited the practice in the last 3 years. The practice believes that this level of service provision is not reaching those at greatest risk of coronary heart disease (CHD) and that more resources than necessary are being used. However, the dilemma is that all the nurses' and GPs' time is currently occupied providing the current level of care. If the practice wants to introduce a new screening strategy it must reduce the level of a particular activity which it already undertakes or replace a service altogether in order to release the necessary resources.

The following discussion will show how the three-step procedure described in Chapter 13 can be used to guide the introduction of this new service.

Step 1: Estimating resources needed

The search

The first step is to collate any relevant published information on resources needed for various types of health checks in general practice. The following electronic bibliographic databases are most likely to contain economic evaluations: MEDLINE, BIDS-EMBASE, BIDS-ISI and the NHS Economic Evaluation database (accessed via the NHS Centre for Reviews and Dissemination web site). The following major medical subject headings should identify relevant studies:

▶ coronary-disease-prevention-and-control;

▶ AND family-practice-economics;

▶ AND mass-screening-economics.

Hand searching recent editions of journals which constitute the best source of economic evaluations will also identify the latest evidence:

▶ *Health Economics*;

▶ *Journal of Health Economics*;

▶ *Health Policy*;

▶ *Journal of Health Services Research and Policy*;

▶ *British Medical Journal*;

▶ *British Journal of General Practice*;

▶ *Public Health Medicine*.

Using this search strategy a cost-effectiveness analysis (CEA) by Field *et al* (1995) is identified which estimates the cost per life year saved for different health-check strategies aimed at reducing coronary risk factors.

Which data to utilise?

For simplicity, I assume that Field *et al* (1995) is the only economic analysis available which examines the cost-effectiveness of CHD screening strategies (although in reality there are a number of studies). The study shows that the most cost-effective strategy for reducing coronary risk factors in men is minimal screening of blood pressure plus taking a personal history of vascular disease ('strategy 1'). Therefore, the practice decides to assess the local resource requirements and benefits of implementing this particular strategy.

Attaching monetary value to a resource is important in determining the relative cost-effectiveness of a treatment. However, I suggest that once an efficient treatment has been identified and is to be introduced, the practitioner would find published estimates of *resource use* more useful than *cost* estimates. As argued in Chapter 13, this is because the latter may not adequately estimate local cost benefits (opportunity costs) or may not use local prices or salary scales. For example, Field *et al*'s (1995) estimated cost per (not discounted) life year gained (£730 for men) for a minimal screening strategy may not accurately represent the opportunity costs to the practice of the resources involved in the screening. In addition, a cost-effectiveness ratio does not provide information on the types and amounts of resource a practice might need, nor the scale of the implementation. Therefore, because I am extracting resource data, I do not adopt the approach that is commonly taken of critically appraising the costing methodology adopted in an economic evaluation using published criteria (Mason and Drummond 1995, Drummond and Jefferson 1996). Instead I will use this paper to:

▶ extract information on the type and amount of resources needed;

▶ make sure all the relevant resources are included and make assumptions about resource use which was not reported or was omitted;

▶ determine whether the type and amount of resources needed are relevant to the practice setting;

▶ estimate total practice resources needed to provide the service to the specified target population.

Extracting information on resource use from study data

Table 14.1 shows information extracted from Field *et al* (1995) (where available) on the resources required per patient for the minimal screening strategy. The initial screening involves taking blood pressure and asking about personal history. For those patients who have a systolic blood pressure >140 mmHg and history of ischaemic heart disease, stroke or transient ischaemic attack, further screening is carried out. This involves screening for smoking, height, weight, diet, family history and cholesterol. The patient is then given the appropriate treatment. Table 14.1 shows the time required to collect information in this second screening phase.

Making sure all the relevant resource information is available

Information on all relevant treatment resources must be collected. These include not only the resources needed for the initial screening outlined above, but also those required to treat the at-risk group, such as drugs (to reduce cholesterol or blood pressure) and/or lifestyle advice. Table 14.1 shows information extracted from Field *et al* (1995) on the amount of resources required to reduce cholesterol levels and to provide lifestyle advice.

Omitted resources: Assumptions made by the practice
Where resources are identified in the study but the amounts required by the intervention are not reported, I need to make assumptions which are relevant to the

Table 14.1. Information extracted from Field *et al* (1995) on resource use for minimal CHD screening ('strategy 1') in men.

Intervention	Population group	Resources required per patient
Initial screening: measure blood pressure, ask about personal history	All men	*[Time to measure blood pressure and ask about personal history not reported]*
Additional screening: smoking, height, weight, diet family history, cholesterol	Systolic blood pressure >140 mmHg, history of ischaemic heart disease, stroke or transient ischaemic attack	16 min nurse grade G time Cholesterol tests
Treatment:		
Drugs to treat raised blood pressure	Systolic blood pressure >140 mmHg	*[Drugs to treat raised blood pressure not reported]*
Lifestyle advice	Cholesterol >8.5 mmol/l	4 × 15 min sessions with nurse with 40 min nurse organisation time
Lipid-lowering drugs	High cholesterol concentration which would not drop below 8.5 mmol/l*	Lipid-lowering drug (simvastatin) involving 9 min of GP time per year

Assumption:
* Estimated in Field *et al* (1995) as 80% of those with cholesterol levels >8.5 mmol/l.

local circumstances of the hypothetical practice. Field *et al* (1995) do not report the time it takes to conduct the minimum screening strategy so the practice might want to use its own estimate of resources needed. Table 14.2 shows that the practice has estimated that measuring blood pressure takes 3 min and asking about personal history takes 5 min.

Field *et al* (1995) also do not report resources used to treat raised blood pressure because these are regarded as a fixed cost common to each of the 5 screening strategies in the paper. However, this means that no information on *absolute* amounts of resources needed to *set up* the screening strategy is provided. The practice must therefore make its own estimation of the amount and type of resources needed to treat raised blood pressure. The practice assumes that to treat raised blood pressure either ACE inhibitors or ß-blockers are used (see Table 14.2).

Omitted resources: Study perspectives
The perspective adopted by those who undertake an economic evaluation is important as it determines which resources are estimated and which are excluded. The viewpoint taken by Field *et al* (1995) appears to be that of a health-care purchaser, so I need to be satisfied that other important resources have not been omitted. A study which takes a societal perspective may include not only NHS resources but also any important and significant use of patients' resources. For example, if I am proposing significantly to increase the frequency of health checks, I must be mindful of the inevitable increase in travel time and costs incurred by patients. To ignore these resources would be to increase the burden on patients, which may impact on attendance rates, reducing the efficiency of the screening programme if those at greatest risk do not attend (Torgerson and Donaldson 1994).

A study may be limited in the length of the follow-up period over which it can estimate cost outcomes. Therefore, I need to be sure that I extract information on or make appropriate assumptions about any resources which might be used or released in the future. For example, I might collect information on treatment resource requirements such as repeat prescriptions for lipid-lowering drugs.

Relevance of study-based resource estimates
I need to assure myself that the amount of resources reported in Field *et al* (1995) is the same as that needed by the practice. The randomised controlled trial reported by Field *et al* (1995) was carried out in five urban general practices in Bedfordshire. I must therefore ascertain that the practices in the trial were similar to the practice which intends to introduce the screening strategy in terms of characteristics of the practice population and available practice resources. The minimal screening strategy requires a qualified grade G nurse to undertake the initial screening which involves measuring blood pressure and taking a personal history. The hypothetical practice employs a grade G nurse, so the type of resources quoted in the study are relevant to this practice setting.

I must also consider other differences between the practice and those which participated in the trial. For example, nurses in the trial may have taken more time to provide lifestyle advice compared with nurses in the practice which intends to

Table 14.2. Estimates of resources required for minimal screening ('strategy 1') for men.

Patient group	Size of patient group	Practice assumptions for resources required but not reported by Field *et al* (1995)	Total resource requirements
Men to be offered minimal screening	750	8 min of nurse grade G time**	100 hours of nurse time
Treatment to at-risk group (lifestyle advice; lipid-lowering drugs; drugs to treat raised blood pressure)	75*	[As in Table 14.1] β-Blockers or ACE inhibitors† [As in Table 14.1]	20 hours of nurse time 75 courses of either ACE inhibitors or β-blockers
Those with cholesterol >8.5 mmol/l	50	[As in Table 14.1]	75 cholesterol tests 8.33 hours of nurse time
Those with high cholesterol concentration whose levels would not drop below 8.5 mmol/l	40**	[As in Table 14.1]	40 courses of lipid-lowering drugs involving 6 hours of GP time

Assumptions:

* 10% of the practice population are assumed to have a systolic blood pressure >140 mmHg.

** The practice assumed that measuring blood pressure takes 3 min and asking about personal history takes 5 min.

† This is an assumption made by the practice about drugs to treat raised blood pressure.

introduce the screening strategy. I could also check that the resource information I extract from the study is not overestimated because of the demands of the research protocol. For example, staff time may be overestimated because the study protocol requires the nurse to spend 30 s per consultation completing a particular data collection instrument. In the study, information on patients' diet is obtained by questionnaire, which may not be the way that the nurse in the hypothetical practice collects dietary information. Whether it takes a longer or shorter time (assuming the same information is collected and it is only the method that differs from the trial's) I must adjust resource requirements appropriately or adopt the method used in the trial practices.

Scale of resource requirements and local clinical risk factors

To keep this example simple, I assume that no additional resources need to be included in the practice's analysis besides those identified in Field *et al* (1995). Also, I assume screening more patients increases resource requirements (e.g. nurse and GP time) proportionately, i.e. there are no economies of scale.

I now have an estimate of what resources are required per patient but I am unsure of the scale of the screening programme I need to implement. For this I need information on the levels of CHD risk factors amongst men in the practice population. If the practice does not have access to this information, then it could use either expert medical opinion or published national or regional estimates of the levels of risk, including those found in the trial. In Table 14.2, hypothetical figures are used as no risk estimates are quoted for men in Field *et al* (1995).

Table 14.2 sets out the resources needed to screen the men aged between 34 and 65 years in the practice population. It shows that approximately 203 hours of nursing time, 6 hours of GP time, 75 cholesterol tests, 75 courses of ACE inhibitors or ß-blockers and 40 courses of lipid-lowering drugs are required as a minimum to screen this particular male population.

Step 2: Identifying where the required resources might be released

In this step the objective is to identify where I might find the resources needed for the new screening strategy. One possible source is the health authority which may be able to reimburse more nursing staff hours or provide additional development monies. These additional resources would have an opportunity cost in terms of the benefit sacrificed as a result of not using this money to fund other treatment. Since the practice has a budget with the PCG based on historical activity, no additional resources are available. Therefore, the only option for the practice is to disinvest in, or replace, current services which deliver less health benefit than would the minimal screening strategy for the same level of resource use.

If the minimal screening strategy only required nursing staff, it would be relatively straightforward to contract or replace other services currently provided by nurses. However, it becomes more complex when a number of resources from a number of different uses need to be released, each with different opportunity costs. In this situation, monetary value acts as a medium of exchange in that it can be used to identify the amount of one resource that can be obtained for another. For example, savings on prescribing and referrals budgets may be used to fund additional nursing time and medication. However, it would be more complex to realise the monetary value of half an hour of GP time. While attaching monetary value to the resources needed can help establish cost-effectiveness in comparison with an alternative service, it does not indicate from where resources might be released.

In this example, I make the assumption that it would not be cost-effective to operate two health-check screening strategies side-by-side. Thus, the practice's previous comprehensive screening policy for male patients is an obvious activity from which resources might be released. I am particularly fortunate in that Field *et al* (1995) compare the minimal screening strategy with a comprehensive health check ('strategy 5'). If I am satisfied that 'strategy 5' is similar or identical to the screening currently carried out by the practice, then I can utilise the appropriate resource data in the same way as in step 1. If the practice's current service is not sufficiently similar to 'strategy 5', then estimates of resource have to be made.

Estimating resources to be released

Table 14.3 shows the available information extracted from Field *et al* (1995) on resources required to provide comprehensive screening to an equivalent male population. Again, because Field *et al* (1995) do not report the time needed to measure blood pressure plus take a personal history or the drugs for reducing blood pressure, the practice's assumptions are stated in Table 14.4. Since Field *et al* (1995) do not report percentages of those with risk criteria, in Table 14.4 I estimate resources released based on assumptions I have already made about the level of CHD risk in the practice population. Whilst these may not be regarded as realistic, they do serve to illustrate the method of applying such evidence in this decision-making context.

Now that I have estimated the resources that could be released, I need to establish whether further resources are required. Table 14.5 shows that by replacing existing comprehensive health checks with minimal screening for all men, not only would there be enough resources to implement the new health checks, but additional resources would also be freed. Approximately 264 hours of nurse time and 6 hours of GP time would be released over time as a result of the service change. There would also be 75 fewer cholesterol tests, 75 fewer ACE inhibitor or ß-blocker prescriptions and 40 fewer courses of lipid-lowering drugs used as a result of the change.

Step 3: Estimating net benefits

Once I have identified which activities might be contracted or altogether substituted for another service in order to release resources, I need to estimate the net benefits that arise from this change. In other words, I need to know that the benefits from minimal screening ('strategy 1') are greater than those that could be achieved from an alternative use of the same resources, such as comprehensive screening ('strategy 5').

Table 14.3. Information extracted from Field et al (1995) on resource use for comprehensive CHD screening ('strategy 5').

Intervention	Population group	Resources required per patient
Initial screening: measure blood pressure; ask about personal history; ask about smoking; measure weight and height; dietary assessment; family history; measure blood cholesterol	All men	*[Time to measure blood pressure and ask about personal history not reported]* 16 min of nurse grade G time Cholesterol tests
Treatment:		
Drugs to treat raised blood pressure	Systolic blood pressure >140 mmHg; history of ischaemic heart disease, stroke or transient ischaemic attack; smokers	*[Drugs to treat raised blood pressure not reported]*
Lifestyle advice		4 × 15 min sessions with nurse with 40 min of nurse organisation time
Lipid lowering drugs*	Body mass index >28; fat intake >110 g per day; first-degree relative with ischaemic heart disease, stroke, or transient ischaemic attack before 60 years; total cholesterol >7.5 mmol/l.	Lipid-lowering drug (simvastatin) involving 9 min of GP time per year

Note:
* 80% of those with cholesterol levels >8.5 mmol/l are given lipid-lowering drugs.

Table 14.4. Estimates of resources released by contracting comprehensive screening ('strategy 5') for men.

Patient group	Size of patient group	Practice assumptions for resources required but not reported by Field et al (1995)	Total resource requirements
Men currently being offered comprehensive health checks	750	[As in Table 14.3] + 8 min of nurse grade G time**	300 hours of nurse time
At-risk group	150*	β-Blockers or ACE inhibitors†	150 cholesterol tests 150 courses of ACE inhibitors or β-blockers
Those with cholesterol >8.5 mmol/l	100	[As in Table 14.3]	166.67 hours of nurse time
Those with high cholesterol concentration whose levels would not drop below 8.5 mmol/l	80	[As in Table 14.3]	80 courses of lipid-lowering drugs 12 hours of GP time

Assumptions:

* The at-risk group, estimated at 20% of the male practice sub-population, is larger than that under 'strategy 1' since there are more risk factors.
** The practice assumed that measuring blood pressure takes 3 min and asking about personal history takes 5 min.
† This is an assumption made by the practice about drugs to treat raised blood pressure.

Table 14.5. Estimates of resources freed-up by substituting 'strategy 5' for 'strategy 1'.

	Resources needed for 'strategy 1'	Resources released by contracting 'strategy 5'	Freed-up resources
Staff time (hours)			
Nurse	203.33	466.67	263.34
GP	6	12	6
Tests and drugs (number)			
Cholesterol test	75	150	75
ACE inhibitor or β-blocker			
prescription	75	150	75
Simvastatin prescription	40	80	40

If I were faced with substituting one activity for another where both used the same amount of inputs, such as nursing time, then the decision to introduce the activity would be a straightforward one of benefit maximisation. It is when the two activities being compared differ in both the amount of resources and the benefits they deliver that the decision becomes more complex.

I assume that the practice adopts an efficient appointment system (Torgerson *et al* 1993), whereby those invited for screening are asked to confirm their acceptance of the appointment and intention to attend by phone. This ensures that the resources to be released will be fully utilised.

I also assume the minimal screening strategy results in the same level of effectiveness as reported in Field *et al* (1995), which in turn assumes that the level of CHD risk in the hypothetical practice and the trial population are the same. Even if this assumption of CHD risk in the hypothetical practice were tenuous by using the 'best' and 'worst' estimates of effectiveness that are reported in Field *et al* (1995), I can account for this uncertainty. Each scenario differs in assumptions about: sustained rate of smoking cessation (10% best – 3% worst); reductions in total cholesterol concentrations in patients with values in the range 7.5–8.5 (20% best – 10% worst) and > 8.5 mmol/l (10% best – 3% worst). Table 14.6 shows the total number of life years gained in the trial population under each strategy and the scenario reported in Field *et al* (1995). I can estimate life years gained per patient by dividing total life years by the number of patients in the trial (n=7840). Using the assumptions already made about the prevalence of CHD risk factors in the practice population, I can estimate, using this per patient benefit figure, the life years gained by the two alternative screening strategies. I have assumed that male patients would *not* necessarily prefer to have improved health in the present rather than the future and I have therefore used (not discounted (Ganiats 1994)) life years gained as quoted in Field *et al* (1995).

As can be seen in Table 14.6, the comprehensive screening strategy delivers approximately twice as much total benefit compared with the minimal screening strategy under the best scenario, and 50% more under the worst scenario. So far, therefore, it appears that by introducing the minimal screening strategy patients will benefit less and the opportunity cost of using these resources in this way is higher because more benefit would be conferred using the comprehensive screening.

Table 14.6. Estimates of life years gained for CHD screening strategies 1 and 5.

Strategy	Effectiveness data extracted from Field *et al* (1995)						
	Discounted life years gained in trial population (n=7840)		Life years gained per patient		Life years gained in practice population (n=750)*		
	Best	Worst	Best	Worst	Best	Worst	
Minimal screening ('strategy 1')	288	109	0.037	0.014	27.55	10.43	
Comprehensive screening ('strategy 5')	628	166	0.080	0.021	60.08	15.88	

Assumption:
* In using the effectiveness data reported in Field *et al* (1995) it is implicitly assumed that the levels of risk in the hypothetical practice (see Tables 14.1 and 14.2) are similar to those in the trial population.

However, the net efficiency of practice health checks would increase because the minimal screening strategy requires substantially fewer resources, i.e. the benefits per unit of resource for the minimal screening strategy are greater than for the comprehensive strategy. As I have argued throughout, cost estimates are useful in ascertaining cost-effectiveness, and the practice could test this assertion by estimating its own costs using local information.

Table 14.6 does not include additional benefits which might arise from this service development. The switch in screening strategies would release practice resources and presumably the practitioner would like to maximise total benefits for the practice population. This requires further work to identify other efficient programmes of care where these resources might be used. Indeed, it might be possible to increase the size of the population receiving the minimal screening strategy using the freed resources. Each individual receives less benefit under the more cost-effective strategy but the benefits are spread more widely. Alternatively, other treatments might be provided. As long as the released resources can be used in another activity, then it is possible that, in conjunction with the minimal screening strategy, total benefits for the practice population will be greater than before.

In this example, the cost-effectiveness of the service development depends on the ease with which freed-up resources are absorbed into other treatments or programmes of care. This should be taken into account during Step 2. If a released resource, such as a specialised piece of equipment, cannot be used in another activity to deliver health benefits (or sold to fund other resources which can), then the cost-effectiveness of the service development may be in jeopardy. Thus, implementing what appear to be 'cost-effective' changes in practice may not be feasible within local resource constraints.

Conclusion

The example described illustrates that:

- economic evaluations can provide information on resources needed for service re-alignment;

- this complex task can be made simpler and more systematic by using the three-step procedure.

The actual details and type of service I have chosen may not be realistic for some practices. However, this does not matter since the purpose of this chapter was to show that it is possible to use a paper reporting trial-based data to estimate the resources that are needed for a new treatment or intervention. Despite using a relatively complex example of a service with multiple inputs, I have also shown that the same study can be used, in conjunction with practice-level knowledge and data, to identify:

- what resources are required;

- where resources might be captured;

- the benefits that arise from the change.

Introducing an intervention which requires only a single resource input would be simpler, especially if the activity being contracted uses the same type and amount of resource.

Invariably, a number of assumptions have to be made in this process but this uncertainty can be explored by systematically varying a particular assumption to demonstrate impacts on cost and effect outcomes. This is a technique widely practised by economists and is termed *sensitivity analysis*. For example, you might vary the assumption of time required to provide the minimal screening between upper and lower estimates, such as 20 and 10 mins, to see if this significantly altered the ease with which resources could be found within the practice.

The approach I have taken in this chapter would require less time, effort and expertise in economic methods of the practitioner than a critical appraisal of the costing methodology adopted in a study. In addition, the information extracted from the study is more relevant at practice level. However, access to bibliographic resources and the time needed to find relevant studies may still be a constraint to the practitioner. In addition, there may be many similar studies that should be taken into consideration. Although I assumed, for simplicity, that there is only one economic study available, some data not reported in Field *et al* (1995) are available in papers detailing the trial results (Imperial Cancer Research Fund OXCHECK Study Group 1994). There are also a number of relevant economic analyses available (Langham *et al* 1996, Wonderling *et al* 1996a,b). Where multiple studies differ in the amounts of resources required for the same treatment, local assumptions should be used in the three-step procedure.

You might argue that a practitioner would save time by extracting economic data from systematic reviews. Whilst this is a valid approach for determining which treatment is more cost-effective than another, there are two reasons why you would still need to obtain individual economic analyses. First, as I have argued in this chapter, data on the *amount of resources* are needed for service implementation and individual studies are more likely to report such detail. Second, whilst it is commonplace to use a statistical technique called meta-analysis to pool *effectiveness data*, there are more difficulties with pooling *cost and resource data* and the techniques are not properly developed yet.

References

Drummond M and Jeffersen T (on behalf of the BMJ Economic Evaluation Working Party) (1996). Guidelines for authors and peer reviewers of economic submissions to the BMJ. *British Medical Journal* **313**: 275–283.

Field K, Thorogood M, Silagy C, *et al* (1995). Strategies for reducing coronary risk factors in primary care: which is most cost effective? *British Medical Journal* **310**: 1109–1112.

Ganiats T (1994). Discounting in cost-effectiveness research. *Medical Decision Making* **14**: 298–300.

Imperial Cancer Research Fund OXCHECK Study Group (1994). Effectiveness of health checks conducted by nurses in primary care: rules of the OXCHECK study after one year. *British Medical Journal* **308**: 308–312.

Langham S, Thorogood M, Normand C, *et al* (1996). Costs and cost effectiveness of health checks conducted by nurses in primary care: the OXCHECK study. *British Medical Journal* **312**: 1265–1268.

Mason J and Drummond M (1995). Reporting guidelines for economic studies. *Health Economics* **4**: 85–94.

Torgerson DJ and Donaldson C (1994). An economic view of high compliance as a screening objective. *British Medical Journal* **308**: 117–119.

Torgerson DJ, Garton MJ, Donaldson C, *et al* (1993). Recruitment methods for screening programmes: trial of an improved method within a regional osteoporosis study. *British Medical Journal* **307**: 99.

Wonderling D, Langham S, Buxton M, *et al* (1996a). What can be concluded from the OXCHECK and British family heart studies: commentary on cost effectiveness analyses. *British Medical Journal* **312**: 1274–1278.

Wonderling D, McDermott C, Buxton M *et al* (1996b). Costs and cost effectiveness of cardiovascular screening and intervention: the British family health study. *British Medical Journal* **312**: 1269–1273.

▶15

Prescribing Dilemmas: A Barrier to Evidence-Based Health

Judith Cantrill

Introduction

General practitioner prescribing accounts for over 80% of the cost of all medicines and 10% of the total NHS budget. In 1997, the net ingredient cost of all prescriptions dispensed in England in primary care was £4367 million, continuing the relentless year-on-year increase of around 9% (Department of Health 1998). In recent years, the pursuit of high quality care and cost containment has focused attention on the problem of inappropriate prescribing (Audit Commission 1994). However, the magnitude of this problem remains largely under-researched and therefore unknown (Buetow *et al* 1993).

There is little published literature seeking to investigate doctors' motivation for inappropriate prescribing. However, prescribing without pharmacological justification was recognised as an area of concern long before the era of evidence-based practice. Harris (1980) published a personal account on the emotional basis of prescribing. Schwartz *et al* (1989) reported the motivations of 141 doctors who were part of a large randomised controlled trial in the US. The commonest reasons offered were patient demand, intentional use of the placebo effect and prescribers' assertions that their own clinical experience indicated that some therapies were beneficial, despite published evidence that this was not the case. Bradley (1992) reported the use of the critical incident technique to analyse 'uncomfortable' prescribing decisions made by 69 doctors in the North of England. He points out:

> 'the main value of this study lies in its exposure of the complexity of decision making that precedes prescribing in general practice.'

Recent research

Two recent qualitative studies conducted in the UK have attempted to explore some aspects of inappropriate prescribing from the GPs' perspective. Weiss and Scott (1997) echoed the views of Bradley when they argued that whilst GPs' use of a prescription may not always conform to the accepted definition of rational prescribing, it is rational behaviour given the context in which prescribing occurs. Their study suggests that this behaviour is a coping strategy to deal with a variety of patient, practice and workload pressures (Weiss and Fitzpatrick 1997). In particular, they urge a recognition of the humanity of the doctor–patient relationship. This sentiment has also been echoed by Butler *et al* (1998) in their study of the rationale for GPs prescribing antibiotics for sore throats, despite well recognised evidence that they are of little therapeutic value. In Butler *et al*'s study, almost all of the 21 GPs felt that prescribing decisions could have an important impact on the therapeutic power of the doctor–patient relationship.

Work conducted at the National Primary Care Research and Development Centre (NPCRDC) has resulted in the development of a set of nine indicators which can be used to measure the appropriateness of long-term prescribing in UK general practice (Cantrill *et al* 1998). Two of the indicators relate to cost, while the remaining seven relate to other dimensions of prescribing, utilising the *British National Formulary (BNF)* as the 'gold standard' (Box 15.1). Subsequently, these indicators have been applied by a pharmacist researcher to the medical records of samples of patients under the care of 24 different GPs in three Health Authorities in England and one Health Board in Scotland. The findings relating to the individual patients were subsequently discussed with each GP by the same researcher. The sample was purposive, with the aim of covering all of the nine prescribing indicators, addressing a wide range of issues with each GP and obtaining a range of views on the same topic. The examples used in this chapter are taken from this study and are used to illustrate some of the dilemmas that GPs encounter in long-term prescribing which may lead to apparently inappropriate decisions.

Box 15.1. Reliable indicators of prescribing appropriateness (Cantrill *et al* 1998)

1. The indication for the drug is recorded and upheld in the *BNF*.

2. The reason for prescribing a drug of limited value is recorded and valid.

3. Compared with alternative treatments in the same therapeutic class, which are just as safe and effective, the drug prescribed is either one of the cheapest or a valid reason is given for using an alternative.

4. A generic product is prescribed if one is available.

5. If a potentially hazardous drug–drug combination is prescribed, the prescriber shows knowledge of the hazard.

6. If the total daily dose is outside the range stated in the *BNF*, the prescriber gives a valid reason.

7. If the dosing frequency is outside the range stated in the *BNF*, the prescriber gives a valid reason.

8. If the duration of treatment is outside the ranges in the *BNF*, the prescriber gives a valid reason.

9. Prescribing for hypertension adheres to the evidence-based guidelines in the *BNF*.

Reasons for inappropriate prescribing

Patient preference or resistance

A recurring theme throughout the interviews was that of perceived patient, or occasionally family, preference to continue with long-term therapy. This encompassed many facets of inappropriate prescribing including (see Box 15.2 for examples):

▶ use of drugs of limited value;

▶ prescribing expensive formulations;

▶ prescribing a branded medicine when a generic was available.

Adequate discussion with patients was widely recognised as one of the keys to influencing change, which although practised by some GPs was not always successful. Several gave detailed accounts of their attempts to persuade patients to change, another rationalised that he learnt from such experiences and tried to avoid similar situations in the future:

> 'The way I tackle this sort of problem is that I take it on board and bear it in mind for fresh prescribing.'

Box 15.2. Examples of patient pressure

Drugs of limited value

> 'I've tried at one stage to persuade this lady to do without [Motival] . . . but she said she couldn't manage.'

> 'I did try to stop it but she had a stroke and it was all the doctor's fault for stopping it [naftidofuryl] . . . you don't argue with the family.'

Generic substitution

> 'I've tried changing to [generic constituents] but she always wants to go back on Frumil.'

> 'Yes, we're trying to do generic substitution . . . We'd consider changing this [Moduretic] to bendrofluazide but it depends very much on the patient and how you put it to them.'

> 'It doesn't matter how long you spend with them or how long you rationalise that something works just as well, they have it in their mind "I want my Zantac".'

Expensive formulations

> 'Changed from MDI [metered dose inhaler] on the request of the patient who has borrowed her friend's diskhaler.'

Other GPs raised their own concerns about individual patients whom they knew well. This was particularly evident in the elderly or those with psychiatric illness, where even small changes to a medication regimen could cause considerable problems. Hence, although it was acknowledged that changes could be made to improve the quality of prescribing, this may produce considerable distress for some individuals:

'He gets very worried and excitable if you attempt to change anything ... even just something minor would cause him a virtual breakdown.'

In contrast, another GP identified a patient with a very different attitude towards his medication:

'He's fairly amenable to tinkering with his pills, so we'll look at that.'

These two contrasting examples would argue for a wide variety of patient characteristics to be taken into consideration when making individual prescribing decisions. There were other examples of where apparently inappropriate prescribing, in this case use of an expensive combination antihypertensive agent, was clearly in the patient's best interest:

'This patient is working and prescription charges here are quite important and he's only paying £5.65 [the prescription charge at the time the study was undertaken] every second month and if I did prescribe separate preparations then it'll double the prescription charges.'

Historical prescribing

In many cases, the decision to initiate the treatment under discussion had been taken several years previously. As would be expected, many GPs recognised that the licensing of new drugs and availability of new evidence had led to changes in their clinical practice and prescribing habits over time. However, many expressed reluctance to change a long-standing prescription unless there was an obvious current clinical need to do so (Box 15.3). The time commitment necessary to effect change was again highlighted, one notable example being benzodiazepine prescribing. Many practices had taken steps to prevent developing new, long-term users, but experienced problems with long-standing patients:

'We have a big problem with long-term hypnotic use. It would take an awful lot of work and it's purely a time and work problem.'

Although recognising the need for change and being aware of current evidence, not all GPs felt able to put this into practice, as exemplified by the dosage recommendations for ACE inhibitors in congestive cardiac failure. Referring to a patient who had been on low-dose captopril for a number of years, a GP commented:

Box 15.3. Examples of historical prescribing

Changing Practice

> 'It [Inderal LA] was popular at the time she was started on it.'

> 'He came to us on it [Berotec] and we haven't changed it ... seems a blast from the past.'

No clinical need for change

> 'The dose [bendrofluazide 10 mg] may not be what we would use now ... I haven't interfered as he is quite well. BP fine and I've just left him on the same treatment.'

Inherited prescribing

> 'He's been on that a long time. This wasn't started by myself and certainly wouldn't be my first choice.'

> 'It's a difficult one ... so you've got someone who's technically asymptomatic, doing very well, but you're now told they have to be on the highest possible dose ... and you find they can't tolerate it because of side effects. It seems a weird way of working.'

Others attributed inappropriate prescribing to decisions made by the patient's previous practice or by another, often now retired, partner. Several GPs acknowledged that this may be compounded by inadequate review of long-term prescribing when patients join a list or a practice:

> 'It is an uncritical acceptance when she first came here. It should have been addressed and reviewed when she first signed on with us.'

This issue of historical prescribing serves as a reminder that any evidence-based guidelines or formularies must be regularly updated to include new data and drug developments. It also emphasises the principle that such guidelines should not focus exclusively on the initial decision to prescribe, but should also incorporate a treatment review.

Hospital-led prescribing

Hospital-led prescribing frequently arose within the context of discussions about the criteria relating to no recorded indication, use of expensive products or formulations, use of potentially hazardous drug combinations, and drug doses outside the *BNF* recommendations (Box 15.4). One GP, acknowledging the instance of inappropriate prescribing under discussion, recognised that he also allowed this to influence his prescribing for other patients:

> 'Huge numbers do come out of [the local] hospital on it and I suppose I've got into the habit because of that. Until the hospital started doing it, we had very few patients on it.'

Box 15.4. Examples of hospital-led prescribing

No recorded indication

> 'He was discharged from hospital on diclofenac ... so I presume it was initiated in hospital for no particular reason and it's just been carried on as a repeat.'

> 'Something that happens a lot is that folk go into hospital and are given aspirin for ischaemic heart disease and the consultant in the hospital says "Oh, you'd better start them on [an H$_2$-antagonist]" and they stay on it, which is a bug bear of mine.'

Expensive formulations

> 'We do have a problem here in that loads of people come back to us from the hospital on it [modified release isosorbide mononitrate] and then we have this hassle about whether we change them onto what's on our practice formulary.'

Potentially hazardous drug combinations

> '... as he was started on it [the combination] in hospital, I assume that they would be aware of that [potential interaction] and have been monitoring it.'

Doses outside BNF recommendations

> 'They [hospital specialists] seem to be a law unto themselves ... they use doses which you would not say were justified.'

This reinforces the rationale of the pharmaceutical industry for discounting drugs for hospital purchasers; namely, the 'knock on' effect of one hospital-initiated prescription. Others clearly felt that changing or questioning hospital prescribing could pose a professional dilemma:

> 'When the hospital consultant recommends a treatment it's difficult ... for us not to prescribe unless there is a very good reason. To some extent we feel obliged to carry on when they have initiated it.'

Taking this dilemma a little further, another GP expressed his concern that ignoring the advice of a hospital prescriber may undermine the patient's faith in their medical carers. He illustrated this with an example he had recently experienced relating to the use of enteric coated aspirin:

> 'I do find it difficult when the hospital does something, then for me to say [to the patient] "I don't believe this". I actually had someone say to me in the last two weeks "They told me it was special aspirin that wouldn't upset my stomach" and I've actually got to counteract that with a definite denial. To suddenly say "No, that's not true, ordinary aspirin is alright". It also reduces their [the patient's] faith in us as they don't know who to believe.'

This provides a clear example of how failure on the part of hospital prescribers to practise evidence-based health (EBH) can have a negative impact on GPs.

The responsibility for hospital-initiated prescribing shifts entirely to the GP when patients are discharged from consultant care, which presents another potential problem area. This may result from either inadequate communication or failure of the GP to recognise the change in responsibility. The following comment referred to a patient who had been initiated on a combination of bendrofluazide, digoxin and verapamil by a cardiologist:

> 'That sort of thing [inadequate monitoring for a potentially hazardous drug interaction] does happen I'm afraid in practice, whereby while they are actually under active hospital management and review, you are assuming all relevant blood tests are being done, but there may be a problem when discharged back to the GP that we don't pick up on the consequences of that ... change of responsibility.'

Repeat prescribing

Although this study inevitably involved some discussions around the GP's original decision to initiate a treatment, its main focus was long-term prescribing. In explaining how inappropriate prescribing may occur within this context, many GPs made unsolicited reference to the process of repeat prescribing. There was a common view that this was a difficult and potentially very time-consuming process to manage:

> 'The problem with repeat prescribing is that it's just ballooned out of hand ... We certainly know we need to address it and I think we need to do that, it just takes time.'

Several expressed unease with the common practice of partners taking it in turns to sign the day's repeat prescriptions. This related both to the volume of prescriptions and taking responsibility for patients who were not under their care:

> 'You can't keep everything in your head and we have so many prescriptions to sign that you can't check everything and a lot of them you don't know.'

> 'I get this pile [of prescriptions], I've not actually seen the patients and I don't feel responsible for them. I don't like the system at all.'

The application of the prescribing indicators constitutes a comprehensive medication review. The NPCRDC research has shown that this is a time-consuming process, a sentiment echoed by the GPs:

> 'The difficulty with all these things is time and reviewing patients, it is far easier to sign a prescription and get them [the patient] out of the room than it is to sit down and review things.'

Another GP was uncertain about his ability critically to review his own prescribing, preferring to have some more independent assessment:

> 'I don't think it's [review of repeat prescriptions] anywhere near as good as sitting down with somebody else and talking through these things ... I'm sure our standard of care would improve greatly.'

The value of independent review was identified by another GP who did not initially feel that the indicators would identify inappropriate prescribing in his patients:

> 'When I saw the list of patients [to be discussed with the researcher], I was quite happy about the prescriptions ... but obviously when you look at them in more detail there are anomalies there that either ought to be checked on, reviewed or even altered.'

These comments may suggest that the review of long-term prescribing, using a case history approach, could provide a tool for education and debate within the context of EBH.

How can these barriers be overcome?

Are we too quick to blame the patient?

Although patient demand has been cited by doctors as an important influence on inappropriate prescribing (Schwartz et al 1989), the evidence that patients' expectations influence GPs' decisions to initiate a treatment is equivocal (Britten and Ukoumunne 1997). Some work has been undertaken to examine whether patients put pressures on their doctors to continue to prescribe, even though the use of the drug is considered by the doctor to be inappropriate. Britten et al (1995) undertook an interview study of 40 patients, all of whom were prescribed drugs which their GP regarded as 'obsolete'. Nineteen patients said that they would consider an alternative medication, but would need assurances from their GP about efficacy and side effects. Barter and Cormack (1996) in a qualitative study of 11 elderly, long-term benzodiazepine users found that 5 wished to stop taking them and that lack of doctor questioning about the medication was taken as indicative of the doctor's approval of their use. In a questionnaire survey of 54 benzodiazepine users in one inner-city London practice (Kendall 1993), 70% of respondents stated that their GP had never suggested stopping their medication. All four doctors in the practice believed that they had encouraged all or most of their patients who were having repeat prescriptions for benzodiazepines to reduce or stop their medication on more than one occasion. These studies suggest that the GP's perspective of what patients want in relation to prescribing may not always be correct.

Do we communicate effectively?

In relation to changing long-standing prescriptions, all the studies in this area clearly show that effective communication is the single most important factor which determines the success of change. Dowell et al (1996) interviewed 17 patients in whom a total of 26 drug changes had been attempted as part of the practice's drive to cut drug expenditure. Although most were willing to try cheaper treatments, they expressed dissatisfaction with the communication they received. Acceptance was also influenced by the doctor–patient relationship; patients who had profound trust in their doctor would accept and rationalise almost any change he made. Conversely, those with little faith in their doctor may fiercely reject any change. Dowell et al concluded:

'Large scale economies in prescribing are feasible for some practices, and patients will tolerate such change if attention is paid to sensitive communication.'

Wood *et al* (1997) also undertook a study of GPs' and patients' perspectives of prescribing changes in one practice in the West Midlands. Interviews with prescribers revealed that they expected a higher level of resistance and complaints from patients than proved to be the case. Overall, there was a high level of patient satisfaction with both GPs and the prescribing change. They concluded:

'We attribute this to the clear and caring way in which the change was communicated to patients.'

Do we have the time?

GPs in the NPCRDC study clearly recognised that effective communication can be time consuming, and even then may not achieve the desired outcome. There was also a sense that GPs felt that their main treatment aim is to manage a patient's day-to-day presenting symptoms, rather than consider longer-term management and mortality. This was exemplified by several GPs' attitudes towards the prescribing of higher dose ACE inhibitors in congestive cardiac failure. In this example, they were aware of the evidence but felt unable or unwilling to apply it in clinical practice. There was a feeling that this could potentially increase their workload for a group of asymptomatic patients, generating more consultations through the need to explain changes, increase doses and manage side effects.

How can we manage hospital-led prescribing?

The influence of hospital prescribers is widely quoted as having an important impact on practice, but has rarely been studied. As government pressure to control drug expenditure continues, the need for effective formulary management becomes paramount. Under the current NHS changes, opportunities arise through primary care groups (PCGs) and the possibility offered by unified drug budgets, to develop collaborative primary/secondary care formularies. However, just like protocols and guidelines, they will only succeed if there is co-operation, ownership and commitment from all involved in the process.

To date, unlike primary care, there has been comparatively little public scrutiny of hospital prescribing, largely because these data are not collected centrally. However, formularies do now operate in almost all UK hospitals with varying degrees of success, and the pressing challenge lies in engaging hospital specialists in justifying their prescribing decisions, particularly those which directly impact on primary care. Justification should include explicit use of EBH, and where this is not adhered to, an explanation should be provided of the rationale.

Can we manage repeat prescribing?

Repeat prescriptions account for at least two-thirds of all GP prescriptions, and represent four-fifths of total drug costs. Systems for managing the demand for repeat prescriptions have emerged without regard to their impact on patient care. As illustrated earlier, this has resulted in a process with which many GPs feel considerable unease. Zermansky (1996) studied the records of 427 patients requesting repeat prescriptions in 57 randomly selected practices in Leeds. For more than half the prescriptions examined, there was no documented evidence in the medical record of a doctor taking an active decision that the drug should be continued long term. Interestingly, he noted that hospital-initiated drugs seemed to be more prone to be added to a patient's medication list without appraisal, suggesting GPs may feel unable or unwilling critically to review the prescribing of hospital colleagues. As discussed earlier, questioning the decision of a hospital prescriber may pose a professional dilemma for the GP.

In over 70% of prescriptions in Zermansky's study, there was no evidence of drugs having been reviewed by a doctor in the previous 15 months. Further, Zermansky felt that reviews tended to focus on drugs being taken for the condition(s) presenting during the consultation, rather than the entire medication regimen. He concluded that, given the nature and pressure of GPs' workload and the length of the average consultation, that this is not a surprising finding. The GPs in the NPCRDC study clearly recognised that effective medication review is a time-consuming process which requires longer or additional consultations and has major workload implications.

The way forward

Clearly, communication between patient and doctor, or doctor and doctor, has to be effective. However, perhaps the most challenging aspect of communication is to ensure that it makes effective use of the evidence. Evidence should be used to involve patients, both in choosing an initial treatment (concordance) and in reviewing the long-term need. At the practice or PCG level, GPs will need to negotiate with colleagues, hospital prescribers and other professionals when developing formularies and guidelines. Informed debate may also be required to agree a management plan for individual patients. Evidence is a powerful negotiating tool, particularly in areas of uncertainty or conflict.

In order to manage their workload, GPs should consider further delegation or devolution of appropriate functions to other health-care professionals. The recent NHS Executive resource document, *GP Prescribing Support* (National Prescribing Centre and NHS Executive 1998), suggests that pharmacists should become more widely involved in medicines management, particularly in the area of organising and reviewing long-term prescribing. The evidence to support this role is reviewed in Chapter 16.

References

Audit Commission (1994). *A Prescription for Improvement: Towards More Rationale Prescribing in General Practice*. London: HMSO.

Barter G and Cormack M (1996). The long-term use of benzodiazepines: patients' views, accounts and experiences. *Family Practice* **13**: 491–497.

Bradley CP (1992). Uncomfortable prescribing decisions: a critical incident study. *British Medical Journal* **304**: 294–296.

Britten N and Ukoumunne O (1997). The influence of patients' hopes of receiving a prescription on doctors' perceptions and the decision to prescribe: a questionnaire survey. *British Medical Journal* **315**: 1506–1510.

Britten N *et al* (1995). Continued prescribing of inappropriate drugs in general practice. *Journal of Clinical Pharmacy and Therapy* **20**: 199–205.

Buetow S, Sibbald B, Cantrill JA (1993). Prevalence of potentially inappropriate long-term prescribing in general practice in the UK. *British Medical Journal* **313**: 1371–1374.

Butler CC, Rollnick S, Pill R, *et al* (1998). Understanding the culture of prescribing: qualitative study of general practitioners' and patients' perceptions of antibiotics for sore throats. *British Medical Journal* **317**: 637–642.

Cantrill JA, Sibbald B, Buetow S (1998). Indicators of the appropriateness of long-term prescribing in general practice in the United Kingdom: consensus development, face and content validity, feasibility and reliability. *Quality in Health Care* **7**: 130–135.

Department of Health (1998). *Statistics of Prescriptions Dispensed in the Community: England 1987 to 1997. Statistical Bulletin 1998/24*. London: Department of Health.

Dowell J, Snadden D, Dunbar J (1996). Rapid prescribing change, how do patients respond? *Social Science and Medicine* **43**: 1543–1549.

Harris CM (1980). Personal view. *British Medical Journal* **281**: 57.

Kendall C (1993). Use of benzodiazepines. *British Journal of General Practice* **43**: 34.

National Prescribing Centre and NHS Executive (1998). *GP Prescribing Support. A Resource Document and Guide for the New NHS*. Leeds: NHS Executive.

Schwartz RK, Soumerai SB, Avorn J (1989). Physician motivation for nonscientific drug prescribing. *Social Science and Medicine* **28**: 577–582.

Weiss M and Fitzpatrick R (1997). Challenges to medicine: the case of prescribing. *Sociology of Health & Illness* **19**: 297–327.

Weiss MC and Scott D (1997). Whose rationality? A qualitative analysis of general practitioners' prescribing. *Pharmacy Journal* **259**: 339–341.

Wood K *et al* (1997). Changing medication: general practitioner and patient perspectives. *International Journal of Pharmacy Practice* **5**: 176–184.

Zermansky A (1996). Who controls repeats? *British Journal of General Practice* **46**: 643–647.

▶16

Role of the Pharmacist in Evidence-Based Prescribing in Primary Care

Mary Patricia Tully and Judith Cantrill

Introduction

The prescribing process

The process of choosing and prescribing the most suitable drug for each individual patient is becoming increasingly complex. Not only are the number and potency of available drugs increasing, but also GPs are being actively encouraged to prescribe in a certain fashion. This method of prescribing is variously called 'rational', 'appropriate', 'cost-effective' and more recently 'evidence based', and the aim is to improve the quality of care and save money, in line with UK government recommendations (Department of Health 1998). It has been suggested that the practice of rational prescribing involves five separate components (Box 16.1), one of which is 'access to independent data on drugs' (Marinker and Reilly 1994). This involves the assimilation and use of an increasingly vast quantity of evidence about the drugs that are being considered, not just for their initiation but also for their long-term use. It places a heavy burden on prescribers to ensure that they are current with the evidence, in addition to the other aspects of patient care that they are expected to deliver.

The process of prescribing can be considered within the continuum of medicines management, starting at the point of the decision about which drug to prescribe and then leading to the act of writing the prescription. This is followed by a review of the prescribing decision, initially during the dispensing process (usually by a pharmacist), and then later when a patient requests further prescriptions and the decision must be

---

Box 16.1. Components of rational prescribing, as suggested by Marinker and Reilly (1994)

▶ A defensible formulation of the patient's problem

▶ Clarity of therapeutic intention

▶ Access to independent data on drugs

▶ Communication with the patient

▶ Follow-up

---

taken as to whether or not to continue the treatment. However, there is evidence to suggest that this decision about long-term use is rarely an active one, neither at the time of the initial prescription nor at later reviews (Zermansky 1996).

Prescribing decision support

Decision-support software, such as that currently being evaluated within the Prescribing Rationally with Decision Support in General Practice Study (PRODIGY)[1], is being increasingly hailed as an effective way of presenting relevant advice to GPs when it is needed (Purves 1998). Currently, this is primarily useful concerning the initial decision to prescribe, rather than any follow-up reviews. An alternative solution is to use advice from other health-care professionals, which has recently been advocated by the NHS Executive.

Pharmacists are becoming increasingly recognised in the primary health-care team, notably within the context of medicines management. Medicines management encompasses all aspects of the use of medicines, from their procurement, to how and why they are prescribed, reviewed and monitored and to how patients use them. Its effective implementation ensures maximum benefit for both patients and the NHS from the appropriate use of medicines. Pharmacists' wider involvement in this process is specifically highlighted in the NHS Executive resource document *GP Prescribing Support* (National Prescribing Centre and NHS Executive 1998). This is defined as 'the use of additional professional input into one or more elements involved in the prescribing process'. Its stated purpose is to help make the prescribing process as efficient and cost-effective as possible.

Both information technology-based and pharmacist-based solutions undoubtedly have their niche in promoting rational prescribing, although as yet little is known about how they will relate to each other. This chapter concentrates on the current evidence on the effectiveness of prescribing support from health-care professionals, specifically pharmacists. However, they (and others) also have a less conspicuous role with decision-support software through their presence on the multidisciplinary teams that prepare the actual recommendations (Purves 1998).

Research

A series of projects, funded by the Department of Health and described in the resource document (National Prescribing Centre and NHS Executive 1998), gives some promising indication that pharmacists can contribute to the achievement of rational prescribing. A second wave of studies, also funded by the Department of Health, has specifically concentrated on prescribing monitoring and review by pharmacists. Unfortunately, most of this work has not yet been published, other than in abstract form. The lack of experimental detail and outcomes data precludes their inclusion, as yet, in the evidence base as to whether this is a valuable use of this particular group of health-care professionals. The detailed results are eagerly awaited. Without such

---

[1] See http://www.schin.ncl.ac.uk/prodigy or contact K Williams at SCHIN, University of Newcastle, Primary Care Development Centre, Newcastle General Hospital NE4 6BE, Tel: 0191 256 3129 for more details.

detail, it is not possible to judge the generalisability or assess the strength of any research conclusions from this Department of Health-funded work. This chapter considers, therefore, only studies published in full and in the public domain.

Dispensing checks

As part of their professional responsibilities, all pharmacists apply a clinical check to prescriptions at the time of dispensing. This ensures, as far as is possible, that there are no interactions with other concurrent medication, contraindications or cautions with a pre-existing disease, nor a need for a change in the formulation or dose of the drug. The legal requirement for this has been tested and upheld by case law in the UK (Anon 1982). Such interventions with less than ideal prescriptions occur routinely. One study, conducted in several London pharmacies, found up to 0.1% of prescriptions required significant interventions, two-thirds of which were judged to be serious or very serious in their potential impact on patient care (Greene 1995). Community pharmacists do not have access to the patient's medical records to perform this role, but may use information that they retain themselves in computerised patient medication records (Rodgers *et al* 1994).

It is only in the past decade in the UK that this method of ensuring safe prescribing, routinely used by pharmacists when dispensing, has been extended to a formal relationship between the pharmacist and prescriber in primary care. Health authorities, health boards or fundholding practices throughout the UK have engaged pharmacists on a contract, part- or full-time basis, in a non-dispensing role. They provide services such as non-patient-specific prescribing advice to the GP or monitoring and review of treatment for selected groups of patients (such as the elderly or those on anticoagulant treatment).

It is not possible in the space of this chapter to do justice to the evidence available for the engagement of pharmacists in the entire prescribing process, from the initial decision through to the continuing review. Therefore, we have decided to concentrate on one particular area: the involvement of pharmacists in the monitoring and review of long-term prescribing for chronic conditions. By this we mean pharmacists who are actively involved in one or more of the following, as part of a *formal* arrangement with the prescriber:

▶ review of part or all of treatment regimen;

▶ treatment initiation or discontinuation;

▶ dosage adjustment;

▶ monitoring of treatment efficacy;

▶ monitoring of adverse drug reactions.

It does not include the routine check or review that accompanies dispensing.

Evidence base for prescribing review by pharmacists in primary care

Search strategy

In order to gather the evidence about the impact of pharmacists providing a monitoring or review service for long-term prescribing for chronic conditions, it was considered necessary to use only those studies where there was an assessment of patient outcomes or the costs of the service provided. Full details of the search strategy and inclusion and exclusion criteria are given in a systematic search and review, conducted by one of the authors, for the Department of Health (Tully and Seston 1998). Box 16.2 gives a brief summary. Studies were excluded if they were published after the end of 1997.

Search results

Seven papers were found of work conducted in community pharmacies (Munroe *et al* 1997, Park *et al* 1996, Shibley and Pugh 1997, Maguire 1994, McKenney *et al* 1973, 1978, Maguire and McElnay 1993) and seven that described work conducted in primary care clinics (Jameson *et al* 1995, Lobas *et al* 1992, Forstrom *et al* 1990, MacGregor *et al* 1996, Grymonpre *et al* 1994, Laucka *et al* 1996, Bogden *et al* 1997). In the UK, primary care clinics are conducted within GP practices. In the USA, they may be separate facilities, run by specific insurance companies and staffed by a group of family practice doctors. In other instances, they are attached to university or veteran affairs hospitals and although resembling outpatient clinics, they provide general health care (or primary care-like service), unlike the clinical specialities offered by outpatient clinics. Whilst there is a wealth of papers that relate to pharmacists working in the hospital outpatient setting, their findings are not neccesarily generalisable to UK primary care, and were thus excluded from this review.

Of the fourteen papers identified, three studies were randomised controlled trials (Park *et al* 1996, Jameson *et al* 1995, Bogden *et al* 1997), five were controlled trials without randomisation (Munroe *et al* 1997, McKenney *et al* 1973, 1978, Forstrom *et al* 1990, Laucka *et al* 1996) and the remainder were before/after studies (Shibley and Pugh 1997, Maguire 1994, Maguire and McElnay 1993, Lobas *et al* 1992, MacGregor *et al* 1996, Grymonpre *et al* 1994). They are of varying methodological quality, but represent the full evidence base for pharmacists reviewing or monitoring long-term medication in primary care.

UK studies

Only two studies were conducted in the UK, one (Maguire 1994, Maguire and McElnay 1993) in a single community pharmacy in Northern Ireland and the other in a single primary care clinic in Scotland (MacGregor *et al* 1996). Five studies were conducted in 2–8 community pharmacies in the USA (Munroe *et al* 1997, Park *et al* 1996, Shibley and Pugh 1997, McKenney *et al* 1973, 1978), five in 1–2 primary care clinics in the USA (Jameson *et al* 1995, Lobas *et al* 1992, Forstrom *et al* 1990, Laucka *et al* 1996, Bogden *et al* 1997) and one in a primary care clinic in Canada (Grymonpre

---

Box 16.2. Sources and search strategy for systematic search and review on the impact of pharmacists' monitoring and reviewing long-term prescriptions in both primary and outpatient care (Tully and Seston 1998).

▶ Databases known to abstract pharmacy practice research, e.g.:
   MEDLINE
   Pharmline
   Excerpta Medica
   International Pharmaceutical Abstracts

▶ Journals known to publish pharmacy practice research:
   American Journal of Health-System Pharmacy
   American Journal of Hospital Pharmacy
   Annals of Pharmacotherapy
   British Journal of Pharmaceutical Practice
   Clinical Pharmacy
   Drug Intelligence and Clinical Pharmacy
   Hospital Pharmacy Practice
   International Journal of Pharmacy Practice
   Journal of Social and Administrative Pharmacy
   Pharmaceutical Journal
   Pharmacy in Practice

▶ Keywords used in search of electronic databases:
   Practice site – *ANY* of: community pharmacy, primary (health) care, family practice, refill clinic(s), ambulatory care, ambulatory clinic(s), outpatient clinic(s), outpatient care, outpatients, follow-up clinic(s)
   AND
   Pharmacist involvement – *ANY* of: community pharmacist(s), clinical pharmacist(s), pharmacies, pharmacy, pharmacy service
   AND
   Research design – *ANY* of: (randomised) controlled trial, random allocation, double or single blind, comparative study, follow-up study, control, controlled study, prospective study

---

et al 1994). As might be expected, therefore, the generalisability of this body of work to the UK setting is limited.

Summary

The interventions provided by the pharmacists in the reported studies varied in frequency, from a single intervention (Grymonpre *et al* 1994, Laucka *et al* 1996) to 3-monthly reviews (Maguire 1994, Maguire and McElnay 1993), and in their scope. Whilst some projects involved a treatment review of all drugs (Jameson *et al* 1995, Lobas *et al* 1992, Grymonpre *et al* 1994, Laucka *et al* 1996), others concentrated on specific conditions:

▶ hypertension (Munroe *et al* 1997, Park *et al* 1996, McKenney *et al* 1973, 1978, Forstrom *et al* 1990);

▶ hyperlipidaemia (Munroe *et al* 1997, Shibley and Pugh 1997, Bogdon *et al* 1997);

▶ diabetes mellitus (Munroe *et al* 1997);

▶ asthma (Munroe *et al* 1997);

or drugs:

▶ theophylline (Maguire 1994, Maguire and McElnay 1993);

▶ warfarin (MacGregor *et al* 1996).

Changes to drugs or dosages were usually recommended to the prescriber, but in two studies (in a community pharmacy-based service to patients with hypertension and in a primary care anticoagulant clinic), the pharmacists made these adjustments themselves, following discussion with the prescribing physician (Park *et al* 1996) or according to a protocol (MacGregor *et al* 1996).

The community pharmacists did not have access to the patients' medical records, but were responsible for collecting their own data to inform their decisions, from prescription forms, patient interviews, or by monitoring clinical parameters such as blood pressure. Pharmacists in the clinics, on the other hand, had access to medical record data, and could interview the patients as desired. In the studies by Forstrom *et al* (1990) and Laucka *et al* (1996), however, the pharmacists only reviewed the prescription and medical notes, *not* the patient.

Analysis of outcomes

Three controlled studies in community pharmacies (Park *et al* 1996, McKenney *et al* 1973, 1978) and one in a primary care clinic (Bogden *et al* 1997) measured clinical outcomes, either following a review of antihypertensive treatment or the full drug regimen. In all cases, significant improvements in the clinical parameters measured were found. For example, the increase in the number of people who were normotensive following the pharmacists' intervention was between 20 and 34.8%. Although less confidence can be placed in the results (as before/after studies are not such a robust research design, being sensitive to, for example, the effects of historical change), a similar significant improvement in most of the measured clinical outcomes was reported in the before/after studies (Shibley and Pugh 1997, Maguire 1994, Maguire and McElnay 1993, Lobas *et al* 1992, MacGregor *et al* 1996).

Changes in quality of life, using common, well validated instruments, were investigated in only two studies, conducted in community pharmacies (Munroe *et al* 1997, Shibley and Pugh 1997). Park *et al* (1996) found a significant improvement from baseline in just the energy/fatigue scale of the Health Status Questionnaire. However, they also reported that the study group had higher scale values at baseline than did the control group (who also showed a small improvement), making it difficult to interpret the implications of these changes. Shibley and Pugh (1997), using a before/after study design and the SF-36 symptom questionnaire, found statistically significant, albeit slight, improvements in the general health scale, vitality scale and role-physical scale compared to baseline. Only two studies, conducted in primary care clinics, compared data on adverse drug reactions with concurrent (Jameson *et al* 1995) or historical (Grymonpre *et al* 1994) controls. Neither found any change in the incidence following the intervention.

The economic analyses that were conducted in this body of work were very limited and mostly considered only differences in the drug acquisition cost between intervention and control groups. Only one study considered this in community pharmacies, using health insurance claim data (Munroe *et al* 1997). They found that the mean monthly cost for medical resources used (adjusted for age, co-morbidity and disease severity) was significantly lower for the intervention group. In the primary care clinics, significant savings were found in two controlled studies (Jameson *et al* 1995, Forstrom *et al* 1990) but not in another (Bogden *et al* 1997). When the cost of the service was taken into account by Lobas *et al* (1992), an annual cost avoidance of $362 per patient (compared to historical controls) was found, although no explicit sensitivity analysis was performed on these data to demonstrate their robustness.

Discussion

The variations in presentation of data, definitions used and methodological quality prevents the use of meta-analyses to calculate the magnitude of overall changes that might be expected. Similar criticisms were made in a Cochrane Collaboration systematic review that also included studies conducted in outpatient clinics (Bero *et al* 1997)

> 'Due to the variability in interventions and outcomes examined in the eligible studies, it was not appropriate to statistically combine the results of the studies.'

However, there does appear to be a trend in the direction of change of the outcomes measured. In summary:

▶ The services provided were consistently accompanied by improvements in the clinical parameters that were measured, regardless of the site of practice or whether or not the pharmacists had access to the patients' medical notes.

▶ Quality of life was assessed in very few studies, but in general, little change was found. Therefore, improvements in clinical parameters do not appear to be at the expense of the patients' overall wellbeing.

▶ Whilst few studies investigated the impact of interventions on the incidence of adverse drug reactions, those that did found no difference.

▶ Drug acquisition costs were the most commonly assessed economic data but, as full details of the data were not always provided, it was not possible to make any judgement as to the overall magnitude of the savings found. However, there was some evidence that savings could be made.

Generalisability

It is important to consider the extent to which the research findings outlined above may be generalisable to primary care in the UK. The interventions provided by the pharmacists in these studies were complex and, from the information given, it was not always possible to deduce the precise nature of the service provided. In particular, we could not necessarily extract from the reports how long pharmacists spent in providing their services, especially for those interventions that might appear, from their description, very similar. In many cases, the work reported was done by a single pharmacist or a small group of dedicated pharmacists, often for relatively short periods. Implementation of the services into routine practice, or even replication of the studies, might be problematic, with no guarantee that similar results would be obtained.

The circumstances under which community pharmacists work in the UK differ from many of those in the reported studies in primary care clinics, particularly with regard to access to patient's medical records. The most relevant work to their practice, unsurprisingly, is that conducted in the mainly USA community pharmacies (Munroe et al 1997, Park et al 1996, Shibley and Pugh 1997, Maguire 1994, McKenney et al 1973, 1978, Maguire and McElnay 1993). In these studies, the pharmacists in the USA, like their colleagues in the UK, did not have access to the patients' medical records. They obtained themselves any information they needed from interviewing or monitoring the clinical parameters of patients in their pharmacy. This represents a duplication of effort and access to medical records is likely to have improved the effectiveness and efficiency considerably. They also used the information that was available from the patients' prescriptions. It is not clear, however, whether they had detailed patient medication records, such as are maintained by many community pharmacies in the UK (Rodgers and Rees 1996). Despite this, the community pharmacists were able to improve the patients' clinical condition by their intervention.

In the studies conducted in primary care clinics (Jameson et al 1995, Lobas et al 1992, Forstrom et al 1990, MacGregor et al 1996, Grymonpre et al 1994, Laucka et al 1996, Bogden et al 1997), the pharmacists had access to the patients' medical records and, hence, greater amounts of information. Here also, pharmacist interventions were able to improve the patients' condition.

A subgroup analysis, comparing community pharmacies with primary care clinics, was not possible for the same reasons as a meta-analysis of the entire evidence base was not possible, i.e. due to the variations in presentation of data and definitions used and methodological inadequacies. Therefore, it is unknown whether access to patients' medical records has any impact on the final patient outcomes.

The future

However, future access to such records may become part of routine practice for community pharmacists. The NHS information strategy plans to provide access for all health-care professionals to patient medical records, by electronic means (via the 'NHSnet'), on a need-to-know basis (National Health Service Executive 1998). Although this will not be fully realised until well into the next decade, it may improve the efficiency with which pharmacists can undertake medication review and remove the barrier of inadequate information. It should be noted that, in common with their medical colleagues, pharmacists have an ethical responsibility to maintain patient confidentiality (Royal Pharmaceutical Society of Great Britain 1998) and routinely have access to patient medical records in secondary care. Nonetheless, there has been resistance to primary care notes being more open to other health-care professionals, from both local medical committees and patient groups.

Against the background of this evidence, it is interesting to note that, in the USA state of Mississippi, it was recently agreed that payment would be made to specially trained community pharmacists to provide a prescription review and monitoring service (Anon 1998). Four diseases were selected for inclusion in this service (diabetes mellitus, asthma, hyperlipidaemia and coagulation disorders), which reflects those conditions that have been previously studied. Pharmacists will be paid for a maximum of 12 visits per patient per year, during which they will evaluate the patient, review the drug therapy with a physician, provide patient education and be required to maintain patient care records. This is being promoted as a way of achieving cost-effective and high-quality care and it is intended that it will be used to evaluate the extent to which these benefits are achieved.

For the past 15 years, in ten states of the USA, there has been direct experience of pharmacists initiating drug therapy, within an organisational framework such as a hospital or clinic and in accordance with agreed protocols (Galt 1995). The recent report of the Crown review of prescribing, supply and administration of medicines has gone some way towards clarifying the legal position of supplying drugs under such protocols in the UK (Review Team for Prescribing Supply and Administration of Medicines 1998). Briefly, these protocols apply to groups of patients (grouped by condition or drug treatment, rather than specifically identified individuals) and permit the supply of named medicines to patients or carers in an identified clinical situation. Pharmacists would, for example, routinely be able to provide and vary the dose of warfarin for patients attending a monitoring clinic, thus improving the efficiency of the service to the patient. It is likely that initially this will become commonplace in primary care clinics, but the possibility exists of such services being provided directly from a community pharmacy.

Conclusion

Currently, there is some evidence to support the role of pharmacists in monitoring and reviewing prescribing in primary care. However, that evidence must be extended, both in quality and in scope. There is clearly a need for:

▶ rigorously designed studies to ascertain the magnitude of the outcomes of prescription review services;

▶ further work to investigate the effect of the pharmacist services on clinical parameters such as adverse drug reactions and, in particular, patient-centred parameters such as quality of life;

▶ detailed economic evaluations;

▶ comparative work on the impact of alternative models of delivering pharmaceutical services and for identical services offered by pharmacists and other health-care professionals;

▶ further work in other disease states and in medication review for vulnerable groups of patients, such as the elderly.

Thus, if a primary care group were to consider involving pharmacists for prescribing support in primary care teams, it would be important to ensure that adequate, rigorous evaluation strategies of such a development were included in the plans. In this way, we could obtain sufficient, reliable data that are relevant to commonplace planning decisions on primary care service development.

References

Anon (1982). Forty per cent of damages in overdose case awarded against pharmacy company. *Pharmaceutical Journal* **228**: 205.

Anon (1998). Medicaid to pay Mississippi pharmacists for disease management. *American Journal of Health-System Pharmacy* **55**: 1238–1239.

Bero LA, Mays NB, Barjesteh K, *et al* (1997). Expanding outpatient pharmacists' roles and health service utilisation, costs, and patient outcomes. In: Bero L, Grilli R, Grimshaw J, Oxman A (Eds) *Collaboration on Effective Professional Practice Module of The Cochrane Database of Systematic Reviews* [updated 1 September 1997]. Available in The Cochrane Library [database on disk and CD-ROM]. The Cochrane Collaboration; Issue 4. Oxford: Update Software. Updated quarterly.

Bogden PE, Koonz LM, Williamson P, *et al* (1997). The physician and pharmacist team. An effective approach to cholesterol reduction. *Journal of General and Internal Medicine* **12**: 158–164.

Department of Health (1998). *A First Class Service. Quality in the New NHS*. London: Department of Health.

Forstrom MJ, Ried LD, Stergachis AS, *et al* (1990). Effect of a clinical pharmacist program on the cost of hypertension treatment in an HMO family practice clinic. *Drug Intelligence and Clinical Pharmacy* **24**: 304–309.

Galt KA (1995). The key to pharmacist prescribing: Collaboration. *American Journal of Health-System Pharmacy* **52**: 1696–1699.

Greene R (1995). Survey of prescription anomalies in community pharmacies: (1) Prescription monitoring. *Pharmaceutical Journal* **254**: 476–481.

Grymonpre RE, Williamson DA, Huynh DH, *et al* (1994). A community-based pharmaceutical care model for the elderly: report on a pilot project. *International Journal of Pharmacy Practice* **2**: 229–234.

Jameson J, VanNoord G, Vanderwoud K (1995). The impact of a pharmacotherapy consultation on the cost and outcome of medical therapy. *Journal of Family Practice* **41**: 469–472.

Laucka PV, Webster WB, Kuch J (1996). Pharmacist review to simplify medication regimens in a VAMC primary care clinic. *Journal of Pharmacy Technology* **12**: 62–66.

Lobas NH, Lepinski PW, Abramowitz PW (1992). Effects of pharmaceutical care on medication cost and quality of patient care in an ambulatory-care clinic. *American Journal of Hospital Pharmacy* **49**: 1681–1688.

MacGregor SH, Hamley JG, Dunbar JA, *et al* (1996). Evaluation of a primary care anticoagulant clinic managed by a pharmacist. *British Medical Journal* **312**: 560.

Maguire T (1994). Plasma levels and therapeutic response: The relevance to community pharmacy. *European Journal of Drug Metabolism and Pharmacokinetics* **19**: 279–281.

Maguire T and McElnay JC (1993). Therapeutic drug monitoring in community pharmacy – a feasibility study. *International Journal of Pharmacy Practice* **2**: 168–171.

Marinker M and Reilly P (1994). Rational prescribing: how can it be judged? In: Marinker M (Ed) *Controversies in Health Care Policies: Challenges to Practice*. London: BMJ Publishing Group, pp 89–110.

McKenney JM, Slining JM, Henderson HR, Devins D, Barr M (1973). The effect of clinical pharmacy services on patients with essential hypertension. *Circulation* **158**: 1104–111.

McKenney JM, Brown ED, Necsary R, Reavis HL (1978). Effect of pharmacist drug monitoring and patient communication on hypertensive patients. *Contemporary Pharmacy Practice* **1**: 50–56.

Munroe WP, Kunz K, Dalmady-Israel C, Potter L, Schonfeld WH (1997). Economic evaluation of pharmacist involvement in disease management in a community pharmacy setting. *Clinical Therapeutics* **19**: 113–123.

National Health Service Executive (1998). *Information for Health: An Information Strategy for the Modern NHS. 1998–2005*. Leeds: NHS Executive.

National Prescribing Centre and NHS Executive (1998). *GP Prescribing Support. A Resource Document and Guide for the New NHS*. Leeds: NHS Executive.

Park JJ, Kelly P, Carter BL, *et al* (1996). Comprehensive pharmaceutical care in the chain setting. *Journal of the American Pharmaceutical Association* **NS36**: 443–451.

Purves IN (1998). PRODIGY: implementing clinical guidance using computers. *British Journal of General Practice* **48**: 1552–1554.

Review Team for Prescribing Supply and Administration of Medicines (1998). *A Report on the Supply and Administration of Medicines under Group Protocols*. London: Department of Health.

Rodgers PJ and Rees JE (1996). Comparison of the use of PMRs in community pharmacy in 1991 and 1995: (1) PMR use and recording of product details. *Pharmaceutical Journal* **256**: 161–166.

Rodgers PJ, Fletcher G, Rees JE (1994). Clinical interventions by community pharmacists using patient medication records. *International Journal of Pharmacy Practice* **3**: 6–13.

Royal Pharmaceutical Society of Great Britain (1998). *Medicines, Ethics and Practice. A Guide for Pharmacists*, Number 20. London: Royal Pharmaceutical Society of Great Britain.

Shibley MCH and Pugh CB (1997). Implementation of pharmaceutical care services for patients with hyperlipidemias by independent community pharmacy practitioners. *Annals of Pharmacotherapy* **31**: 713–719.

Tully MP and Seston EM (1998). *The Impact of Pharmacists Providing a Prescription Review Service. A Report Prepared for the Department of Health*. Manchester: Pharmacy Practice Research Resource Centre.

Zermansky AG (1996). Who controls repeats? *British Journal of General Practice* **46**: 643–647.

▶ 17

Evidence in Practice: A Review of 18 Months of Evidence-Based General Practice

Peter Griffiths

Introduction

The use of evidence-based practice (EBP) in UK general practice is in its infancy. At a recent workshop for GP trainers in the Mersey Deanery there was scepticism about the driving force behind EBP and concern about how time and energy could be found for this new idea. The feeling that a financial or managerial agenda was behind the recent promotion of the concept was strong.

In this chapter I wish to show what one GP trainer working in a group practice in Liverpool achieved over an 18-month period. The only driving forces behind the work were curiosity, a wish to understand more about the concepts involved and how the process could benefit continuing medical education (CME).

The questions

Over this period many questions arose during the course of clinical work; only a small number of these half-formed queries reached the point of being developed into three or four part questions. A total of 36 questions were posed and evidence was uncovered for 20 of these (Box 17.1). The other 16 questions were not addressed because of a lack of time.

One of the first benefits to be found from the EBP approach was that thinking about forming questions helped define the problem. Previously it was common to finish a surgery with a faint feeling of unease, but not knowing exactly why. Thinking about clinical questions helps sort out those issues that may be soluble from those that are not.

Incidentally, the feeling of unease should be common in all medical practice. It is the welcome sign that there is an area of knowledge that needs to be reviewed; the feeling should not be suppressed and should be welcomed by medical teachers and clinicians generally.

The questions concerned a variety of commonly seen conditions in general practice covering a range of specialities (Table 17.1).

Box 17.1. Questions for which evidence was found

1. In a 41-year-old woman with rheumatoid arthritis, what is her prognosis in terms of joint function and pain compared with a woman without rheumatoid arthritis?

2. A 61-year-old woman has back pain, probably due to osteoarthritis of the lumbar spine. Will physiotherapy relieve her pain better than no treatment?

3. A 73-year-old man has had a frontal headache for 4 months and which worsens as the day progresses. He has non-insulin-dependant diabetes and is on verapamil for raised blood pressure. What is the differential diagnosis?

4. A woman aged 64 years developed right tennis elbow 3 weeks ago. How long will it take to resolve if no active treatment is given?

5. Does the MMR injection increase the risk of Crohn's disease in a 4-year-old child being given their second dose?

6. A 60-year-old woman works as a home help. She is worried about the risk of acquiring MRSA from her clients. What are her risks?

7. A 35-year-old pregnant woman has hepatitis C. What are her chances of passing the infection to her baby?

8. A 36-year-old woman has secretory otitis media. Is pseudoephidrine effective in relieving pain and speeding recovery?

9. A 25-year-old woman has ophthalmic shingles. Does acyclovir treatment reduce symptoms and ophthalmic complications?

10. A 23-year-old woman's mother died of ovarian cancer at a young age. Is there an effective screening test that would detect the cancer at an early stage?

11. A 31-year-old woman has pruritis and is 33 weeks pregnant. Is there an intervention that will help?

12. Does improved communication skill improve patient outcome?

13. A 31-year-old man has a cluster variety of migraine. What effective interventions are there?

14. Is fluticasone really any better than beconase for allergic rhinitis?

15. Is there a condition of lymphoedema of the lips caused by streptococcal infection?

16. Does a patient without a spleen (a 48-year-old man) need to continue his penicillin if he has had pneumovax II?

17. Is there a test available locally for α-1-antitrypsin?

18. Could busulphan be responsible for breathlessness in a 78-year-old woman who took it years ago for a blood dyscrasia?

19. Is there an increased risk of Parkinson's disease in a 38-year-old man whose family history is of his father, two uncles and a grandfather having had the disease?

20. Does vasectomy increase the risk of testicular cancer in a 30-year-old man?

Table 17.1. Number of questions by clinical area.

Clinical area	Number of questions
General medicine	17
Obstetrics and gynaecology	4
Rheumatology	3
Dermatology	3
ENT	3
Urology	2
Paediatrics	1
Surgery	1
Communication skills	1

The evidence

Table 17.2. Sources of evidence.

Source	Frequency
BMA OVID MEDLINE	10
Oxford Textbook of Medicine (1996) (OTM)	5
Best Evidence	5
Electronic BNF/DTB/MeReC	2
World Wide Web	1
Local specialist	1
Drug Data Sheet	1
Cochrane Database	1

Table 17.2 shows the sources used to uncover evidence. All of these are either available at the practice or via a phone call; no special trips were required. OVID MEDLINE was available from the consulting room desktop computer via modem, and Best Evidence, Cochrane database and e *BNF* were available in electronic format on the same computer. The *Oxford Textbook of Medicine* was available in hard copy format only. The more observant reader will note that more than one source was used for some questions!

How useful was it?

Simply finding an answer of some kind is not useful in itself. On review it was found that for 18 of the 20 questions (90%) for which evidence was discovered, there was a significant effect on patient care and GP learning. This is a very high percentage and demonstrates the potential benefits of this approach to both patient care and personal professional development.

Example 1

The first example is in fact a question raised by a partner at the practice in response to a question from a patient. The patient, a man in his 30s, asked whether a vasectomy operation would cause an increased risk of testicular cancer in the future. We developed a clinical question as follows:

> Does vasectomy increase the risk of testicular cancer in a 30-year-old man?

The GP who had seen the patient and myself both had no recollection that such effect had been shown, but neither of us felt that this was sufficient basis on which to reassure the patient. As a first step we searched Best Evidence, using the sophisticated search strategy of 'vasectomy'. This was good enough to turn up an interesting article – A long-term study of mortality in men who have undergone vasectomy (Giovannucci *et al* 1992, Anon 1992). To find evidence that had passed through quality filters and had an independent commentary was helpful. The conclusion of the review was (Anon 1992):

> '*Vasectomy does not increase mortality over a 20-year period. That is the main message of this superb epidemiological study of mortality and morbidity. The attractive features of this study are the large number of participants and the long duration of follow-up that included a sizeable group of men followed for >20 years.*'

My colleague felt much happier reassuring the patient on the basis of this information.

> Time taken – 10 min.

Example 2

This example concerned a 41-year-old woman with rheumatoid arthritis (RA) diagnosed 6 years ago. I was concerned about the future course of her illness and wanted to discuss her prognosis; however, my recollection of the prognosis in RA was foggy to say the least. So a question was formulated:

> In a 41-year-old woman with rheumatoid arthritis and possible carpal tunnel syndrome, who is on salazopyrin and ibuprofen, what is her prognosis in terms of joint function and pain compared with a woman without rheumatoid arthritis?

Reference was made to the *Oxford Textbook of Medicine*, which stated:

> '*Of hospital admissions in people with RA only 25% have normal function after 10 years.*'

There was no reference for this assertion, so I decided to carry out a search of MEDLINE. The search strategy was to use rheumatoid arthritis as a MESH term exploded, and cohort studies as a paper type and then combine the searches: this gave 23 articles of which the following was useful – Factors predicting death, survival and functional outcome in a prospective study of early rheumatoid disease over fifteen years (Corbett *et al* 1993).

The abstract proved informative:

> '*Almost 60% of survivors remained with or improved to normal function at 15 years suggesting that morbidity is not as bad as has been suggested in the past.*'

This was interesting as compared with the statement in the *OTM*, and I was able to discuss the prognosis with the patient in a more positive and confident way than if I had relied on the textbook alone. I did not go to the lengths of obtaining the article for critical appraisal so I am making some assumptions about the validity of the research.

> Time taken – 20 min.

Example 3

This is the case of a mother concerned over media reports that MMR injections might be associated with an increased risk of Crohn's disease. This worry took me by surprise, as I had not heard anything about this latest scare story. The question I formulated was:

> Does the MMR injection increase the risk of Crohn's disease in a 4-year-old child being given their second dose?

There was no reference to the topic in the *OTM*, Cochrane database, Best Evidence or e *BNF*. I therefore decided on a MEDLINE search with the strategy of using inflammatory bowel disease as a MESH term exploded and case control as a paper type. The combined searches produced 62 articles, most of which were irrelevant but one was useful – Is measles vaccination a risk factor for inflammatory bowel disease? (Thompson *et al* 1995).

The abstract makes the following statements

> 'The relative risk of developing Crohn's disease in the vaccinated group was 3.01 (95% CI 1.45–6.23). These findings suggest that measles virus may play a part in the development not only of Crohn's disease but also of ulcerative colitis.'

This certainly addressed the problem and having discovered the research unit involved, I was able to ensure that this was their most recent publication of the time (July 1997). I was unsure as to whether the results they were reporting were significant so reference was made to Sackett *et al* (1997) where I discovered that for a case-control study, a relative risk (RR) of <4 should be treated with caution. Thompson *et al* (1995) showed a RR of 3.01 but with a 95% CI of 1.45–6.23). The authors were therefore overstating the strength of their conclusion.

At a further consultation with the mother I was able to discuss the situation in more detail: the parents decided to delay vaccination until further advice was available.

> Time taken – 30 min.

Example 4

Clinical questions can arise from sources other than consultations. This question arose while reading a report in the newspaper entitled 'HRT reduces the risk of heart disease by 50%'. The reduction sounded very impressive and I suspected that I might have some patients consulting about this. A question was formulated:

> In postmenopausal women should HRT be recommended to all to reduce the risk of heart disease?

The newspaper article carried a reference to the article discussed – Postmenopausal estrogen and progestin use and the risk of cardiovascular disease (Grodstein *et al* 1996). As this was obviously an important issue I decided that I would need to see the full paper. The article was in the *New England Journal of Medicine* and a visit to its web site showed that a reprint could be ordered over the Internet for £5.00. The article arrived 2 days later.

A review of the article using one of the checklists in Sackett *et al* (1997) showed that the results could be accepted as valid. The next step was to evaluate if they are important.

> *'Results: We observed a marked decrease in the risk of major coronary heart disease among women who took estrogen with progestin (multivariate adjusted relative risk, 0.39; 95% confidence interval, 0.19–0.78) or estrogen alone (relative risk, 0.60; 95% confidence interval, 0.43–0.83), as compared with women who did not use hormones [corrected]. However, there was no significant association between stroke and use of combined hormones (multivariate adjusted relative risk, 1.09; 95% confidence interval, 0.66–1.80) or estrogen alone (relative risk, 1.27; 95% confidence interval, 0.95–1.69).'*

Again, this percentage looks impressive, but there was a puzzle in that the overall mortality in the HRT group was the same as in the non-HRT group! The reason for this appeared to be the increased rate of breast cancer in the HRT group. The reason for my puzzlement became clear when I realised that the 50% reduction headlined in the newspaper was what is known as relative risk reduction (RRR), and very impressive it sounds. The issue of importance is, however, the absolute risk reduction (ARR), which takes into account the frequency at which the disease actually occurs.

It is because the rate of heart disease in this group of women is low that a 50% reduction does not actually mean much: in order to prevent one cardiac event you would need to treat over 2000 women for 10 years. It then makes sense that such a reduction can be balanced by the increased mortality from breast cancer.

Pleased with my work and analysis I awaited consultations in which I could show off my new found knowledge; no women came to discuss the article! The search has however been very useful in discussing with women the benefits and risks of HRT.

> Time taken – 1 hour 30 min.

Example 5

This example concerns a fairly common condition of general practice, and is included because I had noticed a difference in my practice and that of a colleague. It was routine practice for my colleague to give decongestants to people with secretory otitis media; it was my practice not to. I developed a question around a particular patient as follows:

> A 36-year-old woman has secretory otitis media. Is pseudoephirine effective in relieving pain and speeding recovery?

A search of secondary sources was no help so I did a MEDLINE search using MESH terms and key words: this produced two useful references – Lack of efficacy of a decongestant–antihistamine combination for otitis media with effusion ('secretory' otitis media) in children. Results of a double-blind, randomized trial (Cantekin *et al* 1983) and Prevention and treatment of serous otitis media with an oral antihistamine. A double-blind study in pediatric practice (Klein *et al* 1980).

Despite using various combinations of search terms, these were the only controlled trials I could find relevant to the question (from 1966–1997). Both trials seemed from their abstracts to have been well carried out and neither showed any benefit from decongestants or antihistamines. Both were in children and I could find no trials in adults, but it is probably reasonable to assume that adult results would be similar to those in children.

It was reassuring to me that my practice was in line with available evidence and also showed how little evidence was available for a common primary care problem.

> Time taken – 30 min.

Future ideas

I have found the process described very useful and good for maintaining my professional development; however, at times I would have benefited from the advice and experience of others. The next step I am considering is to set up a small group to work on questions of mutual interest. I am hopeful that this group could include a range of different professionals at different stages of their careers, as the principles involved are applicable to all of us.

Conclusion

The conclusion that I have reached after completing this evaluation is that EBP is a useful component of general practice, continuing education and patient care. It is likely that the full process of obtaining original papers and doing full critical appraisal will be unusual in general practice. This is for good reasons; general practice is different from hospital medicine and public health. We are used to dealing with uncertainty and finding many different ways to assess the importance of information.

As can be seen in the examples, general practice will find sources such as Best Evidence and the Cochrane database extremely useful as quick and reliable methods of finding evidence. It is important that GPs understand the process and concepts involved in appraising evidence, but as generalists it is likely that in most areas we will be able to use the structured work of others.

The process works for areas where we experience a lack of knowledge; the ability of doctors to recognise and acknowledge such areas varies enormously. So we need to develop ways of discovering what it is we do not know as well as addressing things we know we do not know.

The application of the EBP process by GPs should also lead to the identification of important areas where evidence is lacking in primary care.

References

Anon (1992). Does vasectomy affect long-term morbidity? *ACP Journal Club* **117**: 56.

Cantekin EI, Mandel EM, Bluestone CD *et al* (1983). Lack of efficacy of a decongestant–antihistamine combination for otitis media with effusion ('secretory' otitis media) in children. Results of double-blind, randomized trial. *New England Journal of Medicine* **308**: 297–301.

Corbett M, Dalton S, Young A, *et al* (1993). Factors predicting death, survival and functional outcome in a prospective study of early rheumatoid disease over fifteen years. *British Journal of Rheumatology* **32**: 717–723.

Gionvannucci E, Tosteson TD, Speizer FE, *et al* (1992). A long-term study of mortality in men who have undergone vasectomy. *New England Journal of Medicine* **326**: 1392–1398.

Grodstein F, Stampfer MJ, Manson JE *et al* (1996). Postmenopausal estrogen and progestin use and the risk of cardiovascular disease. *New England Journal of Medicine* **335**: 453–461.

Klein SW, Olson AL, Perrin J *et al* (1980). Prevention and treatment of serous otitis media with an oral antihistamine. A double-blind study in pediatric practice. *Clinical Paediatrics* **19**: 342–347.

Sackett DL, Richardson WS, Rosenberg W, *et al* (1997). *Evidence-Based Medicine, How to Teach and Practice EBM*. New York: Churchill Livingstone.

Thompson NP, Montgomery SM, Pounder RE, *et al* (1995). Inflammatory Bowel Disease Study Group, Royal Free Hospital School of Medicine, London, UK. Is measles vaccination a risk factor for inflammatory bowel disease? *Lancet* **345**: 1071–1074.

SECTION 3

EVIDENCE-BASED PRIMARY CARE IN PRACTICE

The following chapters present worked examples of searching for and applying evidence. Many follow the process as it develops, tracing the development of the question, outlining the search strategy and results, then discussing the quality and implications of the evidence obtained. Others adopt a slightly different approach, with an emphasis on summarising the best current evidence.

The purpose of these examples is to provide a number of worked examples to help explain the process both when it is routine, and when it requires modification. A variety of concepts are covered from routine approaches, to decision analysis. We have sought to cover a variety of examples of relevance to different professions in primary care. Certainly, at the time of writing, these examples also serve as useful, relevant summaries for primary care professionals.

Inevitably, these are not systematic reviews, as this is not our purpose. However, at the time of writing, the answers provided are reasonably robust, and provide sufficient detail of the process employed to enable readers to repeat the exercise. We would be surprised if the answers so obtained were always the same. It is quite likely that even if your search results are identical to ours, your access to papers may differ, as may your individual emphasis or interpretation of the evidence. Furthermore, it is to be hoped that good trials and other relevant research will continue to appear in the literature. It is also inevitable that more systematic reviews and meta-analyses concerning topics relevant to primary care will be published, enriching the secondary sources of evidence. All these developments will simplify the process of identifying relevant best evidence.

We hope that readers will also be enthused to seek their own answers, and most importantly, to incorporate the evidence they discover into their practice. It is because we believe that professional satisfaction and clinical care will benefit that we have undertaken this project. Whilst we have attempted to make the following examples from practice reasonably accessible if read in isolation, to save excessive repetition occasional cross-referencing will be required, e.g. to understand the construction of the searches.

▶18

Sore Throat

Trevor Gibbs

Mary was making one of her increasingly common, Friday night visits to the surgery. She had been suffering with a sore throat for the past 2 days, had tried all the medication that doctors had suggested in the past, and was no better. As was usual with Mary, she had an important engagement over the weekend and needed some help.

Examination of Mary's throat was unremarkable; it was slightly red, with a swollen mucosa and she was a little hot. Her '... but I'm desperate Doctor' plea on a Friday night when I was on call over the weekend made me write a prescription for penicillin. Her pleasant exit from the surgery suggested I had done the right thing, but had I really committed the cardinal sin in the eyes of the practice and the health authority whose drug budget I was spending?

The question

Are antibiotics indicated for sore throat and if the answer is no, are there any exceptions?

It is not unusual for this question to arise in practice, especially during this type of consultation. Although the question may arise, it is probably true to say that the enquiry usually stops there and is never pursued. Time, lack of motivation and alternative needs are the usual reasons but not knowing how to progress the question may also be a factor.

Search strategy

An often untapped source of information is the organisation the GP works in, i.e. the surgery. It is always worthwhile discussing the issue with members of the primary care team: it may have been raised before, someone may have already investigated the problem or may be an 'expert' in the field and, most importantly, this is a way of letting others know what you are doing and allows discussion and disagreement to be raised early rather than late.

It should not be expected that GPs are expert in the field of literature searches, evidence-based medicine or similar academic activities. Be prepared to seek out others in the field who are prepared to offer helpful advice.

Try to read around the subject so that you develop a clearer understanding of the subject. A search into a problem is often made less fruitful by not understanding the routine clinical, managerial and occasionally epidemiological implications of the subject.

With this clinical scenario, it is important to learn of the epidemiological picture of the problem, the standard approach to clinical management and to a lesser extent the measured outcomes.

A visit to the books revealed the following information which was helpful for understanding the problem (e.g. Southgate *et al* 1997, Ludman 1997).

▶ Complaints of sore throat are amongst the commonest problems seen in general practice, with an incidence of > 80 per 1000 patients seen.

▶ Controversy over the use of antibiotics is a frequently written about subject.

▶ 70% of sore throats are related to a viral infection, of various types.

▶ The remaining 30% are due to bacterial infections, of which Group A Streptococcus remains the most important.

▶ The incidence of Group A Streptococcus has been rising since the early 1980s both in the USA and to a lesser extent in the UK.

▶ This increased incidence is associated with a more virulent strain, which is also associated with a much severer form of related disease than previously seen.

▶ Clinical features are variable with the diagnosis of viral or bacterial aetiology only moderately reliable.

▶ Diagnostic throat swabs are very uncommon in the UK whilst they are standard practice in the USA.

▶ The reduced prescribing of antibiotics in the USA has been implicated as a cause of an increased incidence of rheumatic fever.

▶ In the period 1977–87, 50 million prescriptions for antibiotics were written (12.5% of all prescriptions).

▶ In the 12 years preceding 1991, there was a 45% increase in the number of antibiotics prescribed.

▶ If overprescribing were reduced, particularly in the area of antibiotics, an estimated £275 million could be saved from the NHS budget.

▶ Prescribing of antibiotics in UK general practice is just as likely to be influenced by social and psychological need as by clinical judgement.

▶ The use of antibiotics far outweighs the incidence of bacterial infection.

It is now important to refine the search. This is made easier by the following.

1. *Identify the key elements in the question*:

▶ sore throat;

▶ antibiotics;

▶ effectiveness.

2. *Consider the relationships between the search elements.* In this case I wish to search all three elements and the relationship between them. Therefore I would use the word 'and' to connect the three, e.g. *sore throat* and *antibiotics* and *effectiveness*, which would produce a very specific search. The use of 'or' to connect the elements would remove duplication in the search. Specifically to remove sub-elements from the search, the word 'not' can be used. Hence, if I wanted to search only adults with sore throat, the search *sore throat* not *children* would be used.

3. *Consider whether the key elements are pure search terms or are too broad.* The word effectiveness is very broad, ranging from clinical effectiveness, managerial effectiveness through to personal effectiveness. The implication is that clinical effectiveness has to be used or clinical outcomes or clinical improvements used instead. The use of the search engine's thesaurus is often of great help at this stage.

4. *Decide upon the size and scope of the search.* In an attempt at both reducing personal effort and increasing the efficiency of the search this stage is important. It will also decide upon which databases are to be used.

The next stage is to commence the search using your newly found information. Most enquiries begin by a visit to the library and dashing straight into searching a specific database. However, it is important to realise that the journals themselves are just as important sources of information.

Search results

Scanning the key journals identified several useful articles.

▶ A randomised controlled trial of antibiotics on symptom resolution in patients presenting to their general practitioner with a sore throat (Howe *et al* 1997). An article written by leading UK practitioners suggesting that antibiotics do improve resolution of sore throat in a specific group of patients (those with a high index of suspicion of bacterial infection).

▶ Open randomised trial of prescribing strategies in managing sore throat (Little *et al* 1997). A trial set in general practice looking at three strategies of management of a sore throat. The conclusions were that prescribing antibiotics only marginally affects resolution of symptoms, enhances patient's belief in antibiotics and affects future consultations in a negative way. It also concluded that psychological factors are important in the decision to see a GP and in predicting the duration of the illness.

▶ Do patients with sore throat benefit from penicillin? A randomized double-blind placebo-controlled clinical trial with penicillin V in general practice (Dagnelie *et al* 1996). A clinical trial from the Netherlands which concluded that antibiotics were only effective if a laboratory diagnosis of bacteria, specifically Group A Streptococcus, was made prior to treatment.

▶ A scoring system for predicting Group A Streptococcal throat infection (Dobbs 1996). Using this diagnostic tool, the authors conclude that significant savings could be made from unnecessary antibiotic prescribing for sore throat.

▶ Sore throat management in general practice (Little and Williamson 1996). Set in the context of recent national guidelines in the *Drugs and Therapeutic Bulletin*, this article concluded that because of the lack of strong evidence in practice, these guidelines were doomed to early failure and may in fact hinder future research in practice.

A search of MEDLINE, using the terms *sore throat* and *antibiotics* and *clinical effectiveness* uncovered 77 papers. However, many were not relevant to the UK or appropriate to general practice and most of the relevant references had already been identified from journal scanning.

Scanning *The Cochrane Library* database for systematic reviews and the Database of Abstracts of Review of Effectiveness (DARE) with the specific key words uncovered what seemed to be the ideal review article – Antibiotic *versus* placebo in the common cold (Arroll and Kenealy 1998). The authors used a search strategy for the years between 1966 and 1997 to uncover data regarding the common cold, including sore throat. Using a collaborative, international approach, all review articles, trials, opinions and letters were collated. Their conclusions were:

▶ Antibiotics appear to have no beneficial effect upon the normal resolution of the upper respiratory tract infection, including sore throat.

▶ Antibiotics should not be given in the first instance as they will not improve symptoms.

▶ Many patients will suffer more from adverse side effects to antibiotics than from the initial illness.

▶ Antibiotics are counter-productive to the development of doctor–patient relationships and lead away from patient independence.

A wealth of further references was held in this database if other evidence was needed.

Conclusion

The practitioner now has the evidence to restrict the prescription of antibiotics for sore throat and to recommend this practice to his colleagues.

As for Mary, there is still work to be done: controlled trials, reviews and guidelines are not the only answer to patient care!

Key points

▶ There is evidence to support decision making for many primary care problems.

▶ Discussion with colleagues is a useful starting point.

▶ Then read round the subject to highlight issues and help with defining the question.

▶ Local experts may be useful sources of advice on evidence and where/how to find it.

▶ Having identified key issues, and defined the question, it is useful to scan the contents/indexes of likely relevant journals from recent years and/or conduct electronic database searches.

▶ Consult secondary evidence sources such as *Cochrane, Bandolier* and *Effective Health Care* bulletins.

▶ Antibiotics are unlikely to have any beneficial effect on the course of uncomplicated upper respiratory tract infection. Indeed resultant adverse effects may worsen the course of the illness.

References

Arroll B and Kenealy T (1998). Antibiotic versus placebo in the common cold. In: *The Cochrane Library*, Issue 4. Oxford: Update Software.

Dagnelie CF, van der Graaf Y, De Melker RA (1996). Do patients with sore throat benefit from penicillin? A randomized double-blind placebo-controlled clinical trial with penicillin V in general practice. *British Journal of General Practice* **46**: 589–593.

Dobbs F (1996). A scoring system for predicting group A streptococcal throat infection. *British Journal of General Practice* **46**: 461–464.

Howe RW, Millar MR, Coast J, *et al* (1997). A randomized controlled trial of antibiotics on symptom resolution in patients presenting to their general practitioner with a sore throat. *British Journal of General Practice* **47**: 280–284.

Little P and Williamson I (1996). Sore throat management in general practice. *Family Practice* **13**: 317–321.

Little P, Williamson I, Warner G, *et al* (1997). Open randomised trial of prescribing strategies in managing sore throat. *British Medical Journal* **314**: 722–727.

Ludman H (1997). *ABC of Otolaryngology*. London: BMJ Publishing Group.

Southgate L, Lockie C, Heard S, *et al* (1997). *Infection*. Oxford: Oxford University Press.

►19

Sinusitis

Mark Gabbay

Background

Patients often consult in primary care concerned about upper respiratory tract infection, and many perceive it as an urgent problem. The conflict between professional reluctance to prescribe antibiotics and patients' apparent belief that antibiotics will effect a cure is well known by those working in primary care. It is commonly considered that acute sinusitis does justify a 10-day course of antibiotics.

The question

In light of the recent Department of Health concern over antibiotic prescribing (Calman *et al* 1998), what is the evidence supporting the prescription of antibiotics in acute sinusitis?

Search strategy

As an exercise I decided to conduct a quick hand search, rather than a formal MEDLINE search. I was interested in primary care studies, and remembered that there had been trials published in the *Lancet* and the *British Journal of General Practice* in 1997. I also scanned recent indexes of the *British Medical Journal* and *Family Practice*, which I deemed to be the other journals most likely to have published trials relevant to primary care. This took 15 min, and I found four relevant papers (the two I remembered plus one I had forgotten I had read, and another I was unaware of).

I also looked at the latest Cochrane database CD-ROM. I searched on the term 'sinusitis'. There were no systematic Cochrane reviews. The DARE section also did not identify any trials other than those I had already identified. The controlled trials register search identified 283 potential references, with abstracts. I worked through these back to 1989, but failed to identify any placebo-controlled trials other than those I had already found from my hand search. The search did identify one review paper I had not seen, and the entry included the full abstract plus a brief commentary, which I was able to print out.

Thus, it seemed that my hand-search strategy, informed by my regular scanning of relevant journals (which I had partly retained in my memory), had proved to be an efficient search strategy on this occasion. I was unsure whether to conduct a MEDLINE search as well. I read the papers I had identified. MEDLINE searches had been undertaken in the recent systematic review I had identified from my hand search, and the results were included in that paper. The Cochrane database included a protocol for a systematic literature review of antibiotics for acute sinusitis by a team from the USA (Williams *et al* 1998). This is a description of work in progress, and summarises the background and search strategies (including MEDLINE) being undertaken, with an estimated date for publication. I decided that as they were planning to complete their review in early 1999, and it was clearly comprehensive, I would await the publication of their work, rather than try and conduct an exhaustive search.

Search results

A quick scan of the titles of the papers identified from the hand search reveals that the results are apparently contradictory.

- Randomised double blind, placebo controlled trial of penicillin V and amoxycillin in the treatment of acute sinus infection in adults (Lindbaek *et al* 1996).

- Primary care based randomised placebo controlled trial of antibiotic treatment in acute maxillary sinusitis (van Buchem *et al* 1997).

- Maxillary sinusitis in adults: an evaluation of placebo controlled double blind trials (Stalman *et al* 1997a).

- The end of antibiotic treatment in adults with acute sinusitis-like complaints in general practice? A placebo controlled double blind randomized doxycycline trial (Stalman *et al* 1997b).

- 10 days of amoxycillin is effective for acute sinusitis (Low and Jea 1997).

Review papers

Both Stalman *et al* (1997a) and Low and Jea (1997) are literature reviews. Stalman *et al* (1997a) conducted a comprehensive MEDLINE and hand search in a number of languages, and searched the Cochrane Collaboration database. They did not seek unpublished studies. Among the 88 clinical trials they identified, the only three that met their criteria were not of high methodological quality and were conducted in the 1970s. They clearly stated their criteria for evaluating the papers they reviewed, and their inclusion and exclusion criteria. This review paper therefore meets the quality criteria outlined in Chapter 2. On balance, they concluded that there was insufficient robust evidence to justify widespread antibiotic treatment for acute sinusitis.

The controlled trials register search on the Cochrane database also suggests that the evidence almost exclusively compares the efficacy of antibiotics with each other, rather than placebo. However, as this review indicates, it is not reasonable to assume that the antibiotics are necessarily responsible for any apparent improvement in symptoms and signs.

The commentary included in the Cochrane database on the paper by Low and Jea (1997) is somewhat equivocal. The paper reports the findings of a consensus symposium largely made up of specialists, and the evidence supporting their conclusions is not particularly strong. Few studies were conducted in primary care and only two were placebo controlled, one in adults and one in children. This is not sufficiently strong evidence to alter my scepticism, based on the Stalman et al (1997a) review.

Trials

The trial by Lindbaek et al (1996) supports the use of antibiotics. They recruited 240 patients from general practice who clinically they concluded had acute sinusitis and referred them for computed tomography of their sinuses. Of the initial referrals, 130 patients were confirmed to have radiographic signs of sinusitis, and these were randomised to receive placebo, amoxycillin 500 mg tds or phenoxymethylpenicillin 1320 mg tds, all for 10 days. Patients were allowed to use decongestants and analgesia as they wished. The paper does not report the differential usage of these ancillary treatments.

Subjects were analysed on an intention-to-treat basis, and subjects and assessors of clinical signs and radiographs were blinded. The trial design also meets the other quality criteria (see Chapter 2). Although a power calculation was reported (180 in total), the recruitment of subjects fell short of this. Despite this, a significant benefit for both antibiotic treatments was demonstrated over placebo on patient- and physician-reported outcomes, time to recovery and radiographic findings. All patients had to be symptomatic for at least a week before they could be recruited into the trial.

The paper fails to justify nasopharyngeal swabs as a confirmation of bacterial sinus infection. The authors do not advocate CT scans as a routine test for such patients presenting in primary care.

There was a marked placebo effect; furthermore, the dosage of phenoxymethylpenicillin far exceeds that recommended in the UK. More than half the antibiotic-treated patients (57%) experienced some side effects, compared to 36% of the placebo group.

You wonder what the results would have been if all 240 patients had been recruited into the trial, which would be more representative of a primary care sample. There is no way of knowing to what extent recovery is due to ancillary treatments such as decongestants as the paper does not report the differential use of these.

The trial by van Buchem et al (1997) does not support the use of antibiotics. Patients considered by primary care physicians to have sinusitis had sinus radiographs. The 214 with radiographic abnormalities confirming the diagnosis were randomised to receive amoxycillin 750 mg tds or placebo for a week. All patients were also advised to use steam inhalations and paracetamol if required. Outcomes were analysed on an intention-to-treat basis. Patients and assessors were blinded to treatments.

There were no significant differences between the treatment and placebo groups, either at treatment end, 2 weeks or 1 year. Radiographs had no prognostic value. There were significantly more side effects (28%) reported among the antibiotic compared to the placebo (9%) group. The gold standard for diagnosis would involve a sinus puncture, but this is not feasible in this type of patient population, and therefore not clinically relevant; indeed, on current evidence, neither is radiographic confirmation. The authors refer to other research suggesting that 19% of patients with a common cold without clinical signs of sinusitis have sinus radiographic abnormalities. There was little evidence of local amoxycillin resistance.

The authors did not find any tendency to development of chronic symptoms in either group. They did note that many patients had signs of frontal sinus infection in addition to maxillary sinusitis. They suggest that there is a clinical continuum of acute rhinosinusitis, and that further research is required to assess whether antibiotics may be useful for patients at the more severe end of the spectrum. In the light of these results, they suggest antibiotics should be restricted to patients with symptoms persisting for at least 2 weeks, as 80% get better in this time without antibiotic treatment.

The trial by Stalman *et al* (1997b) also does not support the use of antibiotics. Patients were recruited into the trial on clinical signs and symptoms, according to the diagnostic criteria of the Dutch College of GPs. Of 607 patients presenting with upper respiratory infections for at least 5 days, 192 fulfilled the study criteria and were randomised to receive doxycycline or placebo. This exceeded the minimum number set in the power calculation of 168. All patients received nasal decongestant drops and steam inhalation. Outcome was analysed on an intention-to-treat basis, and involved patient assessment using a standardised pain questionnaire and measures of activity, and a comparison of clinical assessment at baseline, 10 and 42 days.

There were no significant differences between the outcomes of the treatment or placebo groups. At 10 days, 85% of both groups had improved, 60% being completely cured. Both groups included 10% of subjects still complaining of some symptoms at 6 weeks. Of patients receiving doxycycline, 17% reported side effects, compared to 2% of those on placebo. Compliance with treatment was good in both groups, and usage of inhalation and decongestants was comparable between the groups.

The authors conclude that the ancillary treatments were probably more responsible for improvement than any non-significant advantages conferred by antibiotics.

Potential explanations for conflicting results

Differences in the trial results may be explained by the fact that, in a primary care population, there is no practical way to confirm that patients have bacterial rather than viral sinus infection. Furthermore, it is not possible to exclude the possibility that the differential outcomes in the Lindbaek *et al* (1996) trial were due to decongestants or inhalations. It may be that data on the use of these were edited out of the final paper, but it represents an important potential confounder, which is not discussed in their article. One trial I noted on my Cochrane search was that published in German by Federspil *et al* (1997). The abstract confirmed that the trial was randomised, double blind and placebo controlled, and demonstrated a significant advantage in favour of inhalation of essential oils in the treatment of acute sinusitis.

It may also be that a positive diagnosis of acute sinusitis from a CT scan among patients with symptoms includes a greater proportion of those with bacterial infection.

However, the morbidity among acute sinusitis patients presenting in primary care would not justify radiography or antral punches for diagnostic purposes, except perhaps for those referred for specialist care with prolonged symptoms causing significant problems and resistant to routinely available treatments. Standard radiographs were not shown to have any prognostic value in the van Buchem *et al* (1997) study.

Conclusion

Physicians in the UK have been reminded recently of the risks of excessive antibiotic prescribing, resulting in bacterial resistance, unnecessary side effects and adverse reactions. On the current evidence, I will be recommending decongestants and/or inhalations for symptomatic relief to my patients presenting with acute sinusitis. I will reserve antibiotics for those with significant symptoms persisting for at least 2 weeks despite such treatment. However, I await the results of the impending Cochrane review with interest.

This search represented an interesting exercise in critical analysis and review of available evidence. Others may differ in their judgements and conclusions, but I have tried to demonstrate the process I undertook when reaching my conclusions.

Another lesson from this exercise is that it is worthwhile recording important papers such as these in a card or electronic reference management system, so that if copies were not taken at the time, the relevant journals can be rapidly identified. Furthermore, it may be sufficient to record the main findings and critical appraisal within the indexing system. A similar hand searching of indexes may not always be so effective and rapid on other occasions.

Key points

▶ Scan the most clinically relevant journals for useful papers (see Chapter 2). Copy the articles, or note down their details and index them.

▶ Hand search journals if no relevant indexed articles are identified.

▶ Consult secondary sources of evidence and electronic databases to identify evidence, particularly systematic reviews.

▶ Evidence may be conflicting, so develop critical reading skills. Some apparent contraindications may be due to methodological factors.

▶ Consider relevance of evidence to your clinical circumstances.

▶ Symptomatic relief (inhalations, decongestants and analgesia) should be first-line treatment for sinusitis.

▶ Antibiotics should be reserved for patients whose symptoms persist despite at least 2 weeks of symptomatic treatment.

References

Calman K, Moores Y, Wild JR, *et al* (1998). *Antimicrobial Resistance. Department of Health Letter PL/CMO/98/6*. Wetherby: Department of Health Publications.

Federspil P, Wulkow R, Zimmerman T (1997). Efficacy of myrtol standardised in the therapy of acute sinusitis-results of a double blind, randomised, placebo controlled multicentred trial [in German]. *Laryngo-Rhino-Otologie* **76**: 23–27.

Lindback M, Hjortdahl P, Johnsen UL-H (1996). Randomised double blind, placebo controlled trial of penicillin V and amoxycillin in the treatment of acute sinus infection in adults. *British Medical Journal* **313**: 325–329.

Low DE and Jea DMM (1997). 10 days of amoxycillin is effective for acute sinusitis. *Canadian Medical Association Journal* **156 (Suppl 6)**: 1S–14S.

Stalman W, van Essen GA, van der Graaf Y, *et al* (1997a). Maxillary sinusitis in adults: an evaluation of placebo controlled double blind trials. *Family Practice* **14**: 124–129.

Stalman W, van Essen GA, van der Graaf Y, *et al* (1997b). The end of antibiotic treatment in adults with acute sinusitis-like complaints in general practice? A placebo controlled double blind randomized doxycycline trial. *British Journal of General Practice* **47**: 794–799.

van Buchem FL, Knottnerus JA, Schrijnemaekers VJ, *et al* (1997). Primary care based randomised placebo controlled trial of antibiotic treatment in acute maxillary sinusitis. *Lancet* **349**: 683–687.

Williams *et al* (1998). Cochrane database.

▶20

Depression

Chris Dowrick

The questions?

General practitioners and nurses working in primary care could pose a wide variety of questions about depression. They may begin with fundamental concerns about the exact nature of the condition, at what point (and on what basis) we should differentiate between common unhappiness and a formal depressive disorder, and what are the merits of the various available diagnostic categories. They may wish to consider what factors affect their ability and willingness to diagnose depression, including communication skills, the roles and attitudes of patients, the complex relationship between psyche and soma, and the overall effect of the context within which health professionals and patients meet (Klinkman 1997). They may be interested to know more about the natural history of depression, what factors affect it, and the importance or otherwise of their failure to detect depression (Dowrick and Buchan 1995, Tiemens *et al* 1996). They will probably be uncertain about the most appropriate and effective options for treating depression, including the relative advantages and disadvantages of the plethora of antidepressant drug treatments, and the value or otherwise of the expanding range of psychological interventions.

Consensus statements (Paykel and Priest 1992) and discussion papers (Moore 1997) appearing in the *British Medical Journal* or the *British Journal of General Practice* – journals which the majority of general practitioners receive on a regular basis – are helpful methods of getting started on these issues. However, they should be seen as such: as bases for critical reflection, not definitive and final closed positions.

I will concentrate on the two topics that are most likely to be at the forefront of the minds of busy health professionals:

▶ choice of antidepressant medication;

▶ role of psychological interventions.

I will approach these topics in two ways. For treatments that are common and well established, systematic reviews are probably the most valuable and accessible methods of weighing the available evidence, and this is certainly the approach I recommend in exploring the literature relating to the established antidepressant drug groups, namely tricyclics and selective serotonin re-uptake inhibitors (SSRIs). More provisional approaches, combining reviews, discussion papers and direct searches, are needed when assessing the evidence for less established drug treatments – I take the herbal remedy St John's wort as a case example here – and for distinguishing between the various psychological interventions for depression.

Choice of antidepressant

Pharmacological interventions remain the most popular approach to the management of depressive disorders in primary care (Paykel and Priest 1992). The numbers of prescriptions of antidepressants issued to patients with a diagnosis of depression increased by 33% between 1993 and 1995, with a particularly rapid escalation – 133.8% – amongst the SSRIs (Donoghue *et al* 1996). The relative merits of the wide range of antidepressants may be considered in terms of direct efficacy, side-effect profile, and cost-effectiveness.

There is now substantial agreement that the major antidepressant groups, in particular the tricyclic antidepressants and the SSRIs, if provided in adequate doses and for long enough periods of time (Montgomery *et al* 1993) are of broadly equal efficacy – and better than placebo – in reducing the symptoms of major depression.

The best way for the interested practitioner to make his own mind up on this issue is probably not through electronic searches for original studies, since the available literature is voluminous and overwhelming, but rather by reading the published results of systematic reviews and meta-analyses. Some of these are sent directly to medical practitioners in the mail (and therefore run the risk of being binned unread!), while others can be accessed through MEDLINE or EMBASE, using the key words *depression* and *systematic review*.

The first systematic review to address these questions in the UK was the NHS-funded *Effective Health Care Bulletin* (Freemantle *et al* 1993), which cited 64 randomised controlled trials (RCTs) comparing SSRIs with tricyclics and related antidepressants. Copies of this were sent to all general practices in the UK. It concluded that there:

> 'is no good evidence identifying subgroups of patients with major depression for whom SSRIs may be more effective than other cheaper treatments.'

The Drugs and Therapeutics Bulletin, funded by the Consumers Association and posted directly to all registered medical practitioners in Britain, similarly concluded in 1993 that (Anon 1993):

> 'SSRIs are no more effective than tricyclic antidepressants in the treatment of patients with mild to moderate depression, and are much more expensive.'

A more recent meta-analysis by the North of England Evidence-based Guideline Development Project ('Guidelines Group') (Eccles *et al*, 1999), funded by the Prescribing Research Initiative of the Department of Health, found a marginally greater efficacy for tricyclics, equivalent to about one-third of a Hamilton Depression Rating Scale (HDRS) point.

The 'Guidelines Group' also reported substantial agreement about the relative safety in overdose of different antidepressants, with dothiepin being accepted as the most toxic in overdose (1 fatality per 1750 patients treated for 1 year), while lofepramine and the SSRIs are associated with the smallest risk of fatal poisoning (1 fatality for every 59 000–100 000 patients treated for 1 year). The side-effect profiles of each group of drugs differ substantially but the details of each are generally accepted. It is also generally acknowledged that SSRIs are slightly better tolerated than tricyclics, with an overall 4% reduction in risk of drop out reported by the Guidelines Group.

Much of the debate on the relative merits of these groups of drugs has centred around their cost-effectiveness. This debate can be accessed either through the systematic reviews quoted above, or directly by MEDLINE, EMBASE or BIDS searches using *depression* and *cost effectiveness* as key words.

SSRIs as a group cost 5–6 times more than the tricyclic group. Proponents of SSRIs have argued that this cost differential is more than offset by improved compliance and reduced toxicity rates, and by reductions in costs associated with outpatient and inpatient hospital treatments (Jönsson and Bebbington 1994), but the assumptions behind this analysis have been vigorously contested (Anderson and Tomenson 1995, Woods and Rizzo 1997).

Simon *et al* (1996), in a study funded by Lilly Research Laboratories, compared clinical, functional and economic 6-month outcomes of initially prescribing fluoxetine *versus* imipramine or desipramine in a 'real world' situation in primary care clinics in Seattle, Washington. They found fewer adverse effect reports and lower drop out with fluoxetine, but no overall difference in clinical outcomes or quality of life outcomes. They reported total health-care costs to be approximately equal, with higher fluoxetine drug costs balanced by fewer outpatient visits or inpatient medical and mental health admissions. This pragmatic study provides a useful template for further research to ascertain how valid these findings would be in the context of the very different patterns of health-care utilisation in Britain.

The 'Guidelines Group' has undertaken a detailed cost–benefit analysis of direct costs (drug costs, toxicity admissions and notional lives saved) using 'conservative' and 'optimistic' scenarios. It concluded that on either scenario tricyclics should be used as the routine first-line drug treatment for depression in primary care, with lofepramine as a more cost-effective option than an SSRI if toxic effects of the older tricyclics are perceived to be a problem. However, their analysis did not include an assessment of any *indirect* costs related, for example, to loss of employment or increase in child care payments for depressed individuals or their carers.

Systematic reviews such as these are extremely helpful to the interested practitioner, but they cannot be assumed to provide the definitive answer. First, it is always necessary to note who the funding agent may be for such studies, and to factor this in when exercising critical judgement of the conclusions. Pharmaceutical companies are likely to have agendas which are affected by profit maximisation. Government-funded studies are, conversely, likely to be influenced in part by an awareness of the apparently inexorable escalation of NHS prescribing costs.

Secondly, the great majority of the studies referred to here have been undertaken in psychiatric settings rather than in primary care, and it may not always be straightforward to generalise across discrete patient populations.

Thirdly, people who participate in RCTs are likely to be different from the average primary care attender (Ormel and Tiemens 1995). The former tend to have well-defined diagnostic syndromes, accept their diagnoses and are motivated to change. The latter may have ill-defined or atypical depressive disorders, often have co-existing medical problems, are more reluctant to accept a medical diagnosis and are less inclined to comply with treatment regimens. Therefore, it should not be surprising if the outcomes of antidepressant drug treatment in routine general practice are often somewhat less positive than those found in these clinical trials.

St John's wort

St John's wort is a herbal treatment for depression which is popular in Germany and now merits critical consideration by Anglophone clinicians. Since the literature on this treatment is considerably less well established than for the conventional antidepressants, the best approach to the evidence is through discussion papers and direct electronic searches.

An editorial and a systematic review published in the *British Medical Journal* during 1996 discussed the role that St John's wort might have amongst the portfolio of management options available for the treatment of depression. Linde *et al* (1996) have analysed 23 RCTs. Using the key words 'hypericum', hypericin and 'St John's wort', I searched MEDLINE, EMBASE and BIDS and found one further well-conducted German study (Witte *et al* 1995) and a more recent overview (Volz 1997). Taken together, these studies provide suggestive evidence of the efficacy of hypericin when compared with placebo or with standard (usually tricyclic) antidepressants. Nordfors and Hartvig (1997) have reviewed an overlapping set of studies and calculated that clinically significant improvement was obtained in 61% of patients on low-dose treatment (<1.2 mg hypericum) and in 75% of patients treated with a dose of 2.7 mg.

The side-effect profile of hypericum appears to offer advantages when compared with the older tricyclics in terms of safety, patient tolerance and treatment continuation. Linde *et al* (1996) calculate a (non-significant) difference in pooled drop-out rates due to side effects of 4.0% for hypericum and 7.7% for tricyclics, though I am sceptical that the low drop out in both categories would be replicable in pragmatic 'real life' trials. There are no reports of fatal overdose with hypericum. Its recognised side effects – photosensitivity, gastrointestinal symptoms and sleep disturbances – each appear to affect <1% of patients (Woelk *et al* 1994). It would also appear to have fewer side effects than either lofepramine or the SSRIs, although this has yet to be tested by direct comparison. The side-effect profile of hypericum in the longer term, for example if taken for the 4–6 month period recommended for standard antidepressant medication, remains to be investigated.

De Smet and Nolen (1996) have noted that the criteria used to select cases of depression are very variable across these studies, and that none of the reports has described an homogenous group with major depression defined by standard diagnostic criteria. The longest follow-up period for a trial against standard antidepressants was only 8 weeks, and there have been no reported studies of relapse rates. My own electronic searches have found no reports of trials comparing hypericum with lofepramine or any of the SSRIs, and no reported evaluations of the health economic impact of hypericum. These are important limitations and further research is urgently needed to address them.

My interim conclusion from this evidence is that St John's wort is a useful addition to the range of antidepressant treatments, certainly for cases of mild and moderate depression. It is likely to be popular with patients who are interested in 'alternative' treatments, or who are concerned about the side effects of conventional treatments. It is not yet available on FP10 prescription, which means that interested patients need to be advised about the range of possible preparations and strengths. The need to purchase it directly may limit its usefulness for patients on low incomes.

Psychological interventions

The commonest psychological intervention available in primary care settings is non-directive counselling, and to date it has proved extremely difficult to establish evidence for its efficacy (Corney 1992, Friedli and King 1996, Friedli *et al* 1997). This is due in part to the diffuse nature of the intervention and to consequent and legitimate uncertainty either about what the major components of such therapy are or what a successful outcome should be. It may also be the result of methodological difficulties intrinsic to conducting research in this area (Fairhurst and Dowrick 1996). New approaches to randomisation may prove helpful here (King 1998).

The evidence that is available from RCTs, which are to be found primarily through electronic searches for the original papers rather than through systematic reviews, so far favours focused psychological interventions such as cognitive behavioural therapy and, increasingly, problem-solving treatment. For searches on this topic I recommend adding PsychLit to the list of medical databases. Two large NHS grant-funded RCTs into depression for primary care are currently underway, and preliminary results should be in the public domain later in 1999.

Cognitive behavioural therapy (CBT) is the psychological intervention that has been most extensively researched, and the results of these studies have been summarised by Moore (1997): it is effective as a treatment for major depression in psychiatric settings; it is probably effective in primary care, especially in combination with medication; and it is probably effective in preventing relapse.

Problem-solving treatment (PST) is based on the common observation that emotional symptoms are generally induced by problems of living, and it encourages patients to formulate practical ways of dealing with such problems (Hawton and Kirk 1989). It involves six treatment sessions over 3 months, the first of 60 min and the rest of 30 min duration. It is fully manualised and can be taught easily to a wide range of health and related professionals (Mynors-Wallis *et al* 1997).

PST given by a psychiatrist is more effective than 'treatment as usual' by a GP, in emotional disorders with a poor prognosis (Catalan *et al* 1991). When provided by

GPs in the treatment of depressive disorders, it was as effective as amitriptyline and more effective than a combined drug and psychological placebo treatment (Mynors-Wallis *et al* 1995). When delivered by community nurses in a primary care setting, it was equal in clinical effectiveness, but more cost-effective than GP treatment (Mynors-Wallis *et al* 1997).

PST appears as effective as CBT as a treatment of major depression. However, CBT is usually only administered by psychiatrists or clinical psychologists, needs a prolonged period of training and often involves patients in up to 18 sessions of 45 min duration (Scott 1994). Within the spectrum of psychological interventions for depressive disorders, PST may therefore prove to be a more cost-effective alternative than CBT. It requires less training, less specialist qualification and is less time consuming to deliver. It is more generalisable and feasible in primary care settings.

Long-term studies of the outcome of psychological treatments for depression are rare (Shea *et al* 1992, Ludgate 1994, Scott 1996) and non-existent in the case of PST. Given the demonstrable psychological and health-economic benefits of PST in the short term, there is a clear need to ascertain whether or not such benefits are sustained over longer periods of time (Dowrick *et al* 1998).

It remains important for the critical health professional to bear in mind the fundamental methodological problems of researching this topic, particularly the difficulties of defining outcome measures which are both quantifiable in research terms and at the same time meaningful for the subjects concerned. I would refer

---

Key points

▶ Take time to define answerable questions.

▶ Systematic reviews are probably the most valuable and accessible methods of weighing the evidence for treatments that are common and well established, e.g. antidepressants; the available literature will be voluminous and overwhelming.

▶ A combination of discussion papers and direct electronic searches is recommended when assessing the evidence for less established treatments, e.g. St John's wort and psychological interventions.

▶ Evidence suggests serotonin re-uptake inhibitors (SSRIs) are no more effective than cheaper treatments but there is potential for bias in the agent funding research and the type of person who participates in an RCT, and the fact that most studies are undertaken in psychiatric rather than a primary care setting.

▶ Evidence suggests St John's wort is a useful antidepressant, particularly for mild and moderate depression.

▶ Evidence supports psychological interventions such as cognitive behavioural therapy and problem-solving treatment.

▶ There are fundamental methodological problems associated with researching psychological interventions.

readers who wish to consider these questions in more detail to the papers cited by Klinkmann (1997) and King (1998) and also a seminal discussion paper by Blacker and Clare (1987). Qualitative studies are now needed to bridge this gap, particularly of patients' perceptions of mental health problems, and their views of the best routes to take through health and social care agencies. Finally, we do well to remind ourselves of the dangers of the empirical fallacy, that what cannot be measured cannot be valuable, and of the wisdom of Wittgenstein's (1960) response:

'Whereof one cannot speak, thereof one must be silent.'

References

Anderson IM and Tomensen BM (1995). Treatment discontinuation with SSRIs compared with TCAs. *British Medical Journal* **310**: 1433–1438.

Anon (1993). SSRIs for depression? *Drugs and Therapeutics Bulletin* **31**: 57–58.

Blacker C and Clare A (1987). Depressive disorder in primary care. *British Journal of Psychiatry* **150**: 737–751.

Catalan J, Gath D, Bond A *et al* (1991). Evaluation of a brief psychological treatment for emotional disorders in primary care. *Psychological Medicine* **21**: 1013–1018.

Corney R (1992). The effectiveness of counselling in general practice. *International Review of Psychiatry* **4**: 331–338.

De Smet P and Nolen W (1996). St John's wort as an antidepressant [Editorial]. *British Medical Journal* **313**: 241–242.

Donoghue J, Tylee A, Wildgust H (1996). Cross sectional database analysis of antidepressant prescribing in general practice in the United Kingdom, 1993–5. *British Medical Journal* **313**: 861–862.

Dowrick C and Buchan I (1995). Twelve month outcome of depression in general practice: does detection or disclosure make a difference? *British Medical Journal* **311**: 1274–1276.

Dowrick C, Casey P, Dalgard O *et al* (1998). Outcomes of Depression International Network (ODIN). Background, method and field trials. *British Journal of Psychiatry* **172**: 359–363.

Eccles M, Freemantle N, Mason J (1999). J for the North of England Anti-Depressant Guideline Development Group (in press). North of England Evidence-Based Guideline Development Project: Summary version of guidelines for the choice of antidepressants for depression in primary care. *Family Practice*. 16(2) 103–111.

Fairhurst K and Dowrick C (1996). Problems with recruitment in a randomised controlled trial of counselling in general practice: causes and implications. *Journal of Health Services Research & Policy* **1**: 77–80.

Freemantle N, Long A, Mason A *et al* (1993). *The Treatment of Depression in Primary Care. Effective Health Care Bulletin No 5.* Leeds: School of Public Health.

Freidli K and King M (1996). Counselling in general practice: a review. *Primary Care Psychiatry* **2**: 205–216.

Freidli K, King M, Lloyd M, Horder J (1997). Randomised controlled assessment of non-directive psychotherapy versus routine general practitioner care. *Lancet* **350**: 1662–1665.

Hawton K and Kirk JW (1989). Problem-solving. In: Hawton K, Salkovskis PM, Kirk JW, Clark DM (Eds) *Cognitive Behaviour Therapy For Psychiatric Problems: A Practical Guide.* Oxford: Oxford Medical Publications.

Jönsson B and Bebbington P (1994). What price depression? The cost of depression and the cost effectiveness of pharmacological treatment. *British Journal of Psychiatry* **164**: 665–673.

King M (1998). Mental health research in general practice: from head counts to outcomes. *British Journal of General Practice* **48**: 1295–1296.

Klinkman M (1997). Competing demands in psychosocial care: a model for the identification and treatment of depressive disorders in primary care. *General Hospital Psychiatry* **19**: 98–111.

Linde K, Ramirez G, Mulrow C *et al* (1996). St John's wort for depression – an overview and meta-analysis of randomised clinical trials. *British Medical Journal* **313**: 253–258.

Ludgate J (1994). Cognitive behaviour therapy and depressive relapse. *Behavioural and Cognitive Psychotherapy* **22**: 1–12.

Montgomery S, Bebbington P, Cowen P *et al* (1993). Guidelines for treating depressive illness with antidepressants. *Journal of Psychopharmacology* **7**: 19–23.

Moore R (1997). Improving the treatment of depression in primary care: problems and prospects. *British Journal of General Practice* **47**: 587–590.

Mynors-Wallis L, Gath D, Lloyd-Thomas A *et al* (1995). Randomised controlled trial comparing problem solving treatment with amitriptyline and placebo for major depression in primary care. *British Medical Journal* **310**: 441–445.

Mynors-Wallis L, Davies I, Gray A *et al* (1997). A randomised controlled trial and cost analysis of problem-solving treatment for emotional disorders given by community nurses in primary care. *British Journal of Psychiatry* **170**: 113–119.

Nordfors M and Hartvig P (1997). St John's wort against depression in favour again [in Swedish]. *Lakartidningen* **94**: 2365–2367.

Ormel J and Tiemens B (1995). Recognition and treatment of mental illness in primary care: towards a better understanding of a multifaceted problem. *General Hospital Psychiatry* **17**: 160–164.

Paykel S and Priest R (1992). Recognition and management of depression in general practice. *British Medical Journal* **305**: 1198–2002.

Simon G, Von Korff M, Heiligenstein J *et al* (1996). Initial antidepressant choice in primary care. *Journal of the American Medical Association* **275**: 1897–1902.

Scott J (1996). Cognitive therapy of affective disorders: A review. *Journal of Affective Disorders* **37**: 1–11.

Shea M, Elkin I, Imber SO *et al* (1992). Course of depressive symptoms over follow up. *Archives of General Psychiatry* **49**: 782–787.

Tiemens B, Ormel J, Simon G (1996). Occurrence, recognition and outcome of psychological disorders in primary care. *Psychological Medicine* **153**: 636–644.

Volz H (1997). Controlled clinical trials of hypericum extracts in depressed patients – an overview. *Pharmacopsychiatry* **30**: s72–76.

Witte B, Harrow G, Kaplan T *et al* (1995). Treatment of depressive symptoms with a high concentration hypericum preparation [in German]. *Fortschrift Medizin* **113**: 404–408.

Wittgenstein L (1960). *Tractatus Logico-Philosophicus*. London: Routledge Kegan Paul, p 149.

Woelk H, Burkard G, Grünwald J (1994). Benefits and risks of hypericum extract LI 160: drug monitoring study with 3250 patients. *Journal of Geriatric Psychiatry and Neurolology* **1 (Suppl)**: s34–38.

Woods SW and Rizzo JA (1997). Cost-effectiveness of antidepressant treatment reassessed. *British Journal of Psychiatry* **170**: 257–263.

▶ 21

Anxiety

Mark Gabbay

Background

In the practices I have worked in as an academic GP, anxiety was a common presenting problem (amongst patients, not colleagues). Patient management was often apparently less than satisfactory, and their anxiety would heighten my sense of frustration at times. There were often lengthy waiting lists for counselling and clinical psychology appointments, and I sought to avoid the potentially addictive benzodiazepines. I had been taught about the addiction potential of benzodiazepines, an assertion confirmed by my reading of textbooks and papers and attendance at conferences where personal testimony and research findings had also suggested that short acting ones were more addictive than long-acting ones. So this formed the basis of my question.

The question

What is the effectiveness of treatments for anxiety in general?

Search strategy

To get a general feel for the literature, a PubMed search was conducted through the National Library of Medicine web site, searching on:

    #1 Anxiety in ti   9192 hits (ti = title)
    #2 English language
    #3 Search restricted to the past 5 years.

The search was narrowed further by seeking papers that also contained the following terms in the title:

    #4 management in ti   42 hits
    #5 Primary care in ti   33 hits
    #6 Diagnosis in ti   69 hits

Of the resulting abstracts, 22 papers looked interesting. No systematic reviews or randomised controlled trials were identified by this strategy. The management papers were non-systematic reviews and the primary care ones focused on diagnosis and recognition of anxiety, but again without any clear indication in the abstract of systematic approaches to reviewing the literature. The treatment papers were also non-systematic reviews, but the primary care list contained some potentially interesting papers on prevalence, prognosis and co-morbidity. These were not directly relevant to my question, but were of general interest as an aid to understanding the overall picture.

I repeated the search on the Silver Platter 3.11 CD-ROMs, 1993–1997 (1998 being temporarily unavailable), using MESH terms to look for meta-analyses and systematic reviews. This unearthed a meta analysis comparing the addictive potential of long- and short-acting benzodiazepines, and a further meta-analysis of treatments for panic. I widened the search to include panic and agoraphobia, and also searched PsychLit 1996–1998.

I then searched the Cochrane database. Whilst there were no Cochrane reviews, two of the meta-analyses I had obtained were briefly summarised and reviewed in the database of abstracts of reviews of effectiveness (DARE) section.

Search results

This combined search identified a further 18 promising papers and 2 books. It proved much more effective at turning up meta-analyses of treatments, but they had all been into the treatment of panic disorder and agoraphobia. Furthermore, to my surprise, all the relevant journal volumes that were subscribed to by the library (just over half of the total references I was interested in), were actually available. I am not sure whether this is a sign of misdemeanors in past lives, but it is my usual experience when I search for articles that the only missing volume or issue is the one I want. The most shocking finding is that a paper has been ripped out, presumably to save photocopying costs. The pleasure of finding them all on this occasion reduced my anxiety and paranoid phantasies. This may be a suitable therapeutic approach for academics with library anxiety, though I doubt I will find many references to that on a search.

Neither of the books was available in the library, although I was able to borrow them from a colleague, who also recommended another book, just published. However, the loan was on a strict same-day return basis, the result of past borrowers with apparent memory or transport problems, resulting in gaps on the lender's shelves.

I now had a fairly bewildering variety of papers and book chapters.

Making sense of it all

As a first step I read the abstracts of the papers and chapters. I was then able to make an initial judgement as to their relevance and likely quality. My first impression was that the typical primary care presentation would not necessarily fit into the diagnostic definitions outlined in the papers. Also, it seemed that in the USA (where most of the literature was written), long-term benzodiazepines were an acceptable option. As I began to read the papers it was difficult not to become lost in their apparent complexity. I needed to judge their quality as well as their content. It became clear that I would need to tackle the literature in a logical fashion.

I was struggling to obtain an overview of context and approach from reading the meta-analyses I had found, but was reluctant to turn to non-systematic reviews as they were liable to unduly influence my analysis. I decided to read the comprehensive reviews in the books and then return to the journal articles.

The books

The three books available to me provided a reasonably comprehensive overview of the literature on anxiety:

▸ *Handbook of Psychotherapy and Behaviour Change* (Bergin and Garfield 1994). This seeks to summarise the worldwide clinical research literature on the psychotherapies and contains three particularly relevant sections: Behaviour therapy with adults; Cognitive and cognitive-behavioural therapies; and Medication.

▸ *A Guide to Treatments that Work* (Nathan and Gorman 1998). Another book reviewing research literature and containing two relevant chapters: Psychosocial treatments for panic disorders, phobias and generalized anxiety disorder; Pharmacological treatment of panic, generalized anxiety and phobic disorders.

▸ *What Works for Whom?: A Critical Review of Psychotherapy Research* (Roth and Fonagy 1998). This was written following a Department of Health review into the psychotherapies, headed by Glenys Parry, one of the five contributing authors. This is a UK-based book, again providing a critical summary of relevant literature, and has one particularly relevant chapter: Anxiety disorders: phobias, generalized anxiety disorder, and panic disorder with and without agoraphobia.

I will not attempt to provide a detailed summary of the chapters (as it would take much of the book to do them justice), but I will highlight my main conclusions in a brief review of the chapters in turn.

Behavioural approaches

This contained sections on simple phobias, panic disorder and agoraphobia, social phobia, and generalised anxiety disorder. These give a comprehensive review of the research into behavioural therapies for these problems (422 references, the first author of 31 of which was also the chapter author) and the chapter broadly concludes that there is evidence for the benefits of behavioural approaches for all these conditions. It notes in particular the evidence in favour of therapist guided approaches over self-directed interventions, e.g. pre-recorded relaxation tapes are unlikely to be effective in isolation for generalised anxiety disorder. There seems to be good evidence for the benefits of therapist-guided *in vivo* exposure techniques for the phobias, including panic disorder and agoraphobia.

Cognitive therapies

This covers a similar clinical classification as the above. Evidence is provided supporting cognitive therapies for panic disorder (although there have been few studies of the approach for agoraphobia), generalised anxiety and social phobia. This chapter cites 290 references. There is an element of conflict with some of the above conclusions on the efficacy of cognitive approaches, as the authors assert that much of the early research was poorly designed, and did not utilise what would now be considered an appropriate cognitive approach. They conclude that the relatively negative or neutral findings of past research contrasts with more favourable recent studies, and needs to be interpreted with caution.

Psychosocial treatments

The authors grade the strength of the evidence from 160 references, according to internal and external validity, a model recommended by the American Psychological Association. They also grade the robustness of the research according to a framework outlined in the book's first chapter. They conclude that there is good evidence for cognitive behavioural treatments for panic, but that more research is needed into the efficacy of combined psychological and pharmacological treatments. They also cite good evidence for *in vivo* exposure treatments for social and other phobias. Most approaches are better than placebo for generalised anxiety disorder, the combination of cognitive behavioural therapy and relaxation therapies being particularly effective.

Pharmacological treatments

This chapter does not numerically grade the evidence from187 references. The authors conclude that imipramine and clomipramine are effective in the treatment of panic disorder, but that there are fewer studies of alternative antidepressants, particularly placebo controlled studies. Research supports regimens at full therapeutic doses, as lower doses are less effective. The selective serotonin re-uptake inhibitors (SSRIs) are apparently being increasingly prescribed for anxiety disorders, and there is some placebo-controlled trial evidence in favour of fluvoxamine, paroxetine and sertraline. There is evidence that SSRIs are being preferred for their relatively favourable side-effect profile.

Benzodiazepines (particularly aprazolam, which is the most extensively studied) have been shown to be effective for generalised anxiety. Buspirone is also effective and is favoured over the benzodiazepines as it has less dependency and fewer side effects. Sedating antidepressants have also been shown to be effective. The authors therefore conclude that benzodiazepines should be reserved for special cases. Similar conclusions concerning the positive evidence for antidepressants and benzodiazepines were drawn in the pharmacological treatment section of Bergin and Garfield (1994). It would appear that in the USA at least, the decline in benzodiazepine use is a recent event.

UK evidence review

This provides a particularly useful summary of the diagnostic criteria (DSM IV) adopted for the cited research. This makes it clear that much of what might be termed anxiety disorders in UK primary care settings may be sub-threshold for a formal diagnosis: for example, it is important to note that generalised anxiety disorder is defined as excessive anxiety or worry about a number of life circumstances occurring on most days for at least 6 months.

Many patients with anxiety will have more than one type of disorder, or another mental health problem as well. It is clear that the cited prevalence of co-morbidity varies considerably according to the methodology adopted in the various studies. The chapter ends with a series of bullet points summarising the evidence and its implications. Of note amongst these is the conclusion from the evidence that psychological therapies have lower relapse and drop-out rates than pharmacological therapies. An important implication to draw from their review is that interventions should not necessarily be seen as 'curative'. Many patients in a typical clinical setting will relapse or remain impaired to some extent.

Conclusion

Reading these chapters gave me a fairly comprehensive overview of the evidence I was interested in. I still have some misgivings about the literature searches and potential bias – research viewed as important evidence in some chapters was not even cited in others (although it was published sufficiently in advance of the relevant book's publication). No information was given concerning the methodology of the literature searches, and in most cases, no clear or numerical stratification of the strength of evidence was provided. Instead, the authors may comment briefly about certain aspects of the studies as they are discussed. It is clear, however, that much of the research in this field is flawed in various ways, making interpretation and conclusions difficult.

The journals

Turning to the journal articles, my searches turned up three meta-analyses and one critical literature review of treatments for panic disorder:

▶ A meta-analysis of treatments for panic disorder (Clum *et al* 1993).

▶ A meta-analysis of the treatment of panic disorder with or without agoraphobia: a comparison of psychopharmacological, cognitive–behavioural, and combination treatments (van Balkom *et al* 1997).

▶ A meta-analysis of treatment for panic disorder (Gould *et al* 1995).

▶ Interventions for panic disorder: a critical review of the literature (Acierno *et al* 1993).

I also consulted two literature reviews on the long-term outcome of panic disorders as these might aid my decisions on the best approach:

▶ Long-term outcome of panic disorder treatment, a review of the literature (Milrod and Busch 1996).

▶ Systematic review of the outcome of anxiety and depressive disorders (Emmanuel *et al* 1998).

I also found a paper (Ronalds *et al* 1997) looking at factors influencing the outcome of anxiety and depression in UK general practice. Hallfors and Saxe (1993) have published a meta-analysis of the dependance potential of benzodiazepines.

Below I summarise my main conclusions from these papers.

Treatment

Acierno *et al*'s (1993) paper is not a systematic review, and as a consequence their conclusions must be treated with caution. However, it was instructive to read their comprehensive critical analysis of the methodological approaches of the various studies, most of which they considered flawed. Their discussion helped my understanding of the methodological issues to consider when reviewing such research.

Clum *et al* (1993) conducted an electronic search for controlled studies, supplemented by a hand search of relevant journals up to 1990. They noted that their findings differed in some respects from an earlier review they had published, and that this was in part due to their restricting the more recent review to formal controlled studies (and hence more robust evidence).

van Balkom *et al* (1997) built on the work of others, including Clum *et al* (1993), and conducted an electronic and secondary reference search, without applying quality criteria. They accounted for publication bias by adopting the 'fail-safe N' method, which calculates how many negative studies would be required to negate statistically significant treatment effects. This paper is commented on within the DARE database on the Cochrane CD.

Gould *et al*'s (1995) meta-analysis comes out particularly in favour of cognitive behaviour therapy, noting its long-term benefits.

In general, the conclusions of all these reviews concurred with those contained within the book chapters. Many authors also referred to some studies which demonstrated that group therapy as well as individual work could be effective.

Hallfors and Saxe (1993) confirmed my understanding that shorter half-life benzodiazepines have the greatest dependency potential, and that this is likely to outweigh any apparent reductions in side effects or hangover. They also confirmed the dependency of the entire benzodiazepine group, even after relatively short treatments.

Long-term outcome

Milrod and Busch (1996) report on a comprehensive range of studies (another paper reviewed in DARE), and comment on many methodological flaws contained therein. They felt unable to draw firm conclusions and made recommendations about future studies. Emmanuel *et al* (1998) restricted their comments to the most robust eight papers of the 44 they reviewed, from which they concluded that patients with anxiety did worse than those with depression, and those with both worse than either alone.

Prevalence

I noted that the paper by Emmanuel *et al* (1998) was in a recent supplement of the *British Journal of Psychiatry* on anxiety. The supplement also contained a particularly interesting paper by Weiller *et al* (1998) reporting on their study of the prevalence of anxiety disorders presenting in the primary care services of five European countries.

This confirmed my belief that many primary care patients fail to reach the diagnostic threshold of DSM IV despite considerable disability from their anxiety. Disappointingly, their practitioners frequently failed either to recognise their problem or provide treatment. I noted another paper in the same supplement (which I will not cite out of politeness) which discussed a particular recommended treatment approach. Among the 39 references, 21 included one or more of the authors' names. I wondered if they were aware of Selfcite (Craddock *et al* 1996). Among academics, success and departmental funding is dependent to at least some extent on publications, and citation rates.

Conclusion

I am now more confident that, for most patients, a psychological approach to anxiety should be the first-line treatment, the modality of which depends on the type of anxiety disorder. I can also confidently consider antidepressants rather than benzodiazepines as an adjunctive treatment in more severe cases, or for those not keen on adopting a psychological approach. I am also somewhat reassured that my long-held reluctance to prescribe benzodiazepines is somewhat vindicated, and I feel confident in keeping them as a last resort or for special circumstances. It is clear that whilst there is an abundance of relevant literature, there is a relative lack of well-controlled studies with long follow-up periods and robust methodological approaches. There remains considerable scope for further controlled trials, particularly in non-hospital settings.

With this information, and collected literature, I feel better equipped to suggest treatment options with patients. I also feel able to engage in dialogue with colleagues providing psychological therapies to such patients about their approaches, and their relative merits and supporting evidence. This is particularly useful for practitioners employing other professionals or influencing commissioning of such services. However, it also demonstrates that these allied professionals have a substantial literature available to be searched for evidence. Furthermore, even as a GP and psychotherapist with an interest in mental health problems, I found this a difficult process. In future I would seek to work with a colleague, perhaps a clinical psychologist or psychiatrist to help at an early stage. I would recommend that when searching literature in areas outwith your usual reading or expertise, it is wise to seek guidance and support from those more familiar with the field.

Key points

▶ Get expert help when searching for evidence outside your main expertise.

▶ It may be useful to search databases in addition to MEDLINE, e.g. PsychLit.

▶ In complex and unfamiliar cases, books summarising evidence may be particularly useful to gain a feel for the research. Pay particular attention to search methods and grading of research evidence in such reviews.

▶ There is much relevant literature but few well-controlled studies with long follow-up and robust methodological approaches.

▶ The definition of anxiety in most research is inappropriate to most of the anxiety seen in the primary care setting.

▶ The literature supports a psychological approach as first-line treatment for anxiety.

References

Acierno RE, Hersen M, van Hasselt VB (1993). Interventions for panic disorder: a critical review of the literature. *Clinical Psychology Review* **13**: 561–578.

Bergin AE and Garfield SL (Eds) (1994). *Handbook of Psychotherapy and Behaviour Change*, 4th edn. New York, John Wiley and Sons.

Clum GA, Clum GA, Surls R (1993). A meta-analysis of treatments for panic disorder. *Journal of Consulting and Clinical Psychology* **61**: 317–326.

Craddock N, O'Donovan MC, Owen MJ (1996). Introducing Selfcite 2.0-career enhancing software. *British Medical Journal* **313**: 1659–1660.

Emmanuel J, Simmonds S, Tyrer P (1998). Systematic review of the outcome of anxiety and depressive disorders. *British Journal of Psychiatry* **173 (Suppl 34)**: 35–41.

Gould RA, Otto MW, Pollack MH (1995). A meta-analysis of treatment for panic disorder. *Clinical Psychology Review* **15**: 819–844.

Hallfors DD and Saxe L (1993). The dependence potential of short half-life benzodiazepines: a meta-analysis. *American Journal of Public Health* **83**: 1300–1304.

Milrod B and Busch F (1996). Long-term outcome of panic disorder treatment, a review of the literature. *The Journal of Nervous and Mental Disease* **184**: 723–730.

Nathan PE and Gorman JM (Eds) (1998). *A Guide to Treatments that Work*. Oxford: Oxford University Press.

Ronalds C, Creed F, Stone K, *et al* (1997). Outcome of anxiety and depressive disorders in primary care. *British Journal of Psychiatry* **171**: 427–433.

Roth A and Fonagy P (Eds) (1998). *What Works for Whom?: A Critical Review of Psychotherapy Research*. New York: Guilford Press.

van Balkom AJLM, Bakker A, Spinhoven P, *et al* (1997). A meta-analysis of the treatment of panic disorder with or without agoraphobia: a comparison of psychopharmacological, cognitive-behavioural, and combination treatments. *The Journal of Nervous and Mental Disease* **185**: 510–516.

Weiller E, Bisserbe J-C, Maier W, *et al* (1998). Prevalence and recognition of anxiety syndromes in five European primary care settings. *British Journal of Psychiatry* **173 (Suppl 34)**: 18–23.

22

Headache Diagnosis: When is a Migraine not a Middle Class Tension Headache?

Mark Gabbay and Yenal Dundar

Background

Many patients in primary care report a diagnosis of migraine, made by themselves or health professionals. A proportion will be on repeat prescriptions for analgesia, usually combined with an anti-emetic. The introduction of 5-HT agonists suggests that there may be an effective, if somewhat expensive, management option available for patients with confirmed migraine. *Bandolier* published what they dub as a 'Saturday Night Special' review of drug treatments for migraine in November 1996 (downloadable from their web site at http://www.jr2.ox.ac.uk:80/bandolier). This was so named as they had been unable to identify any systematic reviews of the effectiveness of treatments.

We thought it would be interesting to look at the evidence for the classification of headaches. We had been taught diagnostic parameters as undergraduates, which seemed to have been consistent with our postgraduate reading and learning from various sources. The clinical picture seemed less clear cut, with many patients with 'migraine' seeming to have muscular trigger points, pressure on which seemed to intensify their discomfort. It was also common for patients to complain of gastrointestinal disturbance, but with the other descriptors of the headache being more in line with what we understood to be tension-type headaches.

The question

What are the diagnostic parameters for migraine and how evidence based are they?

Search strategy

This was a MEDLINE CD-ROM search, using the Silver Platter 3.11 system (years 1994–1998 inclusive) and was fairly straightforward.

#1 headache in ti	1226 hits (ti = title, hits = number of references)
#2 diagnosis in ti	24 070 hits
#3 #1 and #2	22 hits
#4 #3 and la=english	13 hits (la = language)

Search results

From reading the abstracts, it seemed clear that the key issue was the International Headache Society (IHS) criteria, which were referred to in Migraine classification and diagnosis: International Headache Society criteria (Olesen and Lipton 1994). This paper outlined the history and development of the classification, and focused on the criteria for migraine. The classification was developed by consensus, and is based mainly on patient history and physical examination and, if indicated, tests to exclude 'secondary headache'. The classification was subsequently incorporated into the international diagnostic system ICD 10, and has been translated into a number of languages. It has also succeeded in becoming the common classification for research into headaches. The group developing the classification were likely to see patients with relatively severe migraine, and may therefore not have reflected the pattern of symptoms amongst the breadth of migraine sufferers seen in primary care (Stewart *et al* 1994). A recent paper considered the IHS diagnostic criteria in the light of consequent research into headaches and suggest an updated diagnostic framework (Solomon 1997). These suggestions simplify classification and some are used in the descriptions below. Solomon (1997) also discusses the research into the validity of the criteria, as do Olesen and Lipton (1994).

Another paper on the same subject was Guidelines for the management of migraine in clinical practice (Pryse-Phillips *et al* 1997), which is also available at: http://www.cma.ca/cmaj.

The criteria

Migraine
The two main forms of migraine described are those with and without aura.
The diagnostic criteria for *migraine without aura* are:

A: At least 5 attacks fulfilling criteria B–D below.

B: Attacks lasting 4–72 hours if unsuccessfully or not treated.

C: Headache having at least two of the following characteristics:

1. Unilateral site. Pain can be bilateral in up to 40% of cases and may spread from one side to another.

2. Pulsating quality. Up to 30% of patients with tension headache may have this, and about half of migraneurs have headaches at least sometimes without throbbing.

3. Intensity moderate or severe, sufficient to inhibit or prohibit daily activity.

4. Aggravated by routine physical activity or movement.

D: At least one of the following coincides with headache:

1. Nausea and/or vomiting (as opposed to anorexia, common in tension-type headaches).

2. Photo- or phono-phobia (osmophobia (phobia ofodours) is also highly sensitive and specific to migraine).

As these symptoms may occur with tension headaches as well, it is useful to classify the severity: in migraine it will be moderate to severe.

E: There should be no evidence of associated organic or systemic metabolic disease (secondary headache).

The diagnostic criteria for *migraine with aura* are:

A: At least 2 attacks fulfilling criterion B below.

B: At least three of the following characteristics:

1. The aura is fully reversible.
2. The aura develops gradually over >4 min.
3. The aura does not last >60 min.
4. The aura is followed by a headache in <60 min, but may occur during the headache.

C: As for E in migraine without aura.

The paper by Pryse-Phillips *et al* (1997) also includes a series of supplementary points from the history, and a list of alarm symptoms and signs. It then goes on to outline the evidence-based recommendations for investigation and treatment.

Tension-type headache

A: At least two of the following pain characteristics:

1. Tightening/pressing quality (not throbbing).
2. Mild or moderate intensity, sufficient to inhibit, rather than prohibit, activity.
3. Bilateral.
4. Not aggravated by routine activity.

B: Both of the following:

1. No vomiting or nausea, but anorexia may occur.
2. No more than one of either photo- or phono-phobia.

C: As for criterion E in migraine without aura.

Mention is made of pericranial muscle tenderness as a potential association.

Cluster headache

A: At least 5 attacks fulfilling criteria B–D below.

B: Severe unilateral orbital, supraorbital and/or temporal pain lasting 15–180 min untreated.

C: Headache associated with at least one of the following ipsilateral (to the pain) signs:

1. Conjunctival injection.
2. Lacrimation.
3. Nasal congestion.
4. Rhinorrhoea.

5. Forehead and facial sweating.

6. Miosis.

7. Ptosis.

8. Eyelid oedema.

D: Attack frequency at least every other day up to 8× a day.

E: As for criterion E in migraine without aura.

Conclusion

This was a fairly straightforward search. There is clearly scope for research to investigate the validity and reliability of these headache classification criteria more fully. We have learnt more about the accepted international classification, and the results of this search will enable a more focused approach to our diagnosis and management of migraine. The journal containing the original publication of the classification was not available at any of the regional libraries, and seemed rather long at 96 pages to order from the British Library. The publications we did have readier access to seemed to fulfil our needs as they contained sufficient information to answer our questions. It is of note that the Canadian guidelines (Pryse-Phillips *et al* 1997) were developed at a consensus conference supported by an unrestricted educational grant from a drug company, which manufactured one of the recommended treatments. However, this seems to be a common occurrence, and was clearly stated in the paper, but it does indicate a potential for bias. This would seem to be another area of primary care where good evidence is relatively thin on the ground.

Key points

▶ There is an accepted international classification for headache.

▶ The validity and reliability of this classification needs to be researched more fully.

References

Olesen J and Lipton RB (1994). Migraine classification and diagnosis: International Headache Society criteria. *Neurology* **44 (Suppl 4)**: S6–S10.

Pryse-Phillips WEM, Dodick DW, Edmeads JG *et al* (1997). Guidelines for the management of migraine in clinical practice. *Canadian Medical Association Journal* **156**: 1273–1287.

Solomon S (1997). Diagnosis of primary headache disorders: Validity of the International Headache Society criteria in clinical practice. *Neurologic Clinics* **15**: 15–26.

Stewart WF, Shechter A, Rasmussen BK (1994). Migraine prevalence, a review of population-based studies. *Neurology* **44 (Suppl 4)**: S17–S23.

23

Mastalgia

Mark Gabbay

Background

Mastalgia presents as painful, tender breasts, often with multiple lumps and is common: it is reported to occur in up to 70% of menstruating women at some time in their lives (Holland and Gateley 1994). It may be cyclical (a patient symptom diary is useful here).

Mastalgia commonly presents a clinical management problem. I have heard many differing anecdotal reports of treatment success and failure, varying from adequate bra support (using a sports bra) by day and night to danazol, bromocriptine, and also homeopathy. I have seen a case of worsening mastalgia disappear overnight for at least a year (when the patient left the practice) following a remedy prescribed by a homeopathist. Some patients are unable to tolerate danazol. A clinical meeting on benign breast disease recommended evening primrose oil as the treatment of choice, with the presentation of research to back up this opinion.

Patient experiences of treatments were contradictory, and I remained at a loss when negotiating management options with patients. They often sought referral for the exclusion of cancer (understandably) and, depending on which clinic they attended, either returned relieved but perhaps disappointed at a lack of clear therapeutic recommendation, or commenced on treatment the benefits of which I was not convinced of based on patient experiences. Meanwhile, the women remained in discomfort if I dithered, or were potentially concerned about side effects if I recommended a more potent therapy. Evening primrose oil seemed to be an attractive treatment option and clearly there was a need for me to look at the evidence.

The question

What is the evidence for the effectiveness of evening primrose oil in the management of mastalgia?

Search strategy

I conducted a Silver Platter 3.11. MEDLINE search using the following MESH terms:

#1 Benign breast*	1 hit
#2 Mastalgia	36 hits

#3 Breast tender*	3 hits
#4 Fibroadenoma-drug therapy	2 hits
#5 Fibroadenoma-therapy	7 hits
#6 #1 or #2 or #3 or #5	49 hits

With this number of papers it seemed reasonable to scan the abstracts rather than narrow the search this turned up seven potentially relevant papers, of which three were available in local libraries and four were not (for one of which only the abstract was in English). Looking at the three available papers, only one focused on a review of treatments – Drug therapy of mastalgia: What are the options? (Holland and Gateley 1994), and the abstracts of the other four suggested that they were unlikely to be sufficiently robust in their approach to be worthwhile ordering from the British Library. This was rather disappointing.

I also searched secondary sources (see Chapter 3), and came across a review on evening primrose oil for cyclical mastalgia (report No 65) done by DEC at its Bristol web site (http://www.epi.bris.ac.uk/rd/publicat/dec   Mellanby et al 1996).

Search results

The answers were conflicting. Holland and Gateley (1994) assert that evening primrose oil is of proven benefit; the DEC report suggests that it is not. The positive recommendation seems to be based on one trial, with some supporting scientific evidence. The DEC report looked at five trials, of varying quality. There is evidence of a marked placebo effect, so they did not feel it appropriate to infer conclusions from open trials. Looking only at controlled trials, the authors of the DEC report concluded that there was no proven benefit, and that a robust, randomised controlled, blinded trial was required. Many of the trials their searches uncovered were from non-peer-reviewed journals and/or sponsored by the manufacturers of the drug. This may reflect a potential publication bias.

The main attraction of the drug is its lack of side effects compared to danazol, bromocriptine or tamoxifen. The reported positive benefits of evening primrose oil are supported by some biochemical theory and evidence. However, the clinical benefits are suggested to be potentially due to a placebo effect.

Conclusion

This was a disappointing result. I am not convinced that there is sufficient evidence to recommend NHS prescription of evening primrose oil, particularly as a first-line therapy, for which the cost of treatment is about £150 for a 6-month course. To put this in perspective, the DEC report estimated that prescriptions of such preparations in their local region cost £1 million in 1995/6.

However, the side-effect profile of danazol and bromocriptine may rule them out for a significant proportion of patients, and tamoxifen is not recommended except under specialist supervision for intractable severe cases. The potential risk of virilising side effects, for example, may not be acceptable to the patient, particularly for those few who may have a permanently changed voice with danazol treatment.

If I restrict my recommendation to suggesting that patients may like to purchase their own evening primrose oil at the recommended doses, this will exclude many patients who are unable to afford the costs.

I was unable to find any published trials of homeopathy for this disorder.

The multicentre trial on bromocriptine seemed to have a robust design (Mansel and Dogliotti 1990), except that the outcome was based on a 3-criteria patient symptom assessment rating scale, as too few completed the more sophisticated assessment. The danazol trial was nearly 20 years ago (Mansel *et al* 1982). One cohort study (Euhus and Uyehara 1997) suggested that depot progesterone contraception may be an effective treatment and that further research is needed. So, I look forward to reading of a randomised controlled trial in the future.

Also, the Cochrane database contains a protocol for an ongoing review of evening primrose oil for the treatment of premenstrual syndrome in general, but no results have been published as yet.

The question for me to consider now is the extent to which I can rely on the considered and published opinions of acknowledged international experts working in the secondary sector. The independent evidence does not support the recommendations of Holland and Gateley (1998); although the evening primrose oil approach seems to be relatively side-effect free, most of the benefits may be a placebo effect. It is a fairly expensive placebo, be it for the NHS or the patient. I look forward to a clearer picture emerging from future literature searches and research.

I can now discuss the options with my patients with a clearer picture of the best current evidence to hand, a perspective on the cost implications of these options, and more knowledge about the prevalence and natural history of the disease. In this way I can hopefully make better informed choices, albeit with some uncertainty, but then that is the art of general practice.

Key points

▶ There is a paucity of evidence and what there is is conflicting.

▶ Beware the 'expert review' paper: its reference to and interpretation of available evidence may be biased and subjective.

▶ Secondary sources of evidence are always worth searching (see Chapter 3).

▶ There is insufficient evidence to recommend NHS prescription of evening primrose oil for mastalgia.

References

Euhus DM and Uyehara C (1997). Influence of parenteral progesterones on the prevalence and severity of mastalgia in premenopausal women: a multi-institutional cross-sectional study. *Journal of the American College of Surgeons* **184**: 596–604.

Holland PA and Gateley CA (1994). Drug therapy of mastalgia: what are the options? *Drugs* **48**: 709–716.

Mansel RE and Dogliotti L (1990). European multicentre trial of bromocriptine in cyclical mastalgia. *Lancet* **335**: 190–193.

Mansel RE, Wisbey JR, Hughes LE (1982). Controlled trial of the antigonadotrophin danazol in painful nodular benign breast disease. *Lancet* **1**: 928–930.

Mellanby A, Best L, Stevens A (1996). *Evening Primrose Oil for Cyclical Mastalgia. Development and Evaluation Committee Report No 65*. Bristol: Wessex Institute for Health Research and Development.

▶ 24

Prostate Screening: A Decision Analysis

Aneez Esmail

Background

In considering an evidence-based approach to clinical problems, generalists are frequently faced with the problem that evidence in the form of clear-cut randomised controlled trials is not readily available. Furthermore, the nature of most trials are such that the results are not always generalisable to the individual case for which the clinician is trying to find evidence to help make a diagnosis or decide a management plan.

However, the advent of the Internet and the increasing accessibility to this medium of information exchange is likely to revolutionise the ability of physicians to obtain information which is up-to-date, easily digestible and which can guide their management plan. The availability of information together with techniques such as decision analysis can potentially revolutionise the information which clinicians can use in order to make judgements. I will demonstrate the potential using the example of prostatic cancer screening.

Cancer of the prostate is the second commonest cancer in men in the UK. There were 13 970 new cases in 1998 and in 1992 there were 9 629 deaths, representing 11% of all deaths from cancer in men. Autopsy series have shown that nearly 30% of men over the age of 50 have evidence of latent prostatic cancer even though only 1% of them have clinically important disease. However, 95% of all new cases of prostatic cancer and 97% of all deaths occur in men over the age of 60. The incidence is highest (age adjusted figures) in black (142 per 100 000) compared to white men (108 per 100 000). Prostatic cancer is a common cancer in men and awareness of the condition is increasing.

Mr Smith is 65 years old and has just retired following 30 years in the Civil Service. He has recently read several newspaper articles on cancer of the prostate where it has been suggested that, because it is a very common cancer in men of his age, he should undergo routine screening. He also saw a television programme on the subject when an eminent urologist was arguing for routine screening on a population basis for all men over the age of 50. His main reasoning was that if caught early, suitable treatment could be instituted and the condition cured. Mr Smith is in good health and decided to come and see me and seek my advice on what to do.

The question

Should a 65-year-old healthy man undergo routine screening for prostatic cancer?

Search strategy

I was sent, completely unsolicited, access to a doctors' guide, address http://www.docguide.com/ Using this site as a gateway, I was able to access a disease reference site and through that found *Cancer Net* which is a site maintained by the National Cancer Institute in the USA with up-to-date information on most cancers. Information is provided on the epidemiology of cancer and on evidence of screening benefit. Critically, it provided up-to-date information on positive predictive values for screening for several diagnostic tests, including digital rectal examination (DRE) and prostatic specific antigen (PSA) screening. This information was down-loaded from the web in <5 min.

Search results

From the National Cancer Institute web site on screening for prostatic cancer, the following information was obtained.

There are two widely accepted methods of screening for prostatic cancer. Digital rectal examination has a sensitivity of 55–69%, a specificity of 89–97%, a positive predictive value of 11–26% and a negative predictive value of 85–96%. The other method relies on a blood test for PSA. The sensitivity of this test is 70% with a positive predictive value of 26–52%. I was given a warning that the positive predictive value will vary considerably depending on the prevalence in the population. Mr Smith, the patient who I am trying to obtain information for is, being white, in the low-risk category.

Prostatic cancer tends to follow a slow benign course and survival depends on the stage of the cancer (whether it is confined locally, has spread to regional lymph nodes or has widespread metastases). A population-based study in Scandinavia has shown that 5-year survival in untreated patients with localised disease was 85–92%, while for regional spread it was 68–82% and for metastatic spread was 22–29%. A 9-year survival of 70% has been reported for untreated locally confined disease. Surgical treatment or radiotherapy is usually considered for locally confined disease and can result in complete cure. However, there is an appreciable mortality and morbidity associated with this intervention. Urinary incontinence can occur in 30–60% of cases, urethral strictures and rectal injury are common and sexual impotence occurs in up to 40% of cases. There is a treatment-related mortality of between 2–8%.

The clinical decision

Mr Smith is completely asymptomatic. If I agree to undertake screening by carrying out both a DRE and a PSA blood test, several outcomes could occur. A standard decision tree is outlined in Figure 24.1. I have not included any of the information obtained from the web site in the decision tree. However, drawing the decision tree has already made clear to me the treatment options that I need to consider in Mr Smith's

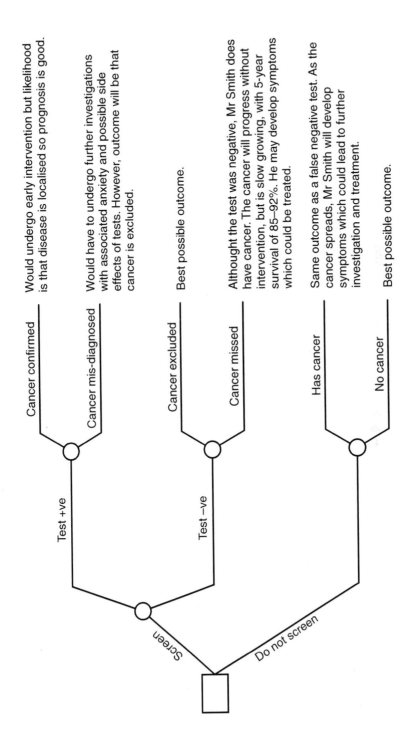

Would undergo early intervention but likelihood
is that disease is localised so prognosis is good.

Would have to undergo further investigations
with associated anxiety and possible side
effects of tests. However, outcome will be that
cancer is excluded.

Best possible outcome.

Althought the test was negative, Mr Smith does
have cancer. The cancer will progress without
intervention, but is slow growing, with 5-year
survival of 85–92%. He may develop symptoms
which could be treated.

Same outcome as a false negative test. As the
cancer spreads, Mr Smith will develop
symptoms which could lead to further
investigation and treatment.

Best possible outcome.

Cancer confirmed

Cancer mis-diagnosed

Cancer excluded

Cancer missed

Has cancer

No cancer

Test +ve

Test −ve

Screen

Do not screen

Fig. 24.1. Should Mr Smith be screened for prostate cancer?

case. Having mapped out the management options I need to have a discussion with Mr Smith as to his own views about the different possible outcomes. In decision analysis jargon, I need to assess Mr Smith's utilities for the various outcomes. However, I am a busy generalist and I present Mr Smith with the following scenario. If I do a test and definitely exclude cancer, then doing the test is the best option. However, if I do a test and find that Mr Smith has cancer, then doing the test would be the worst option, but it would not be disastrous because I may be able to offer treatment. I can tell him that it is a very slow growing cancer and that if he has localised disease the 5-year survival in untreated patients is between 85 and 92%. So I ask Mr Smith to rate the different outcomes as shown in Figure 24.2 on an arbitrary scale from 0 to 1, where 1 is the best outcome of a truly negative test. This discussion where Mr Smith assesses the value to him of the information and/or outcomes resulting from doing a test is very informative both for him and for me.

Using the information that I obtained from the Cancer Net web site and standard decision rules, I can then fill in information. It is beyond the scope of this short chapter to explain in detail how this is done but there are some very useful resources to guide the clinician in simple decision analysis (Richardson and Detskey 1995, Sackett *et al* 1991, Sox *et al* 1988, Weinstein and Fineberg 1980).

Figure 24.3 shows the decision tree with the figures from my researches, best estimates and Mr Smith's utilities included. The junctions represented by a circle indicate a chance node and the boxes a decision node. The probabilities for these nodes are derived by multiplying backwards to the nodes from the end point (where the utility figures are). The chance node probabilities are derived from adding the sums of the probability calculations for each option together. From this you can calculate the

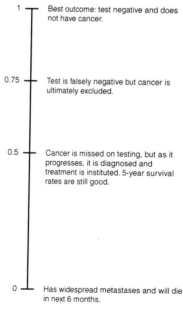

Fig. 24.2. Mr Smith's rating of possible screening outcomes.

decision utilities and get a feel for the relative utility of each decision, in this case whether or not to test. The assumptions of the likely outcome at each junction are derived from the information on tests, prevalence, etc., as explained in Figure 24.3.

Based on the information that Mr Smith has given to me about how he values the different outcomes together with information on positive predictive values for a screening test which includes DRE and a PSA test, I can suggest to Mr Smith that the best decision for him is *not* to have the screening test. In the end the decision is Mr Smith's and I can only advise him, but I can feel that I have done so on the basis of relevant useful information. If as Marshal Marinker says:

> 'The role of GPs is to marginalise danger, explore probability and live with uncertainty'

then I think that I have offered Mr Smith more than the usual 'Well ... perhaps you should and perhaps you shouldn't' type scenario. Using the resources of the Internet to access information rapidly and using simple decision analysis techniques, I would

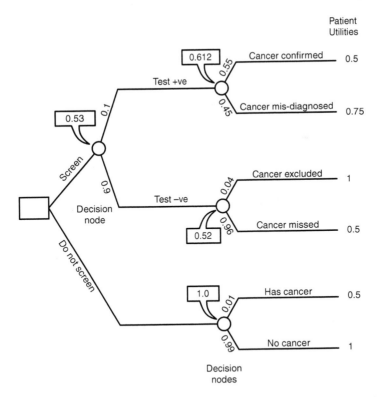

Fig. 24.3. Decision analysis for Mr Smith for prostatic specific antibody and digital rectal examination combined screening. Assumptions: Positive predictive value = 55%; negative predictive value = 96%; prevalence of condition for Mr Smith = 1%; test sensitivity = 97%; therefore total probability of screen positive = 18 per thousand.

argue that Mr Smith has been able to make an informed decision about whether to undergo prostatic screening. My advice based on the simple decision analysis tree (Figure 24.3), was that he should not, and in the end he decided to accept this advice. However, he did so on the basis of information which was almost certainly evidence based.

Conclusion

I could not quite do all the above in one 10 min consultation. I did ask Mr Smith after meeting him for the first time to come back and see me in about 3 weeks by which time I would have had the chance to gather some information and consider the options before discussing them with him. The whole exercise took me about half an hour. The value to me was that in future, when men like Mr Smith come and ask me whether they should have a prostatic screening test, I feel that I can give them an answer based on some form of evidence. Obviously every patient is different and some may value the outcomes differently from Mr Smith but this does not pose a major problem. Most of the calculations can be done with the aid of a calculator and can be altered with different utilities.

Key points

▶ Information in the form of clear-cut randomised controlled trials is not always available directly to underpin decisions in primary care.

▶ Background information is usually available, however, from journals, evidence-based web sites and textbooks.

▶ This information can be used to construct a decision tree to aid decision making and present relevant facts to support negotiated management plans.

References

Richardson WS, Detskey AS for the Evidence Based Medicine Working Group (1995). Users' guide to the medical literature. VII How to use a clinical decision analysis. *Journal of the American Medical Association* **273**: 1292–1295 & 1610–1613.

Sackett DL, Haynes RB, Guyatt GH, Tugwell P (1991). *Clinical Epidemiology: A Basic Science for Clinical Medicine*, 2nd edn. Boston: Little, Brown and Company, pp 139–152 and 238–248.

Sox HC, Blatt MA, Higgins MC, Marton KI (1988). *Medical Decision Making*. Boston: Butterworth-Heinemann.

Weinstein M, Fineberg H (1980). *Clinical Decision Analysis*. Philadelphia: WB Saunders.

▶ 25

Urinary Tract Infections: Test or Treat and How to Treat ?

Yenal Dundar and Frances Mair

Background

Urinary tract infections (UTIs) in adults remain among the most frequently seen clinical problems in primary care. It is estimated that they account for approximately 1.5 million doctor visits and 200000 hospital admissions annually in the UK (Crawford *et al* 1995). Improved management strategies of UTIs could therefore potentially bring about reductions in morbidity and national health care costs.

Age and sex are the well-defined risk factors for acquiring a UTI. In general, the incidence of UTI in adult men is relatively low whereas approximately 50% of women report having had at least one UTI episode in their lives (Barnett and Stefens 1997, Grau *et al* 1997). In a study of university students, the mean incidence of UTI in men was estimated as 5 symptomatic infections per 10000 men enrolled in the university (Krieger *et al* 1993). In a large prospective study of two populations of young sexually active women at a health maintenance organisation and a university health centre in Seattle, Washington, the incidences of symptomatic UTI were 0.5 and 0.7 per person-year respectively (Hooton *et al* 1996). However, the overall prevalence of UTI increases with age for men and women and is nearly equal in the elderly (Lipsky 1989, Nicolle 1994).

The GP regularly has to decide what should be done when confronted by a patient with the characteristic signs of UTI, such as dysuria, frequency, urgency with urination, pyuria and/or haematuria.

Three common approaches to the management of UTI are (MacDonald 1994):

- ▶ treat if the result of an investigation reveals that bacteriological infection is present;
- ▶ treat immediately, ceasing treatment if the result of an investigation reveals that bacteriological infection is not present;
- ▶ treat empirically according to the patient's symptoms and signs.

The question

When a patient presents with characteristic signs of UTI, should we test or treat for UTI?

Search strategy

We decided to explore the existing evidence in this field. Our first step was to establish whether evidence-based guidelines existed.

The web sites listed in Box 25.1 were searched. The key words used were: *urinary tract infections* and *cystitis*, and the former proved more useful.

Box 25.1.   Web sites searched

Agency for Health Care Policy and Research (AHCPR): http://www.ahcrp.gov

Bandolier. http://www.jr2.ox.ac.uk:80/Bandolier

Cochrane Collaboration: http://hiru.mcmaster.ca/cochrane/default.htm

Evidence Based Care Home Page: http://hiru.hirunet.mcmaster.ca/ebm/

Health Information Research Unit: http://hiru.mcmaster.ca/

National Centre for Clinical Audit: http://www.ncca.org.uk

Scottish Intercollegiete Guidelines Network (SIGN): http://pc47.cee.hw.ac.uk/sign/home.htm

---

The Scottish Intercollegiate Guidelines Network web site contained the following two guidelines:

▶ investigation of asymptomatic microscopic proteinuria in adults;

▶ investigation of asymptomatic proteinuria in adults.

However, no guidelines relating to diagnosis and treatment of adult UTI were found using this search strategy.

We next explored MEDLINE using the search terms: *urinary tract infections*, *cystitis*, *diagnosis* and *therapy*. A search of the CD-ROM version for the period 1994 to August 1998 resulted in about 500 references. After limiting our search to those papers relating to adults and in the English language, and excluding articles that did not meet the criteria of applicability, usefulness and relevance, the number of hits came down to about 60 references.

Because systematically reviewed guidelines relating to adult UTI were not identified by this means, we broadened the time period to include the preceding 5 years (1988–1993). This time we accessed an online MEDLINE service. Using the key words *urinary tract infections, diagnosis, economics* and *therapy*, we retrieved 371 papers that were in English and related to humans and selected 53 abstracts to be reviewed based on the criteria outlined above. We also reviewed the reference lists of these papers in order to identify other pertinent research/information in this field. A total of 56 papers appeared to address our clinical question and were obtained for further study. Unfortunately, even this approach did not identify any relevant guidelines.

However, one of the papers (O'Connor *et al* 1996) did identify a guideline addressing the issue of uncomplicated UTI in women which had been produced by the Institute for Clinical Systems Integration (ICSI) in Minnesota. Sufficient information was given to allow the guideline to be accessed on the web. It is posted on the following pages of ICSI's web site: http://icsi.org.guidedev.html and http://www.icsi.org/guideline/chart.html

This guideline was created by a multidisciplinary panel and used the following evidence-grading system:

Grade A: Conclusion based on a randomised controlled trial that has been published in a peer-reviewed journal.

Grade B: Conclusion based on one of the following studies published in a peer-reviewed journal:

> a trial using historical or other non-randomised controls;

> a prospective cohort study;

> a case-control study;

> a meta-analysis.

Grade C: Conclusion based on one of the following:

> an uncontrolled case series;

> expert opinion.

Search results

Approaches to diagnosis of UTI

In everyday practice there is a significant diversity of diagnostic and management strategies for uncomplicated UTI. In order to standardise approaches to diagnosis of UTI and thereby reduce costs, algorithms have been proposed (Hooton and Stamm 1997).

Initial evaluation of uncomplicated UTI is often made on the basis of typical clinical symptoms and signs of infection. The diagnosis is generally confirmed by the presence of pyuria and/or haematuria. Urinalysis to detect pyuria and haematuria is indicated if the symptoms suggest a UTI; however, a definitive diagnosis is confirmed by the identification of significant bacteriuria (Hooton and Stamm 1997).

Tests

Low-power microscopy of a drop of urine and dipstick tests detecting pyuria and nitrites are the most effective and convenient way of diagnosing UTI in primary care practice. In women there is normally no need to send urine samples that do not have significant pyuria for culture. One study of 325 urine samples taken in a general practice to evaluate the practical diagnosis of UTI by various tests showed that in the prediction of a positive culture, sensitivity and specificity of drop method microscopy was 95% and 76%, of leucocyte-esterase estimation 89% and 68% and of nitrite 57%

and 96%, respectively (Ditchburn and Ditchburn 1990). Especially for those who do not have access to a microscope, the combined tests (which detect both nitrites and pyuria by leucocyte-esterase estimation (leucotest)) are helpful in general practice for a rapid diagnosis of UTI (Ditchburn and Ditchburn 1990, Hiscoke *et al* 1990, Carroll *et al* 1992, Jou and Powers 1998). Cloudiness of the urine is not a reliable indicator of UTI (Ditchburn and Ditchburn 1990).

Pyuria is present in almost all women and haematuria in about 50% of those with characteristic symptoms of uncomplicated UTI. Therefore, a urinalysis to look for pyuria can be of great diagnostic value for UTI. Confirmation of haematuria is also important in terms of differential diagnosis as it is not commonly present in women with urethritis or vaginitis (Stamm 1988, Hooton and Stamm 1997). The current consensus is that pre-treatment urine cultures to determine colony counts are unnecessary and not cost-effective in women who have classical symptoms of UTI. An initial culture is unnecessary in symptomatic patients in whom urinalysis results are characteristic of uncomplicated UTI as the therapy is often completed before the results of a urine culture would be available. However, a urine culture should be obtained and further investigation should be considered in patients with persistent symptoms or in those with frequently recurring attacks or symptoms and signs that are suggestive of complicated UTI (Johnson and Stamm 1989, Hooton and Stamm 1997).

In a decision-analysis study, Carlson and Mulley (1985) compared two alternative approaches that included an initial culture for all patients (primary culture) and culture only for patients with symptoms persisting for 2 days after the initial treatment (secondary culture). It was concluded that pre-treatment urine cultures increased the expected cost by about 40% but reduced the overall duration of symptoms by only 10%.

Symptoms and signs of uncomplicated UTI in men are similar to those in women. In a study of otherwise healthy university men (Krieger *et al* 1993), all participants who had symptoms of UTI were shown to have pyuria. In this group the leading symptoms that suggested UTI were dysuria (76%), increased urinary frequency (53%), gross haematuria (42%) and suprapubic pain (13%).

We were unable to identify an optimal, evidence-based diagnostic approach to UTI in men as the number of large randomised studies is limited. However, review of the available data suggests that all UTIs in men should be considered as complicated because of the greater probability of an occult complicating factor. Therefore, routine pre- and post-treatment urine cultures and further investigation are recommended in men with UTI (Hooton and Stamm 1997, Grau *et al* 1997).

Guideline

An algorithmic approach to diagnosing and managing UTI in men was described in a review article of 200 studies by Lipsky (1989). However, this review clearly states that further research is needed for evaluation of appropriate diagnostic strategies for men with uncomplicated UTI.

We identified one evidence-based guideline suggesting the approach outlined in Figure 25.1, which is in line with the evidence presented above based on our literature review. This guideline was used in a study by O'Connor *et al* (1996) based at five

Adult female presents with one or more of the following symptoms:

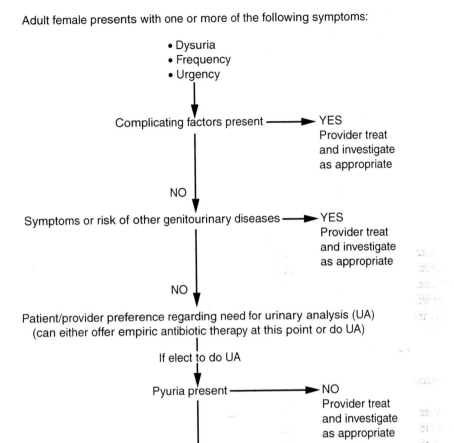

- Dysuria
- Frequency
- Urgency

Complicating factors present ⟶ YES
Provider treat
and investigate
as appropriate

NO ↓

Symptoms or risk of other genitourinary diseases ⟶ YES
Provider treat
and investigate
as appropriate

NO ↓

Patient/provider preference regarding need for urinary analysis (UA)
(can either offer empiric antibiotic therapy at this point or do UA)

If elect to do UA

Pyuria present ⟶ NO
Provider treat
and investigate
as appropriate

↓ YES

Offer short course antibiotic therapy empirically

Fig. 25.1. An approach to the management of uncomplicated UTIs in women (Adapted from a guideline produced by the Institute for Clinical Systems Integration, with permission).

primary care practices of a health maintenance organisation in Minneapolis. The study examined clinical outcomes and costs of care before and after implementation of the ICSI cystitis clinical guideline in female patients with uncomplicated UTI. It was found that use of the guideline resulted in:

▷ a decrease of urine cultures from 70% to 37%;

▷ an increase in the use of the recommended 3-day antibiotic treatment from 28% to 52%;

▷ a reduction in direct care costs for initial cystitis care;

▷ comparable clinical outcomes.

Duration of therapy

Sytematic reviews and studies recommend empiric antibiotic treatment for women with non-complicated UTI. Barry *et al* (1997) found in their cost-utility analysis of office-based strategies that the most cost-effective strategy for uncomplicated UTI in women was empiric antibiotic therapy, regardless of duration. Reviews of published data suggest that 3-day antibiotic regimens are more effective than single-dose regimens. (Rubin *et al* 1992, Hooton and Stamm 1997). Longer courses of a minimum of 7 days' duration are recommended for men with uncomplicated UTI because of possible complicating factors (Hooton and Stamm 1997).

Conclusion

Despite the prevalence of UTIs and their impact on primary care workload, it appears that the evidence base for much of what we do remains inadequate. There appears to be a shortage of high-quality randomised controlled trials on this topic in the primary care setting. Many of the recommendations relating to test or treat issues are based on Grade B or C evidence, which is the best evidence currently available on this subject. It is noteworthy that the suggestions relating to short-course antibiotic therapy are based mainly on Grade A evidence. The current consensus and our key conclusion from the best available evidence is that pre-treatment urine cultures are unnecessary and not cost-effective in women who have classical symptoms of UTI.

Key points

▶ UTIs are common but there is a paucity of high-quality evidence on which to base their management in primary care.

▶ A search of the literature identified an evidence-based guideline for the management of uncomplicated UTI in women.

▶ Pre-treatment urine cultures are unnecessary and not cost-effective in women who have classical symptoms of UTI.

▶ Microscopy and/or 'dipstick' tests for nitrites, leucocyte esterase and haematuria are helpful in confirming the diagnosis.

▶ In women, urine culture should be reserved for complicated UTIs.

▶ Cloudiness of urine is not a reliable indicator of infection.

▶ In men, pre- and post-treatment urine cultures are useful.

▶ A 3-day course of antibiotics for uncomplicated UTI in women is recommended, whereas in men it should be for 7 days.

References

Barnett BJ and Stefens DS (1997). Urinary tract infection: An overview. *American Journal of Medical Sciences* **314**: 245–249.

Barry HC, Ebell MH, Hickner J (1997). Evaluation of suspected urinary tract infection in ambulatory women: a cost-utility analysis of office-based strategies. *Journal of Family Practice* **44**: 49–46.

Carlson KJ and Mulley AG (1985). Management of acute dysruia – a decision-analysis model of alternative strategies. *Annals of Internal Medicine* **102**: 244–249.

Carroll KC, Hale DC, Von Boerum DH, *et al* (1992). Laboratory evaluation of urinary tract infections in an ambulatory clinic. *American Journal of Clinical Pathology* **101**:100–103.

Crawford VLS, McPeake B, Stout RW (1995). Diagnostic regimes for urinary tract infection – are research results applied to practice? *Ulster Medical Journal* **64**: 131–136.

Ditchburn RK and Ditchburn JS (1990). A study of microscopical and chemical tests for the rapid diagnosis of urinary tract infections in general practice. *British Journal of General Practice* **40**: 406–408.

Grau S, Monterde J, Drobnic L, *et al* (1997). Management of urinary tract infections: a comprehensive review. *Pharmacy World & Science* **19**: 236–245.

Hiscoke C, Yoxall H, Greig D, *et al* (1990). Validation of a method for the rapid diagnosis of urinary tract infection suitable for use in general practice. *British Journal of General Practice* **40**: 403–405.

Hooton TM, Scholes D, Hughes JP *et al* (1996). A prospective study of risk factors for symptomatic urinary tract infection in young women. *New England Journal of Medicine* **335**: 468–474.

Hooton TM and Stamm WE (1997). Diagnosis and treatment of uncomplicated urinary tract infection. *Infectious Disease of North America* **11**: 551–581.

Johnson JR and Stamm WE (1989). Urinary tract infections in women: Diagnosis and treatment. *Annals of Internal Medicine* **111**: 906–917.

Jou WW and Powers RD (1998). Utility of dipstick urinalysis as a guide to management of adults with suspected infection or hematuria. *Southern Medical Journal* **91**: 266–269.

Krieger JN, Ross SO, Simonsen JM (1993). Urinary tract infections in healthy university men. *Journal of Urology* **149**: 1046–1048.

Lipsky BA (1989). Urinary tract infections in men – Epidemiology, pathophysiology, diagnosis and treatment. *Annals of Internal Medicine* **110**: 138–150.

MacDonald TM (1994). The economic evaluation of antibiotic therapy: relevance to urinary tract infection. *Journal of Antimicrobial Chemotherapy* **33 (Suppl A)**: 137–145.

Nicolle LE (1994). Urinary tract infection in the elderly. *Journal of Antimicrobial Chemotherapy* **33 (Suppl A)**: 99–109.

O'Connor PJ, Solberg LI, Christianson J, *et al* (1996). Mechanism of action and impact of a cystitis clinical practice guideline on outcomes and costs in an HMO. *Joint Commission Journal on Quality Improvement* **22**: 673–682.

Rubin RH, Shapiro ED, Andriole VT, *et al* (1992). General guidelines for the evaluation of new anti-infective drugs for the treatment of urinary tract infection. *Clinical Infectious Diseases* **15 (Suppl 1)**: 216–227.

Stamm WE (1988). Protocol for diagnosis of urinary tract infection: Reconsidering the criterion for significant bacteria. *Urology* **32 (Suppl)**: 6–12.

►26

Helicobacter Pylori

Mark Gabbay and Yenal Dundar

Background

We qualified at around the time when general surgical lists were likely to include at least one vagotomy and pyloroplasty for peptic ulcer problems. There was interest in the effects of H_2 antagonists on the clinical course of the disease, and new ones were being developed. As our careers continued, peptic ulcer recurrence became an increasing issue, despite the new pharmacological therapies. Many practices today will have proton pump inhibitors (PPIs) high on their list of the top 20 drugs prescribed in terms of costs. In the UK in 1997, £279 million was spent on PPIs. The clinical and economic arguments concerning the 'bottom up' or 'top down' approach to treating dyspepsia are a hotly debated topic (see Eggleston *et al* 1998, and subsequent letters in November and December issues of *Gut*).

Helicobacter pylori infection has assumed an increasing profile in recent years. Issues for debate concern which patients should have an eradication treatment, what regimens should be adopted to do so, and what investigations if any should be conducted in patients suspected clinically of having dyspepsia.

The questions

These grew as we began to try and research a single question:

In a young male of 36 years with probable peptic ulcer, is the treatment of choice a 1-week triple eradication therapy, or should a course of acid suppression therapy be tried first and, as a supplementary question, what tests, if any should be performed?

In trying to pick this out into potentially answerable questions from the evidence we drew up the following list:

► What is *H. pylori* and what is its relationship to gastric and duodenal disease?

► Who should be tested for *H. pylori*, and is it justified as a screening test? Are there any preferences for the types of investigations that should be conducted for dyspepsia, and in which patients?

► Who should be given eradication therapy, and what regimen should we use?

This is a large number of questions and therefore rather outwith the usual evidence-based approach. In writing this chapter we set out to cover areas of uncertainty in clinical practice, as opposed to individual questions. Consequently, the literature coverage is potentially enormous, and liable to be a rather gargantuan task. The rest of the chapter serves to illustrate what you can let yourself in for if you try to bite off rather more than a mere mortal with few resources can chew! Enough to give you ulcers perhaps? It serves to illustrate why evidence searchers should seek to tackle single questions.

Search strategy

The first places we decided to look for guidelines were *Bandolier* and Scottish Intercollegiate Guidelines Network (SIGN): both these electronic ventures proved fruitful. *Bandolier* has a number of review articles on *Helicobacter*, some of which were relevant to each of the questions we posed. Many of them were published 3 or 4 years ago, however. SIGN has some relatively recent guidelines (1996).

Our early optimism was perhaps unfounded and we decided to look at MEDLINE as well. We used the National Library of Medicine web site to search using the Grateful Med search facility and words in title as our criteria, as this is the strategy likely to be used by many readers without easy access to a more sophisticated search engine. This facility has the advantage of accessing the complete MEDLINE database back to 1966.

We searched on:

Helicobacter pylori in title   5 935 hits

We added filters of English language and past 5 years only. We then narrowed the search by limiting papers to those having an additional word in the title. We obtained:

108 hits for diagnosis (with 7 promising abstracts);
48 hits for testing (with 5 promising abstracts);
41 hits for management (with 10 promising abstracts).

We were looking for systematic reviews or randomised controlled trials (RCTs), but many papers seemed to be non systematic reviews or opinion papers.

We also conducted a search at the local university library, using Silver Platter MEDLINE CD-ROMs and confined to 1996 and 1997 (1998 was unavailable). We used this as a worked example with our local medical librarian. We decided to use a MESH term search, limiting publication types.

#1 Helicobacter pylori infections as single MESH search term

This was then limited to include only the following sub-headings:

Diagnosis
Drug therapy
Economics
Epidemiology
Prevention and control
Therapy
This yielded 946 hits. We then added the following limiters:

#2 #1 and la=english   776 hits (la = language of paper)
#3 #2 and tg=human   749 hits (limits references to human research only)

We then tried to limit our search according to the type of paper, which is classified in the 'pt' (publication type) field. We looked at a proportion of the records to get a feel for the sorts of descriptors likely to be useful, and then limited the search according to the publication type descriptors we settled on as being most relevant. This reduced our list to 108 hits described as meta-analyses, systematic reviews and trials, including a variety of sub-categories. Among these, eight seemed to be promising judging by the abstracts.

We also looked at the cross-references in the papers we obtained, and contacted local experts who were able to give us access to systematic reviews of the literature in progress.

It would be tedious to list all the papers in detail, so we will try and summarise the key references, and the conclusions we were able to draw.

Search results

General background to *Helicobacter*

Searching through the material at the *Bandolier* web site (http://www.jr2.ox.ac.uk:80/bandolier), we discovered reviews dating back to 1994 concerning *H. pylori*. The articles titled '*H. pylori* – background', and 'Focus on *H. pylori*', summarise the biological details, the evidence for its implication in causing gastritis, peptic ulcer and gastric cancer, plus brief summaries of the evidence (at that time) about eradication and testing.

Our search highlighted the review paper – Role of *Helicobacter pylori* in gastrointestinal disease: implications for primary care of a revolution in management of dyspepsia (Delaney 1995). Although not a formal systematic review, this sought to summarise the evidence of relevance to primary care at that time (1994). It highlights that much of the available evidence was based on secondary sector research, and therefore may not always be readily applicable in primary care.

The *Bandolier* pages were easy to download and print out, and Delaney's (1995) article was readily available. It does seem clear that whilst *H. pylori* is clearly implicated in causing peptic ulceration, its association with prolonged gastritis is less certain.

We also looked at a variety of abstracts and papers identified from our searches to bring us more up to date. The picture seems to be similarly confused in respect of gastric cancer: whilst there is epidemiological evidence for an association, there is no clear evidence that eradication is likely to be a useful primary prevention strategy (Barbezat 1998).

Danesh and Peto (1998) conducted a meta-analysis which failed to demonstrate any clinically significant association between *H. pylori* infection and coronary heart disease.

There are suggestions that *H. pylori* may protect against oesophageal reflux. It is postulated that the ammonia secreted by the bacteria protects the oesophagus from excess acid (Labenz *et al* 1997). It is suggested that particular strains may protect against oesophageal cancer, so to eliminate infection where the evidence of effectiveness is lacking, may increase the risk of subsequent serious disease (Blaser 1998, Chow *et al* 1998).

It would seem prudent to continue to look periodically for systematic reviews summarising the evidence about the relationship between *H. pylori* and other diseases.

Testing for *H. pylori* in primary care

The current hot debating topic would seem to be what tests, if any, are appropriate for patients presenting with dyspepsia of unknown aetiology? Which patients should be referred for endoscopy? Because of the potential of gastric cancer in the over 45s, it is clear that all new patients in this category should be endoscoped; the evidence surrounding the under 45s remains contradictory.

The literature seems clearly to favour gastroscopy over barium meals. Similarly, whilst the evidence seems to be against near-patient testing for *H. pylori*, due to its relatively low specificity and sensitivity rates compared to laboratory serological tests (Loy *et al* 1996, Anon 1997), the relative benefits of laboratory serological testing, endoscopic biopsies or breath tests remain matters for debate. It does seem clear that after an eradication treatment, only those who remain symptomatic or are in high-risk categories (e.g. history of bleeding or perforation) should have either a breath test or endoscopy (if not already done) to confirm eradication or ongoing disease (Phull *et al* 1996).

The searches identified an interesting discussion paper which we were able to find in the local library, outlining the controversy about testing and eradication in primary care – Testing for *Helicobacter pylori* in primary care: trouble in store? (Foy *et al* 1998). This paper challenges, with apparent justification, the growing received wisdom that all those testing positive for *H. pylori* in primary care should have eradication therapy. The research supporting such an approach has been based in secondary care, where the clinical epidemiology is likely to be considerably different from that pertaining in a primary care setting. Far from reducing endoscopies, the suggestion is that it may increase the need for these in secondary care, and to treat without endoscopy will mean that only the 1:4 *H. pylori*-positive patients who have ulcer dyspesia will be successfully treated. It would seem prudent to await further elucidation of the role of *H. pylori* as a causative, and perhaps protective, agent in disease aetiology.

A cost-effectiveness paper by Briggs *et al* (1996) caused much controversy as demonstrated by the letters pages of the *British Medical Journal* on September 7th of the same year. We are not sure whether the evidence helps us decide whether eradication and treatment is necessarily cost-effective in primary care, but the balance seems to indicate that any savings will take some time to accrue. This may be a good subject for the primary care group to look at in the next year or two, by when hopefully a clearer picture will have emerged from the evidence.

Some preliminary prospective primary care-based research has been conducted (Rosengren and Polson 1996, Hippisley-Cox and Pringle 1997). A recent *British*

Medical Journal editorial (Rauws and Van der Hulst 1998) suggested that patients with uncomplicated peptic ulcer who are under 45 should be entirely managed in primary care by means of *H. pylori* eradication without endoscopy. Commenting on the National Institute of Health (1994) guideline recommendation that all peptic ulcer patients should be tested for *H. pylori* prior to eradication, Greenberg *et al* (1995) argue that the likely 10% false negative rate of even the invasive tests, and their cost, suggests that those with a clear history should proceed to eradication without testing (unless they have additional risk factors).

It is clear that patients over 45 and those with more sinister symptoms, such as bleeding, anaemia, weight loss, dysphagia, palpable mass, etc., should have an endoscopy, and this should be prioritised in those thought to be most at risk of a sinister lesion (alarm symptoms). The problems with the sensitivity and specificity rates of the serological tests for *H. pylori*, and the arguments against blanket endoscopy, suggest that it would be a reasonable approach, based on current evidence, to proceed to eradication without further tests in other patients known to have peptic ulcers.

Eradication regimens

It is of course important to eliminate NSAID use as a causative factor of dyspeptic symptoms. What is clear from our endeavours is that patients with proven, unresolved peptic ulceration should have eradication therapy, if whatever test has been done proves to be positive for *H. pylori*. You may prefer to omit *H. pylori* testing for patients in this category for whom the diagnosis is clear (e.g. under 45s). This will depend on how you interpret the available evidence and apply it to your local circumstances.

It is clear that evidence-based medicine cannot always provide clear-cut answers and can result in a plethora of questions and uncertainty, almost leaving you wishing you had not started. However, it can clarify the issues, and point out where to concentrate enquiries. Either by future searches or focused reading, we should continue to seek further evidence to answer our questions about *H. pylori*. We would hope to see results from primary care-based RCTs of eradication and economic studies as a minimum.

At least we are clear that the group of *H. pylori*-positive patients with recurrent symptoms from proven peptic ulceration should be treated, and that triple therapy is better than double therapy. One-week triple therapy regimens have acceptable success rates in the literature. Which of the regimens to use remains more controversial, and we hesitate to come down in favour of a Bismuth, proton-pump inhibitor or H_2 antagonist-based acid suppression therapy approach. It does seem clear that two antibiotics are better than one, and that metronidazole resistance, which varies, can be at least partly mitigated by concurrent acid suppression. As pragmatic primary care clinicians, we need to consider the regimen most likely to be complied with by our patients, as if patients cannot tolerate the medication, clinical success and any potential prescribing savings will be compromised.

Our search indicated the systematic review – Eradication of *Helicobacter pylori*: an objective assessment of current therapies (Penston and McColl 1997). This reviewed the 352 studies that met the inclusion criteria among over 1 500 considered, up to October 1995. Their conclusion favoured low-dose proton-pump inhibitor-based triple therapy, balancing effectiveness, cost and patient acceptability. At that time there was little published data on H_2 antagonist regimens.

We should be able to reduce long-term acid suppression therapy for patients with a proven ulcer by eradicating *H. pylori*, which the evidence clearly supports. It is also clear that there is little evidence for eradication for patients with non-ulcer dyspepsia.

Guidelines

We came across a few evidence-based and consensus guidelines. SIGN has one on its web site dating from 1996. These guidelines clearly outline and quantify the strength of evidence supporting its recommendations.

In 1997, the Maastricht consensus report (European *Helicobacter Pylori* Study Group 1997) was published, summarising a conference on the management of *H. pylori*. This is fairly comprehensive but gives no clear indication of a systematic evidence review:

> *'Reviews of the latest knowledge in the area were provided by experts in the relevant fields of research before a series of key management questions were posed.'*

This publication resulted in some controversy, e.g. see Heatley (1997), although his views were strongly rebutted in the letters section of the same journal. In the USA, guidelines on *H. pylori* have been published by the National Institute of Health (1994), and on the medical treatment of peptic ulcer disease by the American College of Gastroenterology (Soll 1996). The conclusions of all these guidelines are reasonably consistent, both with each other, and with the findings outlined in this chapter.

Another interesting guideline is that produced by the International Gastro Primary Care Group (Whitaker 1998). This guideline is evidence based and supported by economic models (Haycox *et al* 1998, Duggan 1998, Tosetti and Stanghellini 1998).

Conclusion

The questions remain without definitive answers. Many of the papers we wanted required inter-library loans, a task unlikely to be welcomed by most amateur evidence hunters, stretching both budget and enthusiasm. Furthermore, some of these were subject to lengthy waiting times, and another came with the middle pages missing. Such are the occasional frustrations of retrieving evidence.

There seems to be a clear need for more prospective research (which is likely to be underway) and systematic reviews. Many of the reviews we read were not systematic and therefore it is difficult to rely on their conclusions. Many of the trials seem contradictory, and the more we read, the less clear were our conclusions. We are now fairly convinced that there is good evidence for eradicating *H. pylori* in patients with recurrent ulcer dyspepsia. In primary care it may be reasonable to manage patients with no alarm symptoms and below the age of 45 by eradication of *H. pylori* without confirmatory testing. Patients over 45, or with alarm symptoms however should be prioritised for endoscopy, unless recently done. A 1-week eradication course of acid suppressant plus two antibiotics is probably the best balance between cost, outcome and patient acceptability and thus compliance. We should on balance resist *H. pylori* screening and blind eradication in those without proven ulcer dyspepsia. If symptoms resolve there is little justification for testing for eradication.

We cannot help feeling that we must have missed something somewhere, as the evidence seems often contradictory and confusing. This, however, is perhaps an excellent example of the challenge of evidence-based practice, and of the need for caution. Relying on abstracts alone would probably have led us to erroneous conclusions, and this is not a subject area where you can settle on one or two reviews and feel satisfied that the best evidence has been obtained. We are clearly in the territory of the systematic review, as there are many factions in the field, pharmaceutical and professional, with differing agendas, and a great potential for bias and confusing controversy.

We hope we have clarified the issues a little, and put this subject up as a challenge for your searching and critical analysis skills, but would not recommend it as a place to start.

Key points

▶ Developing clinical issues may prompt a variety of questions.

▶ When searching for evidence, aim to answer single questions.

▶ Beware of relying on abstracts.

▶ Good quality systematic reviews, if available, are useful for complex issues.

▶ Evidence may be difficult to track down and may not be available in local postgraduate or even university libraries.

▶ Many of the trials on *H. pylori* are contradictory and there is a need for more prospective research and systematic reviews in this area, particularly with relevance to primary care.

▶ The relationship between *H. pylori* and peptic ulceration is clear, but less certain for prolonged gastritis and gastric cancer.

▶ Patients with proven recurrent peptic ulceration should have eradication therapy; there is little evidence for eradication therapy for those with non-ulcer dyspepsia.

▶ There is little evidence to justify screening for *H. pylori* in those without proven ulcer dyspepsia.

References

Anon (1997). *Helicobacter pylori* testing kits. *Drugs and Therapeutics Bulletin* **35**: 23–24.

Barbezat GO (1998). Recent advances in gastroenterology *British Medical Journal* **316**: 125–128.

Blaser MJ (1998). *Helicobacter pylori* and gastric diseases. *British Medical Journal* **316**: 1507–1510.

Briggs AH, Sculpher MJ, Logan RPH, *et al* (1996). Cost effectiveness of screening for and eradication of *Helicobacter pylori* in management of dyspeptic patients under 45 years of age. *British Medical Journal* **312**: 1321–1325.

Chow WH, Blaser MJ, Blot WJ *et al* (1998). An inverse relation between cagA+ strains of *Helicobacter pylori* infection and the risk of oesophageal and gastric cardia adenocarcinoma. *Cancer Research* **58**: 588–590.

Danesh J and Peto R (1998). Risk factors for coronary heart disease and infection with *Helicobacter pylori*: meta-analysis of 18 studies. *British Medical Journal* **316**: 1130–1132.

Delaney BC (1995). Role of *Helicobacter pylori* in gastrointestinal disease: implications for primary care of a revolution in management of dyspepsia. *British Journal of General Practice* **45**: 489–494.

Duggan AK (1998). Modelling different approaches to the management of upper gastrointestinal disease. *PharmacoEconomics* **14 (Suppl 2)**: 25–37.

Eggleston A, Wigerinck A, Huijghebaert S, *et al* (1998). Cost effectiveness of treatment for gastro-oesophageal reflux disease in clinical practice: a clinical database analysis. *Gut* **42**: 13–16.

European *Helicobacter Pylori* Study Group (1997). Current European concepts in the management of *Helicobacter pylori* infection. The Maastricht consensus report. *Gut* **41**: 8–13.

Foy R, Parry JM, Murray L, *et al* (1998). Testing for *Helicobacter pylori* in primary care: trouble in store? *Journal of Epidemiology and Community Health* **52**: 305–309.

Greenberg PD, Koch J, Cello JP (1995). Clinical utility and cost effectiveness of *Helicobacter pylori* testing for patients with duodenal and gastric ulcers. *American Journal of Gastroenterology* **91**: 228–232.

Haycox A, Butterworth M, *et al* (1998). Development of an economic model for the management of upper gastrointestinal disease in primary care: preliminary findings. *PharmacoEconomics* **14 (Suppl 2)**: 11–23.

Heatley RV (1997). Dual publication. *Gut* **41**: 595–596.

Hippisley-Cox J and Pringle M (1997). A pilot study of randomised controlled trial of pragmatic eradication of *Helicobacter pylori* in primary care. *British Journal of General Practice* **47**: 375–377.

Labenz J, Blum AL, Bayerdörffer E, *et al* (1997). Curing *Helicobacter pylori* infections in patients with duodenal ulcer may provoke reflux oesophagitis. *Gastroenterology* **112**: 1442–1447.

Loy CT, Irwin CM, Katelaris PH, *et al* (1996). Do commercial kits for *Helicobacter pylori* infection differ in accuracy? A meta-analysis. *American Journal of Gastroentorology* **91**: 1138–1144.

National Institute of Health Consensus Development Panel (1994). *Helicobacter pylori* in peptic ulcer disease. *Journal of the American Medical Association* **272**: 65–69.

Penston JG and McColl KE (1997). Eradication of *Helicobacter pylori*: an objective assessment of current therapies. *British Journal of Clinical Pharmacology* **43**: 223–243.

Phull PS, Halliday D, Price AB, *et al* (1996). Absence of dyspeptic symptoms as a test for *Helicobacter pylori* eradication. *British Medical Journal* **312**: 349–350.

Rauws EAJ and Van der Hulst RWM (1998). The management of *H. pylori* infection. *British Medical Journal* **316**: 162–163.

Rosengren H and Polson RJ (1996). The role of screening for *Helicobacter pylori* in patients with duodenal ulceration in the primary care setting. *British Journal of General Practice* **46**: 177–179.

Soll AH for the Practice Parameters Committee of the American College of Gastroenterology (1996). Medical treatment of peptic ulcer disease. Practice guidelines. *Journal of the American Medical Association* **275**: 622–629.

Tosetti C and Stanghellini V (1998). Management of dyspepsia in general practice: a critical assessment. *PharmacoEconomics* **14 (Suppl 2)**: 57–66.

Whitaker MJ (1998). Consensus guidelines for evaluating and treating patients with upper gastrointestinal symptoms in the primary care setting. *PharmacoEconomics* **14 (Suppl 2)**: 5–10.

▶27

The Trouble with Head Lice

Mark Gabbay and Peter Fink

Background

Conversations about problems of patients presenting with head lice and nits are becoming increasingly common in various practice settings. Indeed it has even been a recent regular agenda item at the local medical committee. The issues seem to be:

▶ Patients seeking appointments for NHS prescriptions of insecticides to treat lice and nits: they often see this as an emergency, as their children are excluded from school if infested.

▶ The suggestion that all members of the family should be treated. NHS prescribing regulations stipulate separate prescriptions for each family member, which presents additional workload to the practice and greater cost to the patients.

▶ Patients' and professionals' concerns about the safety and effectiveness of available treatments.

▶ An apparent plethora of sometimes conflicting advice from various sources including health and education professionals and institutions.

▶ A suspicion that few patients actually follow the recommended treatment regimens.

When these issues were discussed at the committee, different opinions were often expressed.

The question

What are the current official recommended approaches and what evidence is there for the effectiveness and safety of the management options?

Once we had a clearer view of the evidence and the extent to which this matched up with any local or national guidelines, it would be easier to decide on a local strategy and innovation (if any).

Search strategy

We contacted the local public health department for a copy of the latest national treatment guidelines.

We also conducted a MEDLINE (Silver Platter 3.11) search using the following criteria for the years 1992–1998:

#1: head in ti	6299 hits (ti = title)
#2: lice in ti	88 hits
#3: #1 and #2	24 hits
#4: headlice in ti	2 hits
#5: pediculosis in ti	31 hits
#6: #3 or #4 or #5	54 hits
#7 #6 and la=english	42 hits

The abstracts for all these papers were then reviewed and one recent paper was noted which looked promising – Systematic review of clinical efficacy of topical treatments for head lice (van der Stichele *et al* 1995). The listing included four letters in response to the cited systematic review (Burgess 1995, Stallbaumer and Ibarra 1995, Dixon *et al* 1995, Laekeman 1995). All of these were readily obtained from the library.

The other potentially interesting references seemed to be preliminary trials or non-systematic reviews, and as they were not readily available, it seemed unreasonable to order them from remote libraries. Clearly, when conducting electronic searches you are reliant on the accuracy of the cataloguing, and that the titles, key words and abstract content of papers accurately reflect their content and methodological approach. Your approach to the results of such a search, and indeed the methods of conducting a search are dependent on its goal. For our purposes of searching for best evidence, the approach we took is a reasonable one, but is in no way systematic or comprehensive. However it provided us with a reasonable starting point. We were also fortunate in the information forwarded to us from Public Health – Head lice, report for consultants in communicable disease control (Aston *et al* 1998). This report has been made available on the web at: http://www.famenglish.demon.co.uk/phmeghl.htm The report's advisor is cited as Ian Burgess, an author of one of the *British Medical Journal* letters responding to the systematic review we had noted in our MEDLINE search. It seemed we had enough material to start searching for evidence.

We also came across a recent article in our general reading – Treating head louse infections (Anon 1998).

Search results

The systematic review

After reading through the systematic review to ensure it was relevant for our purposes, we then needed to judge if it was reliable (see Chapter 2).

The authors clearly identify the types of papers they were seeking (trials of topical treatments for head lice where scalp inspection was the clinical outcome measure). They identified the MESH keywords used in their searches and the databases searched. They did not restrict the language of publication, and searched for further relevant references from those listed within the papers identified. They contacted 7 'key authors', pharmaceutical companies and a relevant World Health Organization group to seek unpublished trials (to attempt to correct for publication bias). They also conducted hand searches of journals where key references had been published for a year after publication for relevant comments, letters or corrections.

They did not hand-search back issues of potentially relevant journals and books, as they did not believe there was a clearly identifiable group of journals likely to contain relevant material. They did not seek a list of references from the leading researchers and writers in the field, a strategy that has been recommended following a successful trial of such an approach (McManus *et al* 1998).

On balance their search strategy was clearly laid out and seemed reasonably comprehensive. The authors' subsequent published responses to comments on their paper indicated that they had not been notified since the review's publication of any trials that their search had failed to identify.

The authors clearly stated their justification for adopting the chosen clinical outcome. They also clearly identified their quality criteria and how they were derived. Indeed, sufficient detail of these processes was given to enable others to write to the journal criticising aspects of their approach and thus widen the debate. We leave it for interested readers to review the paper and subsequent correspondence for themselves and to form their own judgements.

It is clear that the extent and quality of evidence in this area is disappointing. As one may expect, the authors' conclusions were as a consequence more contentious in the absence of clear, robust research findings. However, the information in the review was relevant to our initial question about current best evidence on management of head lice, at least in respect of topical insecticidals.

The writer of the letter criticising the conclusions of the weighting of the literature review (Burgess) claimed to have conducted one of his own. It was thus possible to contact him to see if his review was published. Following a conversation with a nurse at the entomology centre where he works, it became clear that a further, as yet unpublished, trial were being undertaken, and a list of available literature was sent to us, along with the report of a recent workshop on insecticidal resistance in head lice. A Cochrane review is also being conducted by this group, but was not available at the time of writing.

The public health report

This was wider and more practical in its scope, and asserts that there are many gaps in the research. However, the readers have to take the authors' conclusions on trust as no list of references or supporting evidence is provided. The report makes interesting reading and stresses the importance of treating only professionally verified infestations (observed viable lice), and cautions against relying on second-hand information (the common presentation clinically) or treatment of eggs (nits) in the absence of live lice. This information is also useful to inform our debates, and does seem to outline a reasonable and common sense approach in the current environment of limited supporting research.

Drug and Therapeutics Bulletin

This journal seeks to provide independent reviews of treatment options, and is published by the Consumer's Association for doctors and pharmacists in the UK. The article therein largely draws on the systematic review we had already identified and concurs with its conclusions and the approach recommended in the public health report. It also looks briefly at 'bug busting' (regular systematic combing of hair with a special comb and hair conditioner to remove live lice), an approach which was becoming popular locally, but cites the evidence supporting it as anecdotal.

Conclusion

The main conclusion has to be that our search was disappointing, as there is a paucity of good quality research. We are left with a number of dilemmas. The public health report draws clear conclusions and recommendations, but the absence of supporting references for their conclusions means we have to take on trust their impartiality and comprehensiveness of their literature review. We do have some information on the effectiveness of various insecticides, and are clear that their use should be restricted to treating confirmed cases of louse infection only.

Unfortunately, we are also subject to the concern that absence of evidence of effectiveness is not the same as evidence of ineffectiveness. So we are left not knowing whether the 'bug busting' approach proposed as the first-line management in our local strategy is likely to be effective or not. It certainly runs contrary to the approach recommended by the public health specialists in their report, but as stated above, their recommendations are not supported by references. However, this does not necessarily mean they are erroneous.

The dilemma

The discussions locally amongst various primary care representatives were leading towards a different approach from that recommended in the public health specialists' report. There seemed to be widespread dissatisfaction among health professionals with the status quo. The patients' approach, and indeed that recommended by many professional and schools, did seem at odds with that recommended by the public health report, or indeed the published evidence. Many patients demanded and received prescriptions for unsubstantiated infections (understandably as their children were being excluded from school until 'cured'), or obtained them over the counter at pharmacists. There seemed to be an increasing demand on primary health-care services. Anecdotal reports, including those from GPs treating members of their own families according to the recommendations, revealed that even in the best circumstances insecticides were not always effective. Furthermore, the public perception was that insecticides were potentially harmful, and professionals were becoming concerned that their inappropriate use may be harmful or lead to increasing resistance.

Local approach and audit

This conflict led to a decision to conduct a local audit, with the Multidisciplinary Audit and Quality Forum looking at head lice-related professional activity over the course of 1 month prior to the introduction of the new city-wide, multiagency policy. Data were collected by means of a postal questionnaire. Disappointing response rates indicate that the responses must be interpreted with caution, but they still make disturbing reading. In only 26% of the 421 reported contacts was the patient seen. The most common contact was with a parent (36%), other relative (10%) or teacher (9%), the identity of the contact being unspecified in 16%. Whilst lice or nits were seen in around one-third of cases, lotions were provided for almost three-quarters of contacts. Wet combing was also frequently recommended, particularly by school and practice nurses.

Following this data collection, a city-wide approach was adopted across the relevant professional groups. This involves the recommendation of 'bug busting' as the first-line management strategy, and the restriction of insecticide to cases where such an approach fails. The outcome judged to be of most relevance to the involved professional groups is the frequency of contacts about head lice, rather than a formal epidemiological or direct measurement of the success of treatment. This does increase the potential for confounding factors skewing the data and leading to spurious conclusions. For example, it may be that such an approach has the additional effect of enhancing the appropriate use of insecticides when indicated, and that any reduction in head lice among the population is a result of this rather than the direct effect of the bug-busting approach.

The full results of the subsequent data collection were unavailable at the time of writing. However, the response rate seems to be even less than in the initial data collection. This highlights a common problem in gathering evidence. It may be that the programme has been so successful (which is the anecdotal evidence) that the issue is no longer a professional priority. Unfortunately, completing research questionnaires is rarely high on professionals' priority lists. Due to the initial low response rate, a targeted follow-up audit will be conducted using a fieldworker if necessary. Initial indications are that there is no evidence of an increase in infestations and that the use of lotions has been markedly reduced. More research remains to be done.

Research potential

If the audit confirms an apparent improvement, there is clearly scope for a more formal research project into bug busting as a first-line treatment. The main issue is perhaps which of the potential outcomes should be measured. A biological approach would be to ensure eradication of infestation, an epidemiological one would be reduced incidence or shorter infestation times. You may also want to seek evidence of resistance or side effects. Professional groups and service providers and planners may wish to see reduced workload and more appropriate use of services. There would certainly be a need to convince professional groups such as pharmacists that they should take on the burden implicit in the approach adopted locally, as this entails a switch in who gives advice from doctors and nurses to retail pharmacists. Patients and schools would need to be convinced that lice, rather than nits, are the concern, and that the proposed approach reduces the community and individual infestation rates and duration. Clearly, it would be a Herculean task to devise, finance, and conduct any study to fulfil all the research agendas amongst stakeholders. Perhaps this is why the search for relevant research failed to fulfil our needs!

The clinical relevance of evidence

In practical terms, if the strategy is successful, the professionals associated with its development may not be too concerned about its scientific robustness. They may have some discomfort with its apparent contradiction with the public health report and the consensus-based guidelines contained within it. The strategy can, however, now take account of the review of topical insecticide findings of the systematic review when considering what to recommend for cases where 'bug busting' fails.

We understand that a more scientifically robust study using regular wet combing with conditioner as the control arm has recently been completed, but is not yet in the public domain. We await its publication and that of the Cochrane review with interest.

We hope this chapter not only serves as an example of how to search for evidence, but also leads readers to consider what may be clinically relevant outcomes, and the generalisability of research findings to a clinical environment subject to the vagaries of patient compliance, conflicting opinions, etc.

Key points

▶ Treatments may be recommended in the absence of good supportive evidence.

▶ There is a paucity of high-quality research in this area.

▶ Insecticides should only be used to treat confirmed cases of louse infection.

▶ No evidence of effectiveness is not the same as evidence of ineffectiveness.

▶ Guidelines and recommendations should cite and quantify the strength of supporting evidence.

▶ Pragmatic primary care-based studies may focus on different outcomes from academic research. The results should still be relevant to practical issues and may enhance the opportunities for further research.

References

Anon (1998). Treating head louse infections. *Drug and Therapeutics Bulletin* **36**: 45–46.

Aston R, Duggal H, Simpson J (1998). *Head Lice, Report for Consultants in Communicable Disease Control.* Public Health Medicine Environmental Group.

Burgess IF (1995). Authors differ on assessment of flaws in trials. *British Medical Journal* **311**: 1369.

Dixon R, Eastwood A, Fullerton D *et al* (1995). Review's weaknesses may undermine its conclusions. *British Medical Journal* **312**: 123.

Laekeman GM (1995). Several questions remain. *British Medical Journal* **312**: 123.

McManus RJ, Wilson S, Delaney BC *et al* (1998). Review of the usefulness of contacting other experts when conducting a literature search for systematic reviews. *British Medical Journal* **317**: 1562–1563.

Stallbaumer M and Ibarra J (1995). Counting headlice by visual inspection flaws trials' results. *British Medical Journal* **311**: 1369.

van der Stichele RH, Dezeure EM, Bogaert MG (1995). Systematic review of clinical efficacy of topical treatments for head lice. *British Medical Journal* **311**: 604–608. (Note also their replies to the correspondence in *British Medical Journal* 1995; **311**: 1369–1370 and **312**: 123.)

►28

Leg Ulcers and Fever in Children: Finding Evidence for Non-Medics

Rumona Dickson and Carrie Morrison

This chapter considers two clinical questions that primary care nurses raise and how they may locate the information and research findings needed to answer these questions. It assumes that primary care nurses have access to computers and appropriate databases, the skills and time to do the search and the skills to interpret the findings or access to people who can help them do that (see Chapter 7).

Venous leg ulcer management

Background

In the UK, the management of venous leg ulcers is frequently undertaken by primary care nurses (Fletcher 1996). In our scenario, a primary care nursing team has decided that their management of venous leg ulcers could benefit from an examination of the current research evidence.

The question

What are the most clinically effective means of managing a venous leg ulcer?

Search strategy

With the computer skills and access that our group of primary care nurses have, their search strategy was greatly simplified. Although access to *The Cochrane Library*, MEDLINE and PubMed is available, they also decided to undertake a web search of nursing and paramedical sites of evidenced-based practice. Key words used in the search were: *leg ulcer, venous, stasis, wound care, management* and *treatment*.

Four possible systematic reviews concerning the management of venous leg ulcers were identified. Two of these were located in *The Cochrane Library* (Cullum *et al* 1998, Wilkinson and Hawke 1998), the third was identified on the *Effective Health Care Bulletin* web site (Anon 1997), whilst the fourth was published in the *British Medical Journal* (Fletcher *et al* 1997).

- ▶ Compression bandages and stockings in the treatment of venous leg ulcers (Cullum *et al* 1998).
- ▶ Compression therapy for venous leg ulcers (Anon 1997).
- ▶ A systematic review of compression treatment for venous leg ulcers (Fletcher *et al* 1997).

▶ Does oral zinc aid the healing of chronic leg ulcers? (Wilkinson and Hawke 1998).

Additionally, four protocols for reviews currently being undertaken were identified in *The Cochrane Library*.

▶ Use of drugs in the treatment of venous leg ulcers.

▶ Electrical stimulation for venous leg ulcers.

▶ Laser therapy for the treatment of venous leg ulcers.

▶ Therapeutic ultrasound for venous leg ulcers.

The nurses could easily obtain a copy of the *British Medical Journal* review because the GPs in their practice subscribe to the journal. In fact, they could download it directly off the Internet. They were able to download from the Internet a copy of the report published as an *Effective Health Care Bulletin*. They were only able to read the abstracts of the reviews on *The Cochrane Library* but contacted a colleague who works at the University and who kindly agreed to print a copy of each of these two reviews for them. When they looked at these four reviews, they found that the first three on the list above were the same systematic review published in different formats for different target audiences.

Search results

Having compiled the information relating to their clinical question, the primary care nurses undertook a critical appraisal of their findings. They assessed the quality of the systematic reviews using a checklist provided by Oxman (1994). They concluded that the reviews of effectiveness in the management of venous leg ulcers represent well conducted research with valid findings. The systematic reviews described evidence for the effectiveness of treating leg ulcers with multilayered compression bandaging:

▶ compression bandaging is more effective than non-compression bandaging;

▶ elastic multilayer, high-compression bandaging is more effective than inelastic multilayer compression bandaging.

These conclusions are based on studies in which the outcome is complete healing. This information enables the team of primary care nurses to make a decision to change their current care patterns. However, they are aware of possible inherent drawbacks in implementation. In their search, they also find an implementation report on leg ulcer management (Tinkler *et al* 1999) which outlines some of the difficulties with implementing change in practice. None the less, based on the best available evidence, they begin their task of developing and implementing new practice guidelines advocating the use of compression bandaging regimens in their practice setting.

Non-pharmacological treatment of fever in children

Background

The treatment of fever in children is a common problem encountered by primary care nurses. Management interventions fall into two categories:

- antipyretics;

- external cooling measures (tepid sponging or unwrapping).

In this scenario, our primary care nurses are interested in the effectiveness of non-pharmacological treatments so that they can provide evidence-based advice to mothers with small children.

The question

What are the most effective non-pharmacological means of managing fever in children?

Search strategy

Following an unsuccessful preliminary search of clinically relevant journals at the university library, the nurses decided to undertake an expanded search using computer databases. The search strategy employed by the team involved examinations of both CD-ROM and Internet databases. These databases were searched to determine the existence of any relevant clinical trials. Key words included *fever, children, non-pharmacological, management* and *treatment*.

Search results

Despite an exhaustive search of *The Cochrane Library*, MEDLINE, PubMed, Internet Grateful Med, HealthSTAR, CINAHL, and 10 nursing and paramedical web sites with associated links, the primary care nurses were unable to find any systematic reviews or randomised controlled trials. However, they did discover that the first systematic review being conducted at the Western Australian Centre for Evidence-Based Nursing and Midwifery is 'The Nursing Management of Fever in Children' (Western Australia Centre for Evidence-Based Nursing 1998). The protocol for this review is available via the Joanna Briggs Institute for Evidence-Based Nursing Internet site (http://www.joannabriggs.edu.au/). This site has links to seven centres for evidence-based nursing in Australia, New Zealand, and Hong Kong, but this protocol is available only to Joanna Briggs web site subscribers (cost Aus$75/year).

However, they were not daunted by this. They made contact, through mail, with the researchers involved in the systematic review and learnt that nine trials have been identified for inclusion in this systematic review. They requested bibliographic details for these trials in order to determine if any preliminary conclusions can be drawn before completion of the review. They obtained copies of these nine reports – no easy task because they had ready access to only two of the journals. The others they obtained from the local university library, the library service at the Royal College of

Nursing and by using the name of a GP in their practice to request the others from the British Medical Association. They decided to use this opportunity to improve their critical appraisal skills and use these reports as a basis for three journal club sessions where the studies were discussed and appraised. The studies however are diverse and our group of nurses did not have the expertise to combine the results. Therefore, they decided to continue to provide their current fever management advice whilst awaiting the conclusions of the team carrying out the systematic review, who are better placed to draw generalisable conclusions from the combined results.

Conclusion

Even if nurses have the necessary equipment to access information, locating this information can often be difficult and time consuming. The two examples in this chapter used a combination of methods to access information. The emphasis leaned heavily towards computer-linked data sources which we believe will be the most useful for nurses now and in the future. Making these resources available and helping nurses develop the skill to use them are the challenges that need to be addressed before attempting to implement evidence-based care within primary care settings.

Key points

▶ Non-medics need access to relevant information resources and training in how to use them and interpret the information obtained.

▶ Evidence for non-medics may not be as plentiful as it is for doctors, or as readily available.

▶ Computer-linked data sources are the most useful for nurses and are being developed.

▶ Compression bandaging is recommended for leg ulcers.

▶ No randomised controlled trials or systematic reviews were identified for non-pharmacological treatment of fever in children; one systematic review is in preparation.

References

Anon (1997). Compression therapy for venous leg ulcers. *Effective Health Care.* August, Vol. 3: 4. World Wide Web: (13/01/99) http://www.york.ac.uk/inst/crd/ehcb.htm.

Cullum N, Fletcher A, Nelson E, Sheldon T (1998). Compression bandages and stockings in the treatment of venous leg ulcers. *The Cochrane Library: Database of Systematic Reviews.* Oxford: Update Software.

Fletcher A (1996). The epidemiology of leg ulcers. In: Cullum N, Roe B (Eds) *Leg Ulcers: Nursing Management.* London: Ballière Tindall.

Fletcher A, Cullum N, Sheldon T (1997). A systematic review of compression treatment for venous leg ulcers. *British Medical Journal* **315**: 576–580.

Oxman A (1994). Checklists for review articles. *British Medical Journal* **309**: 648–651.

Tinkler A, Hotchkiss J, Nelson E, Edwards L (1999). Implementing evidence-based leg ulcer management. *Evidence-Based Nursing* **2**: 6–8.

Western Australia Centre for Evidence-Based Nursing (1998). *Systematic Review of the Nursing Management of Fever in Children.* World wide web: (13/01/99) http://www.health.curtin.edu.au/nursing/wacebn/SysRev.html

Wilkinson E and Hawke C (1998). Does oral zinc aid the healing of chronic leg ulcers? *The Cochrane Library: Database of Systematic Reviews.* Oxford: Update Software.

Heart Failure Guidelines

Frances Mair

Background

Heart failure is a disease that impacts on everyday clinical practice (high volume) and is 'high risk' for patients in that poor management approaches will have profound negative effects on both quality of life and life expectancy. It is therefore a priority for guideline development. Heart failure is a disease of increasing incidence that affects 0.4–2% of the general population and 8–10% of the elderly (Mair *et al* 1996, Wheeldon *et al* 1993). The outlook for individuals suffering from heart failure is extremely poor. Population-based studies suggest that 5-year survival rates are < 50% (Franciosa 1986, Kannel 1989) making the prognosis worse than for many of the common cancers. It is also known to have major adverse effects on quality of life (Grady 1993). The morbidity caused by heart failure is reflected in the workloads of both secondary and primary care with 120 000 hospital admissions per year (McMurray *et al* 1993a) and 14 GP consultations per general medical inpatient stay (Wheeldon *et al* 1993). Consequently, the financial burden upon the NHS is considerable: approximately £360 million is spent annually in the UK (McMurray *et al* 1993b).

Approaches to diagnosis and management of heart failure have altered substantially in recent years. The need to detect heart failure at an early stage in order to slow the progression of left ventricular dysfunction is now emphasised (Dargie and McMurray 1994). Numerous studies have shown that it is very difficult to diagnose mild heart failure accurately on clinical grounds alone (Wheeldon *et al* 1993, Struthers 1996, Remes *et al* 1991) and therefore echocardiography is now viewed as a crucial investigation (The Task Force on Heart Failure of the European Society of Cardiology 1995). Management of heart failure has changed because large scale trials have conclusively shown that treatment of patients diagnosed with left ventricular dysfunction with angiotensin converting enzyme (ACE) inhibitors will decrease morbidity and mortality in mild, moderate and severe heart failure (Consensus Trial Study Group 1987, SOLVD Investigators 1991). Despite the evidence supporting changes in the way patients are treated, it appears that diagnosis remains suboptimal with only a minority of patients in general practice undergoing echocardiography or receiving ACE inhibitor therapy (Mair *et al* 1996).

This chapter focuses on a heart failure guideline for general practice that specifically examines the management of left ventricular systolic dysfunction, as this is the commonest cause of heart failure in the developed world. Furthermore, this type of heart failure has benefited from the greatest advances in research and management.

Development of a heart failure practice guideline

Search strategy

The development of a heart failure guideline that is credible and evidence based is a time consuming process. The creation of such a guideline by an individual practice for its personal use presents a potentially daunting task. Faced with the desire to 'do something' to improve patient management in this area by means of guideline development, it would seem prudent for those members of the primary care team involved first to determine whether heart failure guidelines currently exist. The most time-efficient and straightforward way to approach this is outlined below.

Explore electronic databases such as MEDLINE using the search terms *heart failure* and *guidelines*. To increase the likelihood that identified references will prove useful it is advisable to limit the search to those papers that are: *English language* and *human*. In the first instance, it would seem sensible to use the more recent databases, e.g. those relating to the current and the preceding 3 years (1995–98). The rationale underlying this suggestion is that all guidelines require regular review and modification as new evidence emerges and alters advice on best practice. Thus, a guideline produced 10 years ago, which remains unmodified, is very likely to be outdated and not in keeping with current best evidence.

The proposed search strategy yields in excess of 50 references which represent a selection that can be quickly inspected to determine whether systematically reviewed guidelines exist. Examination of these references indicated that five heart failure guidelines exist. However, this methodology did not locate all the relevant guidelines nor provide full information regarding the guidelines. Some papers identified referred to the use of a specific guideline but did not provide full details of the guideline. Such papers were examined to discover how to locate the guideline. For example, Stomel and Gowman (1996) provided a commentary on the US Agency for Health Care Policy and Research guideline. The Internet, as outlined in the next section, had to be searched to locate the actual guideline. In the same way, Borduas *et al* (1998) commented on the Canadian Cardiovascular Society clinical guidelines but only by searching the web for the Canadian Cardiovascular Society was the information relating to this guideline obtained. In addition, as a guideline for the diagnosis but not treatment of heart failure was noted to have been produced by the European Society of Cardiology, it was decided to do additional specific searches using the terms *heart failure* and *treatment*. Searching for these terms in the title allowed one additional guideline to be identified.

Box 29.1 lists the six guidelines that were identified. If no guidelines had been identified by this means, then it would have been appropriate to search databases over a longer time period, e.g. the preceding 5 years. The search strategy could also have been expanded to include other search terms that are frequently used interchangeably to describe heart failure, e.g. *cardiac failure, left ventricular failure, congestive cardiac failure*, and additional terms such as *management* or *diagnosis*.

Search the key web sites that contain information about practice guidelines. There are a number of such sites (see Chapter 4, Box 4.1). You do not need to have the web addresses for multiple sites as some web sites have links with many or all of the other relevant sites. This makes searching the web for information easier and saves time and effort. Web searching in this manner identified the Agency for Health Care Policy and Research (AHCPR) heart failure guidelines (Konstam *et al* 1994) and allowed direct access to them. An Internet search was performed using the term *Canadian Cardiovascular Society* and the web site (http://www1.ccs.ca/consensus/reports/) relating to that society's consensus reports was identified and the actual guidelines located. No further heart failure guidelines were identified by this method.

Critical appraisal of the literature

Having established that systematic heart failure guidelines exist they should be reviewed in order that judgements can be made as to their validity, and to determine whether or how they could be adapted for local use by the practice. Issues worth considering when reviewing guidelines include:

▶ who was involved in the development of the guideline?

▶ has a systematic literature review been performed?

▶ is there evidence that the identified literature has been critically assessed?

▶ when recommendations are made, is an explanation provided about the strength of evidence supporting the recommendation?

▶ were the guidelines tested (e.g. circulated to potential users of the guidelines and feedback obtained)? (see also Table 4.1).

All six guidelines identified in Box 29.1 were produced by expert panels which based their evidence on systematic reviews of the literature plus expert consensus opinion. The AHCPR panel was multidisciplinary and had a patient representative, whereas the Report of the American College of Cardiology/American Heart Association (ACC/AHA) and the European Society of Cardiology (ESC) had only specialist representation. The working party for the New Zealand guidelines had representation from primary and secondary care but only physician representation. The Canadian panellists, based on the information at their web site, appear to be physicians but their background is not specified.

The AHCPR guideline provides the most explicit information about: how it rated the evidence examined; to what degree each piece of advice on management is based on the evidence or consensus opinion; and if a recommendation is based on evidence it grades the strength of that evidence using the following classification scheme:

A   Good evidence: Evidence from well-conducted randomised controlled trials or cohort studies,

---

Box 29.1.   Heart failure guidelines identified via MEDLINE search

Konstam M, Dracup K, Baker D *et al* (June 1994). Heart failure: Evaluation and care of patients with left-ventricular systolic dysfunction. (Konstam *et al* 1994 for Agency for Health Care Policy and Research).

Guidelines for the evaluation and management of heart failure (American College of Cardiology/American Heart Association Task Force on Practice Guidelines (Committee on Evaluation and Management of Heart Failure) 1995).

Guidelines for the diagnosis of heart failure (The Task Force on Heart Failure of the European Society of Cardiology 1995).

The treatment of heart failure (The Task Force of the Working Group on Heart Failure of the European Society of Cardiology 1997).

New Zealand guidelines for the management of chronic heart failure (The National Heart Foundation of New Zealand, Cardiac Society of Australia and New Zealand and the Royal New Zealand College of General Practitioners Working Party 1997).

Diagnosis and management of heart failure (Canadian Cardiovascular Society 1994).

B   Fair evidence: Evidence from other types of studies,

C   Expert opinion.

Although all the guidelines have been based on systematic, critical analysis of the literature the AHCPR guideline is the one which makes it easiest for the reader to determine the strength of evidence underpinning each recommendation.

It would seem that the guidelines mentioned, particularly the AHCPR guideline, are sufficiently robust for practices to use them as a basis for their own guideline development.

Constructing the guideline

When developing a guideline it is important to identify the key management issues that need to be addressed. Once this has been done, a step-by-step guide can be constructed that guides the health-care provider through the investigation and treatment of a *generic* heart failure patient. Guidelines need to be straightforward and easily understandable. It is therefore useful to develop a single-page algorithm that provides the user with an immediate overview of the guideline. Supplementary accompanying information can be provided: for clarification of specific points; to expand on details of management; or to address special situations. Such additional information should be concise in order to prove practical for everyday use. It should be borne in mind that guidelines are, as their name implies, simply that and are not meant to address every possible clinical circumstance that may present. Guidelines aim to suggest the best management approach for the vast majority of patients suffering from a specific illness based on existing knowledge. Deviation from guidelines may therefore be necessary in some patients in specific circumstances.

In the development of a heart failure guideline, key issues include:

▶ steps necessary for diagnosis;

▶ treatment – who, what, and how?;

▶ follow-up;

▶ referral criteria.

Based on a review of the existing guidelines, and the criteria above, a possible guideline for general practice is shown in Figure 29.1. Once the guideline has been completed, members of the primary care team who will be using it should examine it and give feedback on ease of use, applicability, potential points of confusion or difficulty. The guideline can then be modified as directed by these comments. In this way, a practical, user-friendly guideline can be created. In addition, it is useful to confer with your local primary care group and/or primary care audit group and local cardiologists to ensure that the guidelines developed within the practice are in step with those already in existence, if any, within the community. This is particularly important because the management of heart failure inevitably involves both primary and secondary care providers at some stage and liaison between these parties is important to facilitate continuity in the management approach to this illness.

Keeping up-to-date

Until recently, the received wisdom was that β-blockers were contraindicated in heart failure. However, it has become increasingly apparent that when used in addition to ACE inhibitors, β-blockers can also reduce mortality among patients with left ventricular heart failure. They are not of proven benefit for patients with heart failure due to other causes, so it is important to confirm left ventricular systolic dysfunction prior to their use. More research is needed into the relative effectiveness of this approach among different age groups and disease severity. Current research would seem to support its use in patients under 75 yrs old with milder symptoms due to confirmed left ventricular heart failure. As it is essential that β-blockers, like ACE inhibitors, are started at a low-dose and titrated slowly to maintenance levels over months, many generalists may wish to seek specialist advice prior to their introduction (Cleland *et al* 1999). However, as more evidence is published it is likely that this option will increasingly become part of a primary care approach. This demonstrates the need to keep abreast of evidence relevant to established guidelines, which should be reviewed on a regular basis in the light of such developments.

Audit

Finally, it is extremely important if a practice is planning to implement a guideline that a system for audit and review is built into the implementation strategy in order to ensure that the guideline is successful in facilitating improved management. Criteria

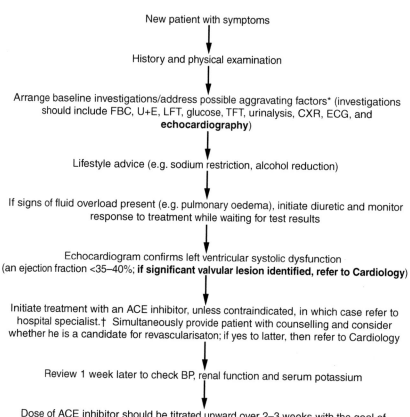

New patient with symptoms

History and physical examination

Arrange baseline investigations/address possible aggravating factors* (investigations should include FBC, U+E, LFT, glucose, TFT, urinalysis, CXR, ECG, and **echocardiography**)

Lifestyle advice (e.g. sodium restriction, alcohol reduction)

If signs of fluid overload present (e.g. pulmonary oedema), initiate diuretic and monitor response to treatment while waiting for test results

Echocardiogram confirms left ventricular systolic dysfunction (an ejection fraction <35–40%; **if significant valvular lesion identified, refer to Cardiology**)

Initiate treatment with an ACE inhibitor, unless contraindicated, in which case refer to hospital specialist.† Simultaneously provide patient with counselling and consider whether he is a candidate for revascularisaton; if yes to latter, then refer to Cardiology

Review 1 week later to check BP, renal function and serum potassium

Dose of ACE inhibitor should be titrated upward over 2–3 weeks with the goal of reaching the doses used in large-scale clinical trials. (U+E's should be rechecked 1 week after each dose increase and the patient assessed for signs of volume depletion; once dose is stabilised, U+Es should be checked at regular intervals thereafter: 3–6 monthly). Refer to Cardiology if symptoms persist, after checking on patient adherence

*Aggravating factors include: various medications, e.g. calcium channel blockers, NSAIDs and corticosteroids; anaemia; arrhythmias such as atrial fibrillation; thyroid disease; and renal failure.
†Contraindications to ACE inhibitor treatment include: mitral/aortic stenosis; history of adverse reaction; K >5.5 mmol/l; creatinine >180 mmol/l; at high risk for postural hypotension (patients with severe heart failure; initial systolic blood pressure <100 mmHg; serum Na levels <135 mmol/l; over 75 years of age; or on high dose of diuretic >80 mg frusemide or equivalent).

Figure 29.1. Example of an evidence-based practice guideline for heart failure.

or markers which would serve as proxy indicators of 'good practice' should be highlighted as outcome measures for audit. In the case of heart failure due to left ventricular systolic dysfunction, key outcome measures might include percentage of patients who have undergone echocardiography and percentage of eligible patients commenced on ACE inhibitors.

Key points

▶ When deciding to implement a guideline, first check if guidelines already exist.

▶ Having identified that guidelines exist, judge their validity and assess how they can be adapted for local use.

▶ Check that a guideline is compatible with others already in existence in the community or secondary care.

▶ Audit care before and after introducing guidelines.

▶ Heart failure is an increasing problem in the community, with considerable morbidity and mortality rates.

▶ Echocardiography is a crucial investigation.

▶ ACE inhibitors are an effective treatment for left ventricular systolic dysfunction.

References

American College of Cardiology/American Heart Association Task Force on Practice Guidelines (Committee on Evaluation and Management of Heart Failure (1995). Guidelines for the evaluation and management of heart failure. *Circulation* 92: 2764–2784 (also published in *Journal of the American College of Cardiology* 1995; 26: 1376–1398).

Borduas F, Carrier R, Drouin D, *et al* (1998). An interactive workshop: An effective means of integrating the Canadian Cardiovascular Society clinical practice guidelines on congestive heart failure into Canadian family physicians' practice. *Canadian Journal of Cardiology* 14: 911–916.

Canadian Cardiovascular Society (1994). Diagnosis and management of heart failure. Canadian Cardiovascular Society – Consensus Development Conference Guidelines. *Canadian Journal of Cardiology* 10: 613–631 and 635–654.

Cleland JGF, McGowan J, Clark A, *et al* (1999). The evidence of ß blockers in heart failure. *British Medical Journal* 318: 824–825.

Consensus Trial Study Group (1987). Effects of enalapril on mortality in severe congestive heart failure. Results of the co-operative north Scandinavian enalapril survival study. *New England Journal of Medicine* 316: 1429–1435.

Dargie HJ and McMurray JJV (1994). Diagnosis and management of heart failure. *British Medical Journal* 308: 321–328.

Franciosa JA (1986). Epidemiologic patterns, clinical evaluation and long term prognosis in chronic congestive heart failure. *American Journal of Medicine* 80 (Suppl 2b): 14–21.

Grady KL (1993). Quality of life in patients with chronic heart failure. *Critical Care Nursing Clinics of North America* 5: 661–670.

Kannel WB (1989). Epidemiological aspects of heart failure. *Cardiology Clinics* 7: 1–9.

Konstam M, Dracup K, Baker D *et al* (1994). *Heart Failure: Evaluation and Care of Patients with Left-Ventricular Systolic Dysfunction. Clinical Practice Guideline No. 11.* AHCPR Publication No. 94-0612. Rockville, MD: Agency for Health Care Policy and Research, Public Health Service, US Department of Health and Human Services.

Mair FS, Crowley TS, Bundred PE (1996). Prevalence, aetiology and management of heart failure in general practice. *British Journal of General Practice* 46: 77–79.

McMurray J, McDonagh T, Morrison CE *et al* (1993a). Trends in hospitalisation for chronic heart failure in Scotland. *European Heart Journal* 14: 1158–1162.

McMurray J, Hart W, Rhodes G (1993b). An evaluation of the cost of heart failure to the National Health Service in the UK. *British Journal of Medical Economics* 6: 99–110.

Remes J, Miettinen H, Reunanen A, *et al* (1991). Validity of clinical diagnosis of heart failure in primary health care. *European Heart Journal* 12: 315–321.

SOLVD Investigators (1991). Effects of enalapril on survival in patients with reduced left ventricular ejection fractions and congestive heart failure. *New England Journal of Medicine* 325: 293–302.

Stomel RJ and Gowman DP (1996). Practice guidelines for the treatment of heart failure: a commentary on the facts you need to know. Agency for Health Care Policy and Research. *Journal of the American Osteopathic Association* **96**: 541–543.

Struthers AD (1996). Identification, diagnosis and treatment of heart failure – could we do better? *Cardiology* **87 (Suppl 1)**: 29–32.

The National Heart Foundation of New Zealand, Cardiac Society of Australia and New Zealand and the Royal New Zealand College of General Practitioners Working Party (1997). New Zealand guidelines for the management of chronic heart failure. *New Zealand Medical Journal* **110**: 99–107.

The Task Force on Heart Failure of The European Society of Cardiology (1995). Guidelines for the diagnosis of heart failure. *European Heart Journal* **16**: 741–751.

The Task Force of the Working Group on Heart Failure of the European Society of Cardiology (1997). The treatment of heart failure. *European Heart Journal* **18**: 736–753.

Wheeldon NM, MacDonald TM, Flucker CJ, *et al* (1993). An electrocardiographic study of chronic heart failure in the community. *Quarterly Journal of Medicine* **86**: 17–23.

▶30

Low Back Pain

Mark Gabbay

> ▶ Example
>
> A bricklayer of 36 attends with low back pain, radiating down to the left knee, which has been present for 5 days. He has not knowingly injured his back, had rested in bed for the 5 days and taken an NSAID when the pain was worst, as was advised to him 4 years ago when he was off work for 6 weeks with a similar problem.

The questions

This case raises a number of questions. About *diagnosis*:

▶ What are the key points from history, including worrying symptoms and signs?

▶ How should I classify low back pain, particularly leg pain?

▶ What are the key points of physical examination?

▶ Should I do any tests, and if so, what, when and in whom?

What should be my first *management plan* options, and what if they do not work? What is the likely *prognosis*.

Search strategy

In the past I had been involved with a bid for waiting list initiative money to treat chronic low back pain in primary care using manipulation and acupuncture. In preparing that bid I had conducted a literature search and became aware of the Clinical Standards Advisory Group (CSAG) report (1994) on back pain. Through conversations with colleagues I had also become aware that the Royal College of General Practice had formed a group to develop guidelines. It seemed as though others may have done the hard work of searching for and critically reviewing the evidence.

I decided to look at the RCGP web site (http://www.rcgp.org.uk). There I was able to view the entire 'acute low back pain management' guidelines (Waddell *et al* 1996) simply by clicking on 'clinical guidelines' on the title page. It is possible to print pages of these, or even the entire document. They are dated April 1998 and so are reasonably up to date.

The introductory chapter explains the methodology of the guidelines development in detail. The participants' backgrounds, the searching methods and strength of evidence criteria are clearly stated. It became clear as I read this chapter that these guidelines were very thorough. They were based on evidence-based material (from both CSAG (1994) and Agency for Health Care Policy and Research (AHCPR) (1994)), plus comprehensive searches on areas of most relevance to primary care assessment and management. The guidelines clearly stated their developmental basis and evidence criteria and standards, and were substantially referenced. As the evidence presented was aimed at typical primary care situations, the evidence was also relevant.

Search results

Using the information on the RCGP web site I was able to answer all of the questions arising from the young bricklayer with the bad back. For each section of the guidelines, the group's view of the strength of the evidence and the main substantive supporting references were made clear.

Diagnosis

Turning first to *diagnosis*, the guidelines follow the AHCPR approach, with minor modifications. Indeed, this diagnostic triage approach is presented as a series of figures and decision trees as appendices to the document. It also seems clear that, at least in primary care, the evidence on appropriate history and examination points is somewhat scanty. However, the guidelines clearly outline the strength of evidence for such clinical assessments and I can confidently summarise the key points from *history* as:

▶ patient's age: simple backache if presentation is between 20 and 55. Watch out for 'red flags', particularly outside these ages;

▶ duration of symptoms;

▶ their impact on activity and work: likely to be mechanical if symptoms vary with time and activity;

▶ description of symptoms: simple backache if lumbosacral/buttocks/thighs;

▶ previous response to therapy;

▶ significant trauma relative to age raises possibility of fracture;

▶ check for psychological and socioeconomic problems, as their presence can complicate assessment and care;

▶ history of cancer, thoracic pain, systemic steroids, IV drug misuse and HIV point to possible serious spinal pathology;

▶ unilateral leg pain, more severe than the back pain, radiating to foot and other unilateral neurological abnormalities, points to nerve root problems.

In terms of *examination*, the guidelines stress:

▶ straight leg raising, which may be normal in the elderly with cauda equina, but otherwise if reduced in extent and reproducing leg pain, indicates nerve root irritation;

▶ ankle and knee reflexes, ankle and toe dorsiflexion and strength, and sensory deficits;

▶ persisting severe lumbar flexion restriction is a 'red flag', as is systemic illness.

You need to exclude cauda equina syndrome, with micturition difficulties, effects on anal sphincter tone, saddle anaesthesia, widespread or progressive motor weakness or gait disturbance. You should also be aware of the other 'red flag' of weight loss and a picture of an inflammatory disorder, such as ankylosing spondilytis.

The guidelines thus point to a clear method of differential diagnosis and *classification*.

The RCGP guidelines follow the tests recommended by the AHCPR. The Royal College of Radiologists' recommendations are based on consensus.

▶ Plain X-rays are not indicated for acute low back pain without 'red flag' signs such as:
 – recent significant trauma;
 – recent mild trauma (if over 50 years);
 – prolonged steroid use;
 – osteoporosis;
 – age >70 years.
 Routine oblique views are not recommended even when an X-ray is indicated.

▶ Tumour or infective aetiology may need ruling out with FBC, ESR and plain X-ray if there is a history of cancer, recent infection, pyrexia, IV drug misuse, prolonged steroids, unexplained weight loss, or if the pain is worse at rest. Indeed, these clinical indications may warrant more detailed investigations such as scans.

Management

This should include a thorough history and brief examination, as above, and reassurance if no serious pathology is suspected (absence of 'red flags'). Patients such as this can be assured that their recovery is likely to be reasonably rapid, information which has been shown to be of benefit. Simple analgesia, such as paracetamol or if necessary a paracetamol/weak opioid combination should be used for pain relief. Whilst there is good evidence that NSAIDs are effective at reducing pain, they are likely to have more side effects. They are less effective for severe root pain. Similarly, whilst muscle relaxants and strong opioids have been shown to be effective for acute low back pain, they also have relatively more side effects, and have not been consistently shown to be superior to simple analgesia or NSAIDs.

There is evidence against bed rest and in favour of continuation of ordinary activity, which if graduated over a few days has been shown to have a better long-term outcome. Patients should be advised to return to work as soon as possible. There is weak evidence in favour of manipulation and exercises, and whilst physical therapies may provide symptomatic relief, there is no convincing evidence they improve outcomes. Traction and corsets have not been shown to be of benefit. There is inconclusive evidence in favour of TENS, shoe insoles, trigger point or ligamentous injections and acupuncture. There is evidence against narcotics or benzodiazepines for longer than 2 weeks, colchicine, traction with bed rest, systemic steroids, a plaster jacket, and manipulation under a general anaesthetic.

Prognosis

The guidelines summarise the evidence on *prognosis* as follows (adapted from CSAG (1994) report):

- psychosocial problems can worsen outcome and are important at a relatively early stage;
- risk factors for chronicity include:
  - previous low back pain and also recent time off work with it;
  - radiating leg pain, reduced straight leg raising and other signs of nerve root involvement;
  - poor physical strength and fitness;
  - personal and work problems;
  - heavy smoking.

These guidelines have thus answered all the questions I posed about an hypothetical manual worker with acute low back pain, a common occurrence in practice. The evidence, whilst not always of the highest standard, can be relied upon as the best available. The evidence is targeted at primary care, and the methodology whereby it was sought, collated and assessed is clearly stated. Furthermore, the guidelines contain material in a form which can be readily adapted to guidelines suitable for local use.

Additional questions

Below is a list of potential additional questions arising from the simple case of low back pain.

Clinical findings

- How useful is the finding of decreased straight leg raising as a diagnostic test for a herniated intervertebral disc?
- How important is a contralateral restricted straight leg raising? How does it compare with other neurological signs or vertebral tenderness, for example?

Simply asking what signs and symptoms are diagnostic of a prolapsed disc would be much more difficult to search on. It needs breaking up into more specific questions, and perhaps comparisons.

Aetiology

▶ Are certain occupations related to increased incidence or relapse rates ?

▶ Is a family history of low back pain related to incidence, severity or recurrence rates (three different questions)?

Differential diagnosis

▶ Does the presence of radiating pain beyond the knee differentiate between neurological and mechanical low back pain? This question may be easier to answer than what signs and symptoms differentiate between mechanical, neurological and malignant causes of low back pain.

Diagnostic tests

▶ How useful is a plain X-ray of the lumbo-sacral spine compared to no X-ray? What are the indications for a plain X-ray?

Prognosis

▶ Is the prognosis of low back pain dependent on the frequency and/or duration of recurrence? Is the duration of symptoms related to the prognosis? 'What is the likelihood of this patient getting back to work within 6 weeks?' is another form of question which may be amenable to an evidence-based medicine approach.

Therapy

▶ How does the efficacy of bed rest with specific exercises compare with graduated normal activity as the appropriate advice on mobilisation?

▶ Which is the most effective type (e.g. regular NSAID compared to PRN simple analgesia), dose and duration of drug treatments? This is more likely to lead to an answer than the vaguer 'What are the most effective treatments?'

▶ You could look at other specifics, such as acupuncture, manipulation, etc.

Prevention

▶ Do back exercises prevent recurrence?

▶ Can the avoidance of poor lifting practices reduce the primary incidence in those at risk?

Self improvement

➤   Am I better reading an orthopaedic textbook or evidence-based guidelines on the diagnosis and management of low back pain?

Many of these questions would be difficult to answer from the RCGP guidelines and would require more specific literature searches. Some questions are, however, answerable from the material included in the guidelines. If an apparently relevant topic or question is not mentioned in a set of guidelines, it is not always apparent whether this is because it is an ineffective intervention or strategy, or just outwith the guideline's focus. This is why separate searches would be required to answer many of the questions about back pain outlined above.

A recent comprehensive systematic review of treatments for acute and chronic low back pain summarises English language published trials of treatments up to September 1995 (van Tulder et al 1997). This is a useful adjunct to the guidelines, as it also considers chronic low back pain, and may include some evidence published too late to be incorporated into the RCGP guidelines (although this is being updated in 1998/9). van Tulder et al (1997) acknowledge the limitations of their search strategy (English language and electronic search only), but their review is comprehensive in its breadth of topics. It provides useful summaries of the evidence on analgesia, NSAIDs, muscle relaxants, epidural injections, bed rest and exercise approaches, back schools, manipulation, TENS, traction, and behavioural therapy for acute back pain. It similarly covers drug therapy, epidural injections, manipulation, back schools, biofeedback, exercise, traction and orthoses, TENS and behavioural therapy for chronic low back pain.

Work continues to be published about back pain. Indeed, a recent paper on prognosis (Croft et al 1998) has shed doubt on some of the RCGP guideline's conclusions about prognosis. They express concerns that the methods used to collect data in previous studies on the prognosis and natural history of low back pain may not represent the wider perspective, and suggest that the common pattern is one of acute exacerbations of a chronic grumbling problem. They also challenge the outcome of no longer presenting to services as a sign of recovery, and assert that most patients continue to have some difficulties but fail to report them. Chew and May (1997) present qualitative data about the consequences of chronic back pain, and the effects they have on the patient/professional relationship.

Thus it seems that evidence is often in a state of flux and liable to change with time. This is why it is necessary to check on recent evidence. Indeed, substantive guideline committees will tend to re-visit the literature on a regular basis, and alter their guidelines as indicated by any new and better evidence. However, I hope that it is clear that the information from a systematic literature review often will have been collected and critically assessed by reliable bodies, and that secondary sources, such as these guidelines, can be a valuable and time-saving resource, which may also have a considerable impact on clinical practice and planning.

Key points

► Check to see if evidence-based guidelines are available to answer your question.

► Ensure that you can critically evaluate the quality of the guidelines, in particular the strength of evidence supporting their conclusions.

► RCGP guidelines give evidence-based recommendations for diagnosis, management and prognosis of acute low back pain.

► Remember that evidence will often change with time and the literature should be revisited on a regular basis, checking for systematic reviews.

References

Agency for Health Care Policy and Research (1994). *Management Guidelines for Acute Low Back Pain*. US Department of Health and Human Services.

Chew AC and May CR (1997). The benefits of back pain. *Family Practice* **14**: 461–465.

Clinical Standards Advisory Group (1994). Back Pain: Report of a Clinical Standards Advisory Group on Back Pain. London: HMSO.

Croft PR, Macfarlane GJ, Papageorgiou AC, Thomas E, Silman AJ (1998). Outcome of low back pain in general practice: a prospective study. *British Medical Journal* **316**: 1356–1359.

van Tulder MW, Koes BW, Bouter LM (1997). Conservative treatment of acute and chronic nonspecific low back pain: A systematic review of randomised controlled trials of the most common interventions. *Spine* **22**: 2128–2156.

Waddell G, Feder G, McIntosh A, Lewis M, Hutchinson A (1996). Low back pain evidence review. London: Royal College of General Practitioners.

▶31

Asthma

Mark Gabbay

Background

The practice nurse has suggested to the practice manager that we need to address the issue of insufficient nebulisers in the practice. The problem is that they are lent to patients and not returned and the doctors on call forget them in their cars for days on end, and then there are none left in the treatment room.

I remembered a pharmaceutical representative telling me that there was evidence that large spacer devices could deliver drugs to the lungs as effectively as nebulisers in acute asthma, so I decided to conduct a search.

The question

How do large spacer devices and nebulisers compare in the delivery of drugs in acute asthma?

Search strategy

Having recently discovered how to access a CD-ROM copy of the Cochrane database remotely, I decided to practise searching it using this as an example. I was fortunate therefore to discover the following – Comparison of holding chambers and nebulisers for beta-agonists in acute asthma (Cates 1998).

I also came across another couple of items in the asthma section which caught my eye, but more of them later.

Search results

Cates (1998) is a Cochrane review and thus pretty robust in its methodology. The Cochrane Airways Review Group Trials Register was searched (as was the general Cochrane Trials Register), and then secondary references were sought from identified primary papers. The information assessed in the review included both published and unpublished data, and in all languages.

The criteria for assessing the quality of the papers is clear, and papers were independently judged according to standardised criteria, one reviewer was blinded to identifying data to minimise bias, and the agreement between the assessors was measured using the kappa coefficient. The results were statistically analysed, according to the standardised Cochrane approach. It is not surprising that there is little to fault here, as the Cochrane Collaboration works hard to maintain high standards in the quality of its reviews.

Of 113 abstracts identified from the initial searches, 45 were selected for potential inclusion in the review: of these, 13 were of a sufficiently robust design to be included in the final analysis. The agreement between reviewers was high.

This review concludes that:

- For adults the choice of delivery method should reflect patient preference, local circumstances and economic considerations, as there is no apparently significant difference between the two delivery methods in the clinical outcomes assessed.

- For children, the clinical outcomes were no worse with holding chambers, and the incidence of side effects and length of stay in A&E was lower with them compared to wet nebulisers. Oxygenation was better with holding chambers than nebulisers.

- It is suggested that repeated treatments of β-agonists (4 puffs into a holding chamber, or 1 respule) and repeated as necessary at shortish intervals (15 min). As it is impossible accurately to predict the quantity of medication any patient may need, this strategy enables titration of drug dosage according to the individual patient's response.

- High-dose oral steroids should continue to be used early to treat the exacerbations.

- There are some limitations in the quality of the current best available evidence, particularly with respect to children with acute exacerbations, and in community settings.

Relevance and implications for practice

Only one of the studies included in the review was conducted in the community, the rest being hospital based. However, it is probably the case that within the UK at least, increasingly severe exacerbations are managed in the community, rather than in hospital. The severest cases were excluded from these studies, but as these would almost certainly necessitate emergency referral to hospital anyway, this is less of a problem.

It would seem reasonable to prescribe appropriate holding chambers for patients prone to exacerbations, and to keep a supply in doctors' on-call bags and the emergency room. Thus, wet nebulisers can be reserved for patients who are unable to tolerate the holding chamber, who should be few in number.

There is a need for further community-based research and studies of patient satisfaction with the two devices.

What else caught my eye?

I noted two other Cochrane reviews in my 'asthma' search relevant to topics that had recently cropped up in my clinical practice.

Influenza immunisation

Young asthmatics were regularly requesting influenza immunisations. It was not practice policy to provide them in otherwise healthy asthmatics under the age of 65. I wondered if we were justified in this, particularly as this caused friction in some consultations. Cochrane came to the rescue in the shape of – Influenza vaccination in asthma: efficacy and side effects (Cates *et al* 1998).

Cutting to the chase, there is a lack of sufficiently robust or large studies; however, those that have been done fail to provide evidence that influenza vaccination provides a protective effect, and indeed one study has shown a small increased risk of exacerbation in the week following immunisation. It is as yet unclear whether this is because there has been insufficient research (i.e. insufficient sample size in well designed studies) to enable confident conclusions to be drawn, or whether there is no significant protective effect. However, it seems reasonable to continue with the practice policy of not offering influenza immunisation to otherwise well adult asthmatics below 65 years of age.

Homeopathic management

I had recently been involved in a prolonged discussion with a parent expressing serious doubts about conventional medical treatment for their child's asthma, preferring instead a homeopathic approach, which she assured me was more effective and less prone to side effects. Other patients had given similar reports in the past, so I was intrigued to notice another Cochrane review – Homeopathy for chronic asthma (Linde and Jobst 1998).

This review had searched the databases of the Glasgow Homeopathic Library and the Münchener Modell (University of Munich), in addition to the standard Cochrane databases and secondary searches. Five trials were identified, among which 3 were deemed suitable for inclusion, although there were methodological deficiencies.

Unsurprisingly perhaps, the authors concluded that despite some evidence of benefits among the homeopathically treated groups, the methodological problems rendered the results insufficiently reliable. Furthermore, in practice homeopathists adopt an holistic approach rather than following generalisable regimens. They go on to suggest research approaches to investigate the subject further, and highlight two potentially promising ongoing studies.

Key points

▶ The Cochrane database is a useful place to search for evidence.

▶ A systematic Cochrane review comparing drug delivery devices is available.

▶ In general, holding chambers should be prescribed for asthmatics and wet nebulisers reserved for those who cannot tolerate holding chambers: they are much cheaper than nebulisers and are prescribable.

▶ Influenza vaccination does not have a protective effect for asthmatics.

References

Cates CJ (1998). Comparison of holding chambers and nebulisers for beta-agonists in acute asthma. In: *The Cochrane Library*, issue 4. Oxford: Update Software.

Cates CJ, Jefferson TO, Bara AL (1998). Influenza vaccination in asthma: efficacy and side-effects. In: *The Cochrane Library*, issue 4. Oxford: Update Software.

Linde K and Jobst KA (1998). Homeopathy for chronic asthma. In: *The Cochrane Library*, issue 4. Oxford: Update Software.

▶ 32

Secondary Prevention of Coronary Artery Disease

Peter Bundred

Background

Coronary artery disease remains the single largest cause of premature death in the UK. Epidemiological data suggest that approximately 25% of patients who have a myocardial infarction die within 48 hours of the initial event and the survivors are at >3-fold greater risk of developing a further infarct in the next 5 years (Shaper *et al* 1985). In a typical primary care group of 100 000 patients, each year 400 patients will have a myocardial infarction and 100 of these will die almost immediately. A further 4000 patients will be receiving some form of medication for the management of angina. In the primary care group there will be approximately 8000 patients who are potentially at high risk of having a myocardial infarction. A large proportion of these individuals would benefit from lifestyle modification and optimal medical interventions.

The objective of secondary prevention is therefore to slow down the development of the disease and thereby reduce both fatal and non-fatal consequences (Pyorala *et al* 1994). Since most of these patients will be managed in primary care, the secondary prevention of their disease is the responsibility of the members of the primary care team.

The challenge

In 1996 the British Cardiac Society published the results of a study, which examined the extent to which coronary risk factors were being measured, recorded and managed in clinical practice. The ASPIRE study (Action on Secondary Prevention through Intervention to Reduce Events) found that there was a considerable potential to reduce the risk of further major ischaemic events in patients with established coronary disease. It was suggested that this reduction in risk could be achieved by effective interventions aimed at improving lifestyle, the rigorous management of hypertension and raised cholesterol and the appropriate use of prophylactic drugs (ASPIRE Steering Group 1996).

The evidence

The evidence for the secondary prevention of coronary artery disease is extensive and continues to grow. In a recent review article Mehta and Eagle (1998) carried out a MEDLINE review between 1980 and 1997. They searched on acute myocardial infarction with an emphasis on secondary prevention. This produced more than 3 000 articles. Moher (1995) has published a review entitled *Evidence of Effectiveness of Interventions for Secondary Prevention and Treatment of Coronary Heart Disease in Primary Care*. A very comprehensive review of existing evidence has been published by the British Cardiac Society in conjunction with the British Hyperlipidaemia Association, the British Hypertension Society and the British Diabetic Society (Woods *et al* 1998).

The Internet is increasingly being used to disseminate information and there are a number of important general sites that relate to the secondary prevention of coronary artery disease. The Agency for Health Policy and Research in the USA has recently published a very comprehensive document entitled *Cardiac Rehabilitation (Clinician's Guide)* which covers most aspects of secondary prevention and which can be accessed on the Internet (http://text.nlm.nih.gov/: then by searching for the document once logged onto their site). *Bandolier*, the Oxford-based journal which publishes on the Internet, had a recent review on all aspects of cardiac rehabilitation: this can also be accessed on the Internet (http://www.jr2.ox.ac.uk:80/Bandolier/band9/b9-3.html).

The evidence for the effectiveness of secondary prevention can be subdivided into two parts. First, evidence that lifestyle modification improves survival and secondly, evidence that appropriate medical treatment is beneficial to patients who have coronary artery disease.

Lifestyle modification

From a primary care standpoint, modification of sub-optimal lifestyle can be achieved through active participation of the primary care team and close liaison with the cardiac rehabilitation team. The evidence for each of the modifiable elements contributing to coronary artery disease has been well documented.

Smoking

The effect that cigarette smoke has on the coronary arteries has been reviewed (Bartecchi *et al* 1994). A large study in China suggests that worldwide the number of people who smoke is increasing (Liu *et al* 1998); in the UK approximately 30% of the population are smokers. However, there is evidence that the adverse effects of smoking are quite quickly lost and therefore it is a priority to get patients who have a history of coronary artery disease to stop smoking.

A number of strategies have been developed to assist smokers to give up the habit. A MEDLINE search of review articles on smoking cessation between 1995 and 1998 revealed 49 articles. This included a British review which examined the efficacy of interventions intended to help people stop smoking (Law and Tang 1995). Although counselling and support are important, only 2% of smokers receiving this intervention had not relapsed after 1 year. Nicotine-replacement therapy helped 13% of patients stop smoking and is particularly effective in those individuals who have nicotine dependence. The authors conclude that smokers who intend to stop smoking should be given support and encouraged to use nicotine replacement therapy.

Diet and lipid lowering

There are two outcomes required from dietary interventions in the secondary prevention of coronary artery disease. First, obesity (BMI >30 in men and >27 in women) is a risk factor, although the direct relationship between obesity and coronary artery disease is not proven. *Weight reduction* will have an effect on other risk factors such as blood pressure, lipid profile and glucose tolerance and should form part of the strategy for secondary prevention of coronary disease (Pyorala *et al* 1994).

Of more importance is the *reduction in the levels of low-density lipoproteins* by dietary and drug interventions. The pathophysiology of the effects of cholesterol in the development of coronary disease has been reviewed (Levine *et al* 1995). There is considerable evidence that reduction in the levels of low-density lipoprotein with an increase in the levels of high-density lipoprotein reduces the risk of developing coronary events (Scandinavian Simvastatin Survival Study Group 1994). A MEDLINE search covering the years 1995–1998 for review articles on coronary artery disease and lipid reduction produced 126 articles.

Reduction in cholesterol levels can be achieved by reducing the intake of saturated fats in the diet. However, the use of the HMG co-A reductase inhibitors (statins) has been shown to be highly effective in the secondary prevention of coronary artery disease in patients who have increased levels of low-density lipoproteins (Shepherd *et al* 1995). In 1997, the Standing Medical Advisory Committee produced guidelines for the use of statins in the secondary prevention of coronary artery disease (Jones 1997). For patients who have established coronary disease these can be summarised as follows:

➤ consider other methods of reducing the risk of coronary heart disease before prescribing statins;

➤ prescribe statins to those who have had a myocardial infarction and have total cholesterol of 4.8 mmol/l or more, or have angina and a total cholesterol of 5.5 mmol/l or more.

Exercise and cardiac rehabilitation programmes

In a randomised clinical trial of cardiac rehabilitation, Oldridge *et al* (1988) showed that patients who had been actively involved in an exercise programme had a lower mortality when compared to the controls. Hardman (1996) reviewed the evidence for the positive effects of physical activity in the management of patients with atherosclerotic, metabolic and hypertensive diseases. He showed that long-term adaptions to regular exercise resulted in improved blood pressure, glucose/insulin dynamics and lipoprotein metabolism, as well as a general feeling of wellbeing.

In 1998 the NHS Centre for Reviews and Dissemination published an *Effective*

Health Care Bulletin devoted to cardiac rehabilitation. The reviewers identified some 215 systematic reviews from computer-based searches. They summarised their findings as follows:

▶ Cardiac rehabilitation can promote recovery, enable patients to achieve and maintain better health, and reduce risk of death in people with heart disease.

▶ A combination of exercise, psychological and educational interventions is the most effective form of cardiac rehabilitation.

▶ Exercise improves physical aspects of recovery at no additional risk, but as a sole intervention it is not sufficient to reduce risk factors, morbidity or mortality.

▶ Current provision is growing rapidly but there is wide variation in practice, management and organisation of services. Many patients who might benefit do not receive cardiac rehabilitation.

▶ Many of the problems experienced by people with heart disease are not due to physical illness but to anxiety and misconceptions about their health. Health professionals should provide accurate information that can be understood by patients.

Diabetes mellitus

Patients with diabetes are at much greater risk of developing heart disease. Risk factor management in patients with both conditions becomes a priority. Turner *et al* (1998) showed that in patients with type 2 diabetes, four modifiable risk factors should be targeted: increased levels of low-density lipoprotein, decreased levels of high-density lipoprotein, raised blood pressure and smoking.

As well as targeting concomitant risk factors in diabetic patients, glycaemic control should also be reviewed. Intensive therapy has been shown to reduce the incidence of microvascular-related events in type 2 diabetics (UK Prospective Diabetes Study Group 1998). The primary care team should aim to lower the Hb A1 level to as close to normal levels as possible.

Pharmacological interventions

There is an increasing body of evidence that suggests that there are a number of drugs that positively improve both morbidity and mortality in patients with coronary disease.

Aspirin

The use of low-dose aspirin as an antiplatelet therapy in the management of patients who have had a coronary event is well described (Antiplatelet Triallists Collaboration 1994). The pathophysiology of this action is reviewed in Patrono (1994). The NHS Centre for Reviews and Dissemination published an *Effective Health Care Bulletin* on aspirin in myocardial infarction in 1995. It showed that if aspirin is started immediately after a myocardial infarction is suspected, a considerable reduction in immediate mortality could be obtained. It also showed that for every 86 patients at high risk of myocardial infarction who receive aspirin for 2 years after an acute episode, one death would be prevented. Despite the level of evidence showing the positive effects of aspirin in the secondary prevention of coronary disease, many patients who have no contraindications are not prescribed this drug (McCallum *et al* 1997).

β-Adrenergic blockers

There have been a number of randomised clinical trials that have shown improved survival in patients with coronary artery disease managed on this group of drugs (Yusuf *et al* 1985). β-Blockers effect the heart by reducing myocardial workload and oxygen consumption by reducing the heart rate, blood pressure and contractility, as well as decreasing the risk of ventricular fibrillation. Treatment with intravenous drugs should be started within 24 hours of the acute episode and should continue indefinitely with oral preparations (Ryan *et al* 1996). Despite the strength of the evidence for the use of this class of drugs in the secondary prevention of coronary disease, <50% of patients in one American study were prescribed a β-blockers (Gottlieb *et al* 1998). This figure is much lower in the UK, especially for the use of intravenous β-blockers in the immediate post-infarction period (Owen 1998).

Angiotensin-converting enzyme (ACE) inhibitors

Patients who have evidence of left ventricular dysfunction following a myocardial infarction have increased risk of death. Those individuals who have a left ventricular ejection fraction of <30% have a 4-fold increase in mortality over patients with an ejection fraction of >40%. ACE inhibitors have been shown to be of great benefit in patients with left ventricular dysfunction, especially in those with an ejection fraction of <40% (The Acute Infarction Ramipril Efficacy (AIRE) Study Investigators 1993). They have also been shown to be effective in reducing ischaemic events after myocardial infarction (Pfeffer *et al* 1992). In a recent Scottish study, less than half of the patients who had evidence of heart failure following a recent myocardial infarction were being prescribed an ACE inhibitor (Campbell *et al* 1998).

Conclusion

The evidence supporting secondary prevention in patients following myocardial infarction is very strong. There are now many hundreds of clinical trials which have shown that both lifestyle modification and pharmacological interventions reduce subsequent mortality and improve the quality of life in these patients. The ASPIRE Steering Group (1996) highlighted the need for improved management of patients with a history of coronary disease. In Campbell *et al*'s (1998) study of secondary prevention of patients in general practice, <70% were taking aspirin, <35% were taking a long-term β-blocker and <50% were on ACE inhibitors.

The opportunities for the prevention of premature death from coronary artery disease in primary care groups are enormous. With approximately 8 000 patients requiring secondary prevention it should not be difficult to apply the currently available knowledge on this subject. However, if the evidence-based approach to secondary prevention is to succeed, greater efforts will need to be made in changing the attitudes of both primary and secondary care clinicians. The publication of academic books and papers on the subject of evidence-based medicine will do little in themselves to change the behaviour of the practising doctor – unless they result in evidence dissemination and change routines. Actions speak louder than words!

Key points

▶ Coronary artery disease remains the single largest cause of premature death in the UK.

▶ It is worthwhile consulting secondary sources of evidence, including those on the Internet.

▶ In important areas such as this, systematic reviews are likely to be available and may well be easier to consult than the vast literature.

▶ There is strong evidence that lifestyle modification and pharmacological interventions reduce mortality and improve quality of life in patients with a history of coronary disease.

▶ The evidence supporting interventions is overwhelming. The important and crucial response from clinicians is to act on the knowledge and intervene. This will prevent premature deaths and reduce morbidity amongst our patients.

References

Antiplatelet Trialists Collaboration (1994). Collaborative overview of randomised trials of antiplatelet therapy – Prevention of death, myocardial infarction, and stroke by prolonged antiplatelet therapy in various categories of patients. *British Medical Journal* **308**: 81–106.

ASPIRE Steering Group (1996). The British Cardiac Society survey of the potential for secondary prevention of coronary disease: ASPIRE (Action on Secondary Prevention through Intervention to Reduce Events); Principal results. *Heart* **75**: 334–342.

Bartecchi C, Thomas D, Schrier R (1994). The human cost of tobacco use. *New England Journal of Medicine* **330**: 907–912.

Campbell NC, Thain J, George Deans H, *et al* (1998). Secondary prevention of coronary heart disease: baseline survey of provision in general practice. *British Medical Journal* **316**: 1430–1434.

Gottlieb SS, McCarter R, Vogel R (1998). Effect of beta-blockade on mortality among high-risk and low-risk patients after myocardial infarction. *New England Journal of Medicine* **339**: 489–497.

Hardman AE (1996). Exercise in the prevention of atherosclerotic, metabolic and hypertensive diseases: A review. *Journal of Sports Sciences* **14**: 201–218.

Jones AF (1997). Statins and hypercholesterolaemia: UK Standing Medical Advisory Committee guidelines. *Lancet* **350**: 1174–1175.

Law M and Tang JL (1995). An analysis of the effectiveness of interventions intended to help people stop smoking. *Archives of Internal Medicine* **155**: 1933–1941.

Levine GN, Keaney JF, Vita J (1995). Cholesterol reduction in cardiovascular disease: Clinical benefits and possible mechanisms. *New England Journal of Medicine* **332**: 512–521.

Liu BQ, Peto R, Chen ZM *et al* (1998). Emerging tobacco hazards in China: 1. Retrospective proportional mortality study of one million deaths. *British Medical Journal* **317**: 1411–1422.

McCallum AK, Whincup PH, Morris RW, *et al* (1997). Aspirin use in middle-aged men with cardiovascular disease: are opportunities being missed? *British Journal of General Practice* **47**: 417–421.

Mehta RH and Eagle KA (1998). Secondary prevention in acute myocardial infarction. *British Medical Journal* **316**: 838–842.

Moher M (1995). *Evidence of Effectiveness of Interventions for Secondary Prevention and Treatment of Coronary Heart Disease in Primary Care. A Review of the Literature.* Anglia and Oxford Regional Health Authority.

NHS Centre for Reviews and Dissemination, University of York (1995). Aspirin and myocardial infarction. *Effective Health Care Bulletin* **1**: 1–4.

NHS Centre for Reviews and Dissemination, University of York (1998). Cardiac rehabilitation. *Effective Health Care Bulletin* **4**: 1–12.

Oldridge NB, Guyatt GH, Fischer ME, *et al* (1988). Cardiac rehabilitation after myocardial infarction: combined experience of randomised controlled trials. *Journal of the American Medical Association* **260**: 945–950.

Owen A (1998). Intravenous β blockade in acute myocardial infarction (editorial). *British Medical Journal* **317**: 226–227.

Patrono C (1994). Aspirin as an antiplatelet drug. *New England Journal of Medicine* **330**: 1287–1294.

Pfeffer MA, Braunwald E, Moye LA *et al* for the SAVE Investigators (1992). Effect of captopril on mortality and morbidity in patients with left ventricular dysfunction after myocardial infarction. Results of the survival and ventricular enlargement trial. *New England Journal of Medicine* **327**: 669–677.

Pyorala K, Debacker G, Graham I, *et al* (1994). Prevention of coronary heart disease in clinical practice: Recommendations of the task force of the European Society of Cardiology, European Atherosclerosis Society and European Society of Hypertension. *European Heart Journal* **15**: 1300–1331.

Ryan TJ, Anderson TL, Antman EM *et al* (1996). ACC/AHA guidelines for the management of patients with acute myocardial infarction: A report of the American College of Cardiology and American Heart Association Task Force on Practice Guidelines (Committee on Management of Acute Myocardial Infarction). *Journal of the American College of Cardiology* **28**: 1328–1428.

Scandinavian Simvastatin Survival Study Group (1994). Randomised trial of cholesterol lowering in 4444 patients with coronary heart disease: the Scandinavian simvastatin survival study (4S). *Lancet* **344**: 1383–1389.

Shaper AG, Pocock SJ, Walker M, *et al* (1985). Risk factors for ischaemic heart disease: the prospective phase of the British regional heart study. *Journal of Epidemiology and Community Health* **39**: 197–209.

Shepherd D, Cobbe SM, Ford I for the West of Scotland Coronary Prevention Group (WOSCOPS) (1995). Prevention of coronary heart disease with pravastatin in men with hypercholesterolaemia. *New England Journal of Medicine* **333**: 1301–1307.

The Acute Infarction Ramipril Efficacy (AIRE) Study Investigators (1993). Effect of ramipril on mortality and morbidity of survivors of acute myocardial infarction with clinical evidence of heart failure. *Lancet* **342**: 821–828.

Turner RC, Millns H, Neil H AW *et al* (1998). Risk factors for coronary artery disease in non-insulin dependent diabetes mellitus: United Kingdom prospective diabetes study (UKPDS: 23). *British Medical Journal* **316**: 823–828.

UK Prospective Diabetes Study (UKPDS) Group (1998). Intensive blood-glucose control with sulphonylureas or insulin compared with convential treatment and risk of complications in patients with type 2 diabetes (UKPDS 33). *Lancet* **352**: 837–853.

Woods D, Durrington P, Poulter N, *et al* (1998). Joint British recommendations on prevention of coronary heart disease in clinical practice. *Heart* **80 (Suppl 2)**: S1–S29.

Yusuf S, Peto R, Lewis J, *et al* (1985). Beta blockade during and after myocardial infarction: An overview of the randomized trials. *Progress in Cardiovascular Disease* **27**: 335–371.

▶ Epilogue

Mark Gabbay

The concept of evidence-based health (EBH) may be a fashionable one, but it is likely to be increasingly incorporated throughout health-care training, practice, service development and delivery. Remember, such an approach is only part of the science and art that is health care. At best it provides good quality information to professionals, planners and patients to aid their decision making, enhances the quality of care and hopefully the confidence and satisfaction of practitioners. It may even help improve the cost-effectiveness of health care as a side effect.

I hope that readers now understand the concepts, hopefully rendering EBH less mysterious or threatening. This book should also arm you with the knowledge to help resist pressures to practice in new ways that are not based on evidence. Now you too can hold your own in debates with managers, purchasers, pharmaceutical representatives, etc. The other consequence, of course, is that you are less content to accept your own prejudices and long-standing practices, unless you can justify their continuance.

A major aim of this book was to familiarise readers with the concepts of EBH and its potential relevance and impact on family medicine and primary care. I believe EBH has relevance for all the team, not just the GPs. We also sought to present a series of examples from practice, demonstrate the techniques and process, and provide some answers. The answers by definition will not necessarily remain true, and readers should check their current validity – this after all is the basis of the evidence-based approach. We hope that in addition to having an overview of the concepts, and some new knowledge, readers will also have retained their interest in the subject. It was not our intention to dampen enthusiasm!

Hopefully, some readers will begin to explore the evidence as it pertains to their clinical work, using it as a way of learning and improving their practice and patient care. Our aim in introducing the principles of EBH, and outlining skills such as searching the literature for more information, should enable those now sufficiently interested and stimulated to explore the evidence in more detail. Some will go on to introduce EBH to colleagues and students, and even into their consultations at times. Indeed our students and practitioners in training will benefit from helping us in our evidence hunting and interpretation, as will we from their efforts, and the process of teaching them. Courses in developing and passing on such skills are burgeoning.

Good luck with your future evidence hunting, hopefully it will prove to be worthwhile and enjoyable. I welcome feedback on this book.

▶ Appendix: Useful Sources of Evidence for Primary Care

Alastair McColl

This appendix presents some of the many sources of evidence relevant to primary care that are available in printed form, CD-ROM or on the world wide web. These sources may help to make evidence more easily available. They may also help critically appraise the quality and relevance of this evidence when attempting to use it in primary care.

The Cochrane Library

The Cochrane Library is published quarterly on CD-ROM and the Internet (http://www.cochranelibrary.net/), and is distributed on a subscription basis. It is a worldwide initiative with over 4000 collaborators (97% voluntary). There are 44 review groups and 14 Cochrane centres around the world.

The Cochrane Library includes:

▶ *The Cochrane Database of Systematic Reviews* – a growing collection of regularly updated, systematic reviews of the effects of health care. They mainly review randomised controlled trials. Evidence is included on the basis of explicit quality criteria and data are often combined statistically, with meta-analysis, to increase the power of the findings of numerous studies which are each too small to produce reliable results individually.

▶ *Database of Abstracts of Reviews of Effectiveness* – critical assessments and structured abstracts of good systematic reviews published elsewhere which have been critically appraised by reviewers at the NHS Centre for Reviews and Dissemination at the University of York.

▶ *The Cochrane Controlled Trials Register* – bibliographic information on over 132 000 controlled trials.

The Cochrane Database of Systematic Reviews
Examples of reviews relevant to primary care include:

▶ Antibiotic *versus* placebo for acute otitis media in children

▶ Antibiotics for acute bronchitis

▶ Antibiotics for the symptoms and complications of sore throat

▶ Vitamin C for the common cold

▶ Acupuncture for the treatment of asthma

▶ Family therapy in the treatment of childhood asthma

- Homeopathy for chronic asthma

- The effectiveness of corticosteroids in the treatment of acute exacerbations of asthma: a meta-analysis of their effect on relapse following acute assessment

- The effects of limited (information only) patient education programmes on the health outcomes of adults with asthma

- Conservative management of mechanical neck disorders

- The effectiveness of transcutaneous electrical nerve stimulation (TENS) and acupuncture-like transcutaneous electrical nerve stimulation (ALTENS) in the treatment of patients with chronic low back pain

- Effectiveness of different strategies for inviting women to participate in breast cancer screening

- Audit and feedback to improve health professional practice and health-care outcomes

- Effectiveness of hospital at home compared to in-patient hospital care

- Interventions to assist patients to follow prescriptions for medications

- Interventions to change collaboration between nurses and doctors

- Local opinion leaders to improve health professional practice and health-care outcomes

- Outreach visits to improve health professional practice and health-care outcomes

- Printed educational materials to improve the behaviour of health-care professionals and patient outcomes

- Nimodipine in the treatment of primary degenerative, mixed and vascular dementia

- The efficacy of piracetam in patients with dementia or cognitive impairment

- The efficacy of tacrine in Alzheimer's disease

- Antihypertensive drug therapy in the elderly

- Antihypertensive therapy in diabetes mellitus

- Diabetes care: the effectiveness of systems for routine surveillance for people with diabetes

- Carbamazepine *vs* valproate monotherapy: an individual patient data meta-analysis

- Efficacy of yoga in the treatment of epilepsy

- Cervical smear collection devices: how effective are they at detecting endocervical cells and dyskaryosis?

- Effectiveness of bladder training for the treatment of urinary incontinence

- The effectiveness of oral contraceptive pills *versus* placebo or any other medical treatment for menorrhagia

- Effectiveness of co-ordinated multidisciplinary in-patient rehabilitation for elderly patients with proximal femoral fracture

- Vitamin D and vitamin D analogues in the prevention of fractures in involutional and post-menopausal osteoporosis

- The comparative efficacy of non-aspirin non-steroidal anti-inflammatory drugs for the management of osteoarthritis of the knee

- Analgesia and anti-inflammatory therapy in osteoarthritis (OA) of the hip

The database also lists protocols for over 200 systematic reviews in progress.

Database of Reviews of Effectiveness

These abstracts are also available on http://nhscrd.york.ac.uk/
Published papers relevant to primary care summarised on this database include:

- Physician advice for smoking cessation

- A meta-analysis of the effectiveness of acupuncture in smoking cessation

- Effectiveness of training health professionals to provide smoking cessation interventions

- Nicotine replacement therapy for smoking cessation

- Systematic review of interventions in the treatment and prevention of obesity

- A systematic review of the effectiveness of promoting lifestyle change in general practice

- Shared care for diabetes: a systematic review

- Diabetes care: the effectiveness of systems for routine surveillance for people with diabetes

- Promoting weight loss in type II diabetes

- Group education interventions for people with low back pain: an overview of the literature

- Conservative treatment of acute and chronic nonspecific low back pain

- Paracetamol with and without codeine in acute pain

- Corticosteroid injections for lateral epicondylitis: a systematic overview

- The management of menorrhagia

- Treating menorrhagia in primary care: an overview of drug trials and a survey of prescribing practice

▶ Management of chronic pelvic pain in women

▶ A reassessment of efficacy of the yuzpe regimen of emergency contraception

▶ Brief interventions and alcohol

▶ Effectiveness of physician-based interventions with problem drinkers: a review

▶ The efficacy of treatments in reducing alcohol consumption: a meta-analysis

▶ The treatment of depression in primary care

▶ Are SSRIs a cost-effective alternative to tricyclics?

▶ Is counselling in primary care growing too fast? A clinical, economic and strategic assessment

▶ The effectiveness and cost-effectiveness of counselling in primary care

▶ The effect of on-site mental health workers on primary care providers' clinical behaviour

▶ The efficacy of psychosocial treatments in primary care: a review of randomized clinical trials

▶ An overview of family interventions and relapse on schizophrenia: meta-analysis of research findings

▶ A review of randomized trials of psychiatric consultation-liaison studies in primary care

▶ Differentiation of dementia and depression by memory tests

▶ Cholesterol lowering with statin drugs, risk of stroke, and total mortality: an overview of randomised trials

▶ A meta-analysis of cholesterol lowering trials

▶ Aspirin and other antiplatelet agents in the secondary and primary prevention of cardiovascular disease

▶ The primary prevention of myocardial infarction

▶ Implications of the primary prevention trials against coronary heart disease

▶ Evidence of effectiveness of interventions for secondary prevention and treatment of coronary heart disease in primary care

▶ Primary care management of acute herpes zoster

▶ Clinical efficacy of antimicrobial drugs for acute otitis media

▶ The efficacy of influenza vaccine in elderly persons: a meta-analysis and review of the literature

▶ Should general practitioners refer patients directly to physical therapists?

▶ Organisation of asthma care: what difference does it make?

▶ Screening and self examination for breast cancer

▶ A meta-analysis of nurse practitioners and nurse midwives in primary care

▶ Capitation, salaried, fee for service and mixed systems of payment and the behaviour of primary care physicians

▶ Impact of mass media on health services

▶ A systematic review of near-patient testing in primary care

▶ Effectiveness of hospital at home compared to in-patient hospital care

▶ A meta-analysis of 16 randomised controlled trials to evaluate computer-based clinical reminder systems

Effective Health Care Bulletins

Effective Health Care Bulletins are based on a systematic review and synthesis of research on the clinical effectiveness, cost-effectiveness and acceptability of health service interventions. All health authorities receive copies to distribute to GPs in their area. They are available on http://www.york.ac.uk/inst/crd/ehcb.htm

Bulletins relevant to primary care include:

▶ The management of subfertility

▶ The treatment of persistent glue ear in children

▶ The treatment of depression in primary care

▶ Brief interventions and alcohol abuse

▶ Management of menorrhagia

▶ The prevention and treatment of pressure sores

▶ Benign prostatic hyperplasia: treatment for lower urinary tract symptoms in older men

▶ Management of cataract

▶ Preventing falls and subsequent injury in older people

▶ Preventing unintentional injuries in children and young adolescents

▶ Preventing and reducing the adverse effects of unintended teenage pregnancies

▶ The prevention and treatment of obesity

▶ Mental health promotion in high-risk groups

▶ Compression therapy for venous leg ulcers

▶ Management of stable angina

▶ Cholesterol and coronary heart disease: screening and treatment

▶ Pre-school hearing, speech, language and vision screening

▶ Deliberate self-harm

Bandolier

Bandolier is produced monthly in Oxford for the NHS R&D Directorate. It contains 'bullet points' (hence *Bandolier*) of evidence-based medicine. *Bandolier* is available free on http://www.jr2.ox.ac.uk:80/Bandolier/ or a printed version is available on subscription.

'Bullet points' relevant to primary care include:

▶ ACE inhibitors in CHF

▶ Angina

▶ Calcium channel blockers

▶ Cholesterol lowering in CHD and statins

▶ Cholesterol screening

▶ Exercise and intermittent claudication

▶ Smoking cessation

▶ Nicotine replacement: patches, sprays, inhalers and gum

▶ Diabetes care

▶ Analgesics for dysmenorrhoea

▶ Alternatives for the menopause and menopausal decisions

▶ Stress urinary incontinence in women

▶ Antimicrobials for cystitis

▶ Giving birth at home

▶ Clinical scoring for alcohol abuse

▶ Benzodiazepine reduction by GPs

▶ Counsellors in primary care

▶ Suicide prevention

▶ Childhood asthma

▶ Ménière's disease

▶ Parkinson's treatment

▶ Drug treatments for migraine

- Bell's palsy

- GI complications and NSAIDs

- Constipation

- Laxatives

- Acid suppressing prescribing

- *H. pylori* and ulcers

- Back pain and back pain guidelines

- Intra-articular shoulder injections

- Nitroglycerin patches for shoulder pain

- Diagnosis of acute sinus infections

- Glue ear

- Acute otitis media

- Tonsillectomy for sore throats

- Acyclovir and post-herpetic neuralgia

- Verrucas and games

- Freezing warts

- Dog bites – antibiotic prophylaxis

- Nitpicking head lice

- Allergy screening

- Alternative medicine studies

- Dandruff

- Erectile dysfunction treatments

- Falls in the elderly

- Near patient testing

- Nutritional assessment tools for nurses

Journals

Of course there are many regular journal with sources of evidence relevant to primary care.

The bi-monthly *Evidence-Based Medicine* provides summarised 'value-added' abstracts and commentaries by a clinical expert on a wide range of recent papers in other journals. Most of the summaries are on therapeutic interventions and only some are relevant to primary care.

The *Journal of Family Practice* is available on http://jfp.msu.edu/ Its web site contains *Evidence-Based Practice*, a monthly newsletter, and *Patient Orientated Evidence that Matters* (POEMS). Each month it reviews and critically appraises over 80 journals to identify the 8 articles with patient-oriented outcomes that have the greatest potential to change the way primary care clinicians practice.

A list of the contents of the *British Journal of General Practice* and some of the editorials are available on http://www.rcgp.org.uk/publicat/journal/index.htm

The *British Medical Journal* is available on http://www.bmj.com/index.shtml and has a search facility.

The Lancet is available on http://www.thelancet.com/ with limited access to non-subscribers.

Bulletins and journals sent to all UK general practitioners

The following are sent to all UK GPs and attempt to summarise evidence. Each provides an annual index of the topics covered.

▶ The fortnightly *Drug and Therapeutic Bulletin* is commissioned and researched by the Association for Consumer Research. A team of 'impartial editors' aims to provide the 'best available advice on treatment'. (For details on how they produce articles, see *Drug and Therapeutic Bulletin* 1997; **35**: 73–74 or their web site at http://www.which.net)

▶ *The Prescribers' Journal* is compiled by a 'representative Committee of Management supported by an Advisory Panel'. Its articles are commissioned and peer reviewed. The journal is published quarterly.

▶ The *Medicines Resources (MeReC) Bulletin* is the main output of the National Prescribing Centre in Liverpool. This monthly bulletin focuses 'directly on the information needs of GPs and aims to facilitate high-quality, cost-effective prescribing.

Other useful sources of evidence available on the world wide web

NHS Centre for Reviews and Dissemination at the University of York

The NHS Centre for Reviews and Dissemination (CRD) is a facility commissioned by the NHS Research and Development Division to produce and disseminate reviews concerning the effectiveness and cost-effectiveness of health-care interventions (http://www.york.ac.uk/inst/crd/welcome.htm).

The following databases are available:

▶ *Database of Abstracts of Reviews of Effectiveness (DARE)* (see above).

▶ *NHS Economic Evaluation Database* – contains structured abstracts of economic evaluations of health-care interventions.

▶ *Health Technology Assessment Database* – contains abstracts produced by INAHTA (International Network of Agencies for Health Technology Assessment) and other health-care technology agencies.

Agency for Health Care Policy and Research

The US (AHCPR) web site on http://text.nlm.nih.gov/ contains its evidence reports and supported guidelines. These include the following topics relevant to primary care with many sources of evidence:

- Acute pain management

- Alzheimer's disease

- Benign prostate hyperplasia

- Cataract

- Depression

- Heart failure

- Low back problems

- Otitis media

- Smoking cessation

- Unstable angina

- Urinary incontinence

ScHARR 'Netting the Evidence' web site

The University of Sheffield School of Health and Related Research (ScHARR) 'Netting the Evidence' web site (http://www.shef.ac.uk/~scharr/ir/netting.html) has an excellent and comprehensive list of web sites with sources of evidence some of which are relevant to primary care.

Evidence-based health teaching packages available on the Internet

Evidence-based teaching packages
Centre for Evidence-Based Mental Health Toolkit
http://www.psychiatry.ox.ac.uk/cebmh/toolkit/index.html
The Clinician's Lament: How Do I Keep up with the Literature?
http://www.nyam.org/library/ebm/index.htm
Clinical Epidemiology & Evidence-Based Medicine Glossary
http://www.vetmed.wsu.edu/courses-jmgay/GlossClinEpiEBM.htm
Evidence-Based Healthcare: A Resource Pack
http://drsdesk.sghms.ac.uk/Starnet/pack.htm
Evidence-Based Medicine Powerpoint
http://www.health.usyd.edu.au/ebm/PPTPRES/
Introduction to Information Mastery
http://www.familypractice.msu.edu/InfoMastery/
On the Need for Evidence-Based Medicine: Some Problems and Some Solutions
http://www.med.usf.edu/CLASS/Gene/Presentation/sld00l.htm

RES&WCE – How to Find the Evidence
http://www.shef.ac.uk/~scharr/reswce/rescwce.htm
SUNY Health Sciences Evidence-Based Medicine Course
http://courses.hscbklyn.edu/ebm/ebmtoc.htm
University of Illinois
http://www.uic.edu/depts/lib/health/ebm.html

Scenarios
Centre for Evidence-Based Mental Health Teaching Scenarios
http://www.psychiatry.ox.ac.uk/cebmh/toolkit/scenarios.html
Educational Scenarios for Teaching EBM
http://cebm.jr2.ox.ac.uk/docs/scenarios.html
McMaster – Therapy Scenarios
http://hiru/hirunet.mcmaster.ca/ebm/workshop/therapy/default.htm

Checklists/Worksheets
CASP Checklists
http://www.ihs.ox.ac.uk/casp/workshops.html
Centre for Evidence-Based Medicine Teaching Resources
http://cebm.jr2.ox.ac.uk/docs/teachingresources.html
Evidence-Based Medicine Toolkit
http://www.med.ualberta.ca/ebm/ebm.htm
User Guides to the Medical Literature
http://hiru.hirunet.mcmaster.ca/ebm/userguid/default.htm

Web sites particularly relevant to nurses

Rumona Dickson and Carrie Morrison

The Cumulative Index to Nursing & Allied Health Literature (CINAHL)
This is available on CD-ROM and may also be accessed through PubMed. It provides access to nearly all English-language nursing journals and 13 journals from associated health areas.

Evidence-Based Nursing

This on-line edition of the journal published by the Royal College of Nursing and the *British Medical Journal* requires a subscription in order to obtain access to its contents (http://www.bmjpg.com/data/ebnpp.htm). The journal reports on studies and reviews relating to the nursing role in evidence-based care whilst summarising these reports in abstract form.

Hardin Meta Directory – Nursing

Web links to evidence-based sites for nurses are provided by this web site created and maintained by the Hardin Library for the Health Sciences, University of Iowa (http://www.lib.uiowa.edu/hardin/md/nurs.html).

Joanna Briggs Institute for Evidence-Based Nursing

The Joanna Briggs Institute has taken the effectiveness of nursing as its central focus by following the processes developed by the Cochrane Collaboration and the NHS Centre for Reviews and Dissemination. Each of its seven collaborating centres conducts systematic reviews according to their specific interests. Access to the reviews is only available through subscription (http://www.joannabriggs.edu.au/).

Nursing & Health Care Resources on the Net

Web links to evidence-based sites designed for nurses and allied health professionals are available from this University of Sheffield web site (http://www.shef.ac.uk/~hcon/).

Sigma Theta Tau International Registry of Nursing Research

This registry of nursing research is restricted to subscribers. It provides information on nurse-researchers, abstracts of their studies, as well as related projects and programmes (http://www.stti.iupui.edu/research/).

University of York – Centre for Evidence-Based Nursing

Part of the UK's national network of centres for evidence-based practice, this web site provides web links to full-text, evidence-based health-care articles (http://www.york.ac.uk/depts/hstd/centres/evidence/ev-intro.htm).

If you are fortunate enough to work for the NHS in the West Midlands, its library service provides access to a special selection of OVID features that include the major databases as well as access to 15 on-line nursing journals (P Priory, personal communication).

▶ Index